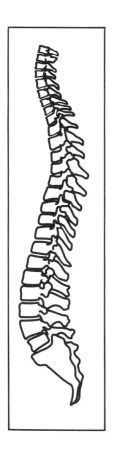

THE AGING SPINE

Essentials of Pathophysiology, Diagnosis, and Treatment

Scott D. Boden, M.D.

Department of Orthopaedic Surgery
George Washington University School of
Medicine and Health Sciences
Washington, D.C.

Sam W. Wiesel, M.D.

Professor and Chairman
Department of Orthopaedic Surgery
Georgetown University School of Medicine
Washington, D.C.

Edward R. Laws, Jr., M.D.

Professor and Chairman
Department of Neurological Surgery
George Washington University School of
Medicine and Health Sciences
Washington, D.C.

Richard H. Rothman, M.D., Ph.D.

James Edward Professor and Chairman
Department of Orthopaedic Surgery
Jefferson Medical College of the
Thomas Jefferson University
Chairman of the Rothman Orthopaedic Institute,
Pennsylvania Hospital
Philadelphia, Pennsylvania

1991
W.B. SAUNDERS COMPANY
Harcourt Brace Jovanovich, Inc.

Philadelphia ■ London ■ Toronto ■ Montreal ■ Sydney ■ Tokyo

W. B. SAUNDERS COMPANY
Harcourt Brace Jovanovich, Inc.
The Curtis Center
Independence Square West
Philadelphia, PA 19106

Library of Congress Cataloging-in-Publication Data

The aging spine : Essentials of pathophysiology, diagnosis, and
    treatment / Scott D. Boden . . . [et al.].
        p.   cm.
    ISBN 0-7216-3538-5
    1. Spine—Diseases—Age factors.   2. Spine—Aging.   3. Geriatric
orthopedics.   I. Boden, Scott D.
    [DNLM: 1. Spinal Diseases—diagnosis.   2. Spinal Diseases—in old
age.   3. Spinal Diseases—therapy.   WE 725 A267]
RD768.A35   1991
617.3′75—dc20
DNLM/DLC   90-8884

Editor: Edward H. Wickland, Jr.
Developmental Editor: Kathleen McCullough
Designer: Joan Wendt
Production Manager: Ken Neimeister
Manuscript Editor: Ellen Murray
Illustration Coordinator: Peg Shaw
Indexer: Julie Figures

The Aging Spine   ISBN 0-7216-3538-5

Printed in the United States of America

Last digit is the print number: 9 8 7 6 5 4 3 2 1

This book is authored by three generations of spine surgeons and therefore is dedicated to our teachers, our colleagues, and our pupils.

This book is also dedicated to Mary, my wife, for her critical editorial judgment, her patience, and especially her energy and encouragement during the preparation of this work.

S.D.B.

Foreword

In our industrialized societies, people live longer and can stay active well into the eighth and ninth decades. By doing so, they not only achieve better health for themselves, but they also are less of a burden for society. With the development of joint arthroplasty, a diagnosis of osteoarthritis of the hip or knee no longer means a life of diminished activity. Unfortunately, the success achieved with peripheral joint disease has not been mirrored in the management of older patients suffering from common painful disorders in the axial skeleton.

The success of total hip and knee replacements has actually served to increase the need for effective treatment methods for spinal disorders, in particular those of the lumbar spine. Therefore, this book on the aging spine by a team of internationally known authorities is very timely indeed. Although much is still to be learned, the authors present a clear, succinct, and up-to-date text that will guide the reader in finding the best way to treat the aging patient population in the 1990s. The authors discuss the specificity and sensitivity of diagnostic tests and examine both proven and unproven methods of treatment in each region of the spine.

In particular, the text can be recommended for its clear presentation of steps in differential diagnoses, which are of particular importance in this age group. In addition, the reader will gain a sound understanding of the essentials of the pathophysiology, diagnosis, and management of spinal disorders in the aging population. Several chapters are devoted to a comprehensive, yet succinct, review of infection, tumors, hematologic disease, and metabolic disorders.

There is often little to be gained from surgery in the older patient and this makes a thorough understanding of all diagnostic and treatment options essential. Hence, this is a book not only for orthopedists, but for all practitioners confronted with spinal complaints in older people.

ALF L. NACHEMSON, M.D.
GOTHENBURG, SWEDEN

Preface

The population of people over the age of 60 is increasing at a rapid rate. This group is universally affected by some degree of degenerative change, and thus the complaints of neck pain and back pain are common. Two decades ago, these patients were told that little could be done for their pain and that they should simply decrease their activity level. Today, however, with increased emphasis on physical fitness, the uniform prescription of decreased activity level is not well accepted, nor is it indicated.

The purpose of this monograph is to focus on the basic pathogenesis of the most common problems of the aging spine and to present an organized approach to their diagnosis and treatment. Most patients can expect significant improvement, and certainly the majority should be able to function as active citizens in daily life.

In spite of the plethora of studies in the literature, surprisingly little is known about the true cause of degenerative spine problems. Current concepts of the biochemical, biomechanical, and histologic aspects of spinal aging and degeneration are presented. A succinct description of the key points of the history, physical examination, and diagnostic evaluation is specifically for the cervical, thoracic, and lumbar regions. The topics included here are those that primarily affect the aging spine and should be considered in a differential diagnosis of neck or low back pain in adults. A special effort has been made to distinguish pathologic changes seen with normal aging from abnormalities more likely to be clinically significant.

It is hoped that after reading this text, the physician will be able to take an organized clinical approach to the older patient with neck and back pain. It will also be appreciated that there are many questions yet to be answered. This volume is intended to be a starting point for those dealing with this increasingly important group of patients.

SCOTT D. BODEN, M.D.
SAM W. WIESEL, M.D.

Acknowledgments

The authors wish to acknowledge the contributions of several individuals without whom this project could not have been accomplished. The chapter on metabolic bone disease was co-authored by Dr. Frederick S. Kaplan of the University of Pennsylvania. Dr. Kaplan is an associate professor of Orthopaedic Surgery and Medicine and chief of the Metabolic Bone Disease Unit; his expertise in this field is greatly appreciated. Dr. Neil Shonnard is a Spine fellow at Thomas Jefferson University and co-authored Chapters 3 and 4 dealing with examination and imaging of the cervical spine. We thank Dr. David Borenstein for his invaluable assistance with preparation of the chapter on arthritis of the spine. The authors also appreciate the efforts of Dr. David O. Davis and Dr. Henry H. Bohlman for supplying several important radiographs. Similarly, the authors are indebted to Dr. Morrie E. Kricun for allowing us to reproduce many of the superb radiographs from his book on spinal imaging. All of these individuals, as well as their assistants and others who were not specifically mentioned, were an essential part of this work and deserve our sincere appreciation. Finally, our thanks go to Mr. Edward Wickland and the entire editorial and production staff at W. B. Saunders Company, whose guidance and patience made this project an enjoyable and worthwhile experience for all.

Contents

Anatomy and Physiology

CHAPTER 1

Anatomy of the Spine

The structure of the spine is quite complex. To diagnose and treat this area effectively, one must have a thorough knowledge of the normal anatomy. Consequently, this chapter presents a working description of the anatomy as a keystone on which to build as the various pathologic entities affecting the aging spine are presented.

BONE ARCHITECTURE OF THE VERTEBRAL COLUMN

There are 33 vertebrae in the human spine: 7 cervical vertebrae, 12 thoracic vertebrae, 5 lumbar vertebrae, a sacrum of 5 fused segments, and a coccyx of 4 fused segments. With the exception of the first and second cervical vertebrae, the vertebral bodies are separated by intervertebral discs, which account for one fourth of the total length of the vertebral column.

The typical vertebra consists of a body and a neural arch, which enclose an area known as the vertebral canal through which the spinal cord passes. The arch is composed of two pedicles, which form its sides, and the lamina, which forms the roof. A spinous process projects dorsally from the midline of the lamina. Extending laterally from the junction of the lamina and pedicles are the transverse processes. Projecting upward from the junction of the pedicles and the lamina are the superior articular processes, and projecting downward, the inferior articular processes. These processes form synovial joints between two adjacent vertebrae. This means that articulations are found between the articular processes and the intervertebral discs of any two typical vertebrae.

On the lower border of each pedicle is a deep notch and on the upper border a smaller notch, which together form the intervertebral foramen. These foramina are longer in their vertical dimension than in their horizontal one. Through these intervertebral foramina pass the spinal nerves, which usually occupy the superior portion of the foramina.

Cervical Vertebrae

The bony elements of the cervical spine consist of seven vertebrae. Between each vertebral body below the second vertebra is interposed an intervertebral disc. From cephalad to caudad the size of each subsequent vertebra increases progressively. The third, fourth, fifth, and sixth vertebrae exhibit identical anatomic features and are designated typical vertebrae (Fig. 1–1). The first, second, and seventh vertebrae possess distinct anatomic features not encountered elsewhere in the spine and are therefore called atypical vertebrae.

The body of a typical vertebra is elongated transversely so that its width is approximately 50 percent greater than its anteroposterior dimension. The upper surface is concave from side to side, and this concavity is deepened by an uncinate process, which is a bony protuberance projecting upward from the posterior lateral aspect of the rim of the body. The upper surface is also convex in the anteroposterior direction. The lower surface of the vertebral body is convex from side to side and concave in the anteroposterior direction. A prominent inferior overhanging lip is noted on the anteroinferior surface of the vertebral body. The inferior and slightly posterolateral aspects of the first vertebral body are beveled and lie in apposition to the uncinate process of the body, below which they form the bony components of the so-called joints of Luschka.

The pedicles are short and bear superior and inferior articular processes. The articular processes of the superior facets face upward and posteriorly, whereas those of the inferior articular facets face downward and anteriorly. On either side of the body are situated the transverse processes. The anterior portion of the transverse process is developmentally a rib, whereas the posterior portion is a true transverse process. These portions fuse, but between them persists the transverse foramen, which allows for passage of the vertebral artery. The transverse processes contain a gutter running obliquely from back to front for the spinal nerves. Posteriorly the laminae terminate in a short, slender spinous process that is bifid.

The atlas, or first cervical vertebra, possesses no vertebral body (Fig. 1–2). The bone that is where the body would be is joined to that of the second cervical vertebra, the axis, to form the odontoid process, or dens. The atlas consists of an anterior and posterior arch, called the heavy lateral masses, that bear the superior and inferior articular surfaces. The superior facets articulate with the occiput, and the inferior facets with the axis. Spanning the lateral masses anteriorly is the slender anterior arch, which lies in front of the dens. It has on its internal surface a facet for articulation with the dens and in the front, an anterior tubercle for muscular

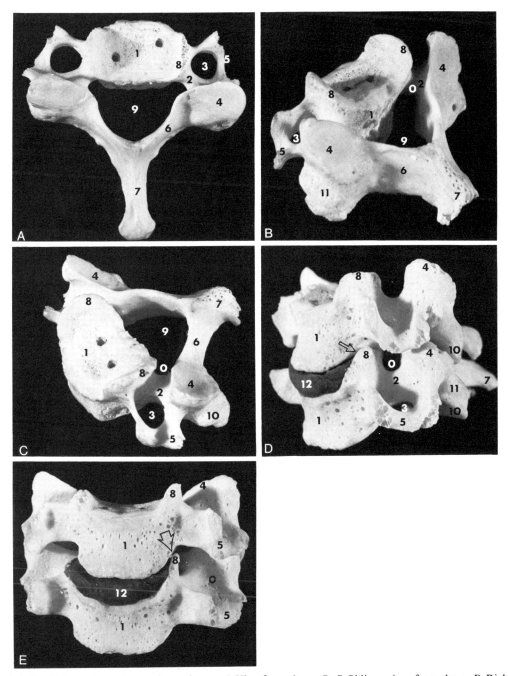

Figure 1-1. Cervical vertebrae. Anatomic specimens. *A,* View from above. *B, C,* Oblique views from above. *D,* Right posterior oblique view (C5–C6). *E,* Frontal view (C5–C6). *Key:* 0 = neural foramen; 1 = vertebral body; 2 = pedicle; 3 = foramen transversarium; 4 = superior articular facet; 5 = transverse process; 6 = lamina; 7 = spinous process; 8 = uncinate process; 9 = spinal canal; 10 = inferior articular facet; 11 = articular pillar; 12 = intervertebral disc; *arrow* = uncovertebral "joint." (From Kricun ME: Imaging Modalities in Spinal Disorders. Philadelphia, W.B. Saunders, 1988.)

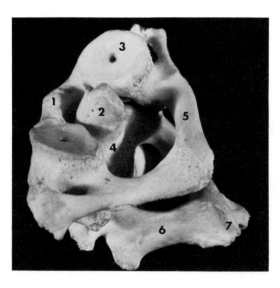

Figure 1–2. Atlas and axis. Anatomic specimen demonstrating the relationship of the bony structures. *Key:* 1 = anterior arch of C1; 2 = odontoid process; 3 = superior articular facet of C1; 4 = body of C2; 5 = lamina of C1; 6 = lamina of C2; 7 = spinous process of C2. (From Kricun ME: Imaging Modalities in Spinal Disorders. Philadelphia, W.B. Saunders, 1988.)

attachments. The posterior arch is longer and bears a small posterior tubercle in place of a spinous process. On its upper surface are found sulci for the vertebral arteries.

The second cervical vertebra, also known as the axis, is identified by the projection of the odontoid process or dens that develops from the embryologic body of the first vertebra. The dens is continuous with the body of the second vertebra. Its spinous process is massive, elongated, and bifid. The superior articular surfaces are large and face upward, posteriorly and laterally. They are placed on heavy masses arising from the body and pedicles.

The seventh cervical vertebra is considered atypical because of its particularly long and unbifurcated spinous process, which is known as the vertebra prominens. The seventh cervical vertebra also has a small transverse foramen since it does not usually transmit the vertebral artery.

Thoracic Vertebrae

There are 12 thoracic vertebrae, which increase in size from cephalad to caudad. They are unique in that each side of the body has facets for articulation with the heads of the ribs (Fig. 1–3). Their anterior height is 1 to 2 mm less than their posterior height; this difference accounts primarily for the thoracic kyphosis. The body surfaces above and below are essentially flat.

The laminae are long and overlap the laminae of the adjacent vertebrae. The spinous processes are long and slender and also tend to overlap the adjacent spinous process. The superior articular facets face posteriorly, upward, and laterally; the inferior articular facets face anteriorly, inferiorly, and medially. The long heavy transverse processes bear facets on their lateral anterior surfaces for articulation with the tubercles

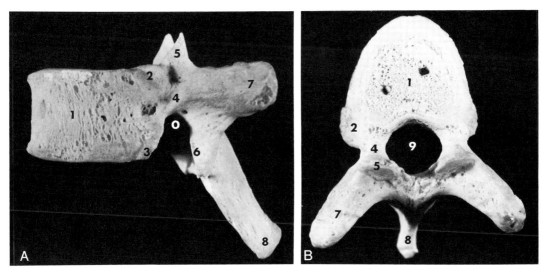

Figure 1-3. Thoracic vertebra (T8). Anatomic specimen. *A,* Lateral view. *B,* View from above. *Key:* 0 = neural foramen; 1 = body; 2 = superior demifacet for head of rib; 3 = inferior demifacet for head of rib; 4 = pedicle; 5 = superior articular facet; 6 = inferior articular facet; 7 = transverse process; 8 = spinous process; 9 = central spinal canal. (From Kricun ME: Imaging Modalities in Spinal Disorders. Philadelphia, W.B. Saunders, 1988.)

of the ribs. These vary somewhat in the first, eleventh, and twelfth thoracic vertebrae. The body of a thoracic vertebra may exhibit half of a facet at both its upper and lower borders for articulation with the head of the rib. The arrangements of these facets also vary at the cranial and caudal extremes of the thoracic spine.

Lumbar Vertebrae

The lumbar vertebrae are very large and heavy (Fig. 1–4). The bodies are wider in the transverse direction than in the anteroposterior direction. The last three lumbar vertebrae tend to have less height anteriorly than posteriorly and are therefore slightly wedge-shaped when viewed from the side. The pedicles are massive and exhibit a shallow superior vertebral notch and a deep inferior vertebral notch. The transverse processes are long and delicate, being flattened in their anteroposterior direction. On the dorsal surface of the base of each transverse process is an accessory process.

The laminae are directed caudally from their attachment to the pedicle, forming a V shape. The spinous processes are broad and massive with a prominent thickening of the tip. The superior articular processes arise at the junction of the laminae and pedicle and have on their posterior borders a mammillary process. The articular surfaces of the superior articular processes face medially and backward. In succeeding vertebrae they tend to face more posteriorly and less medially. The inferior articular process is essentially a mirror image of the adjacent superior articular process with respect to its direction.

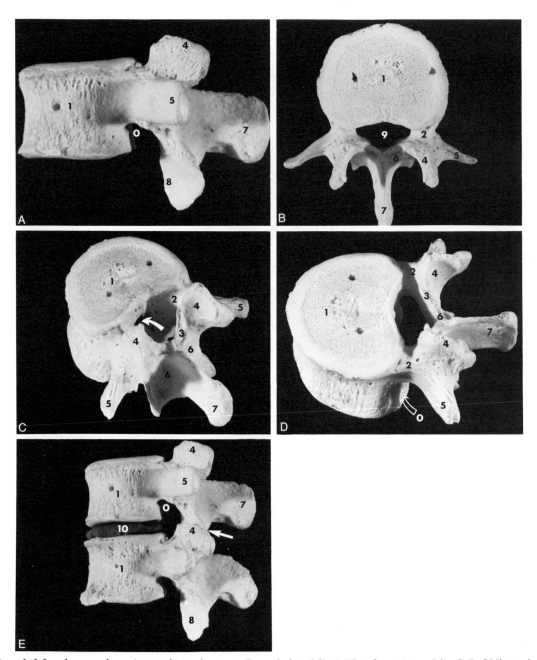

Figure 1–4. Lumbar vertebrae. Anatomic specimens. *A,* Lateral view (L2). *B,* View from above (L2). *C, D,* Oblique views from above (L2). *E,* Lateral view of L2 and L3. *Key:* 0 = neural foramen: 1 = body; 2 = pedicle; 3 = pars interarticularis; 4 = superior articular facet; 5 = transverse process; 6 = lamina; 7 = spinous process; 8 = inferior articular facet; 9 = central spinal canal; 10 = intervertebral disc; *straight arrow* = apophyseal (facet) joint; *curved arrow* = basivertebral groove. (From Kricun ME: Imaging Modalities in Spinal Disorders. Philadelphia, W.B. Saunders, 1988.)

The Sacrum

The sacrum is composed of five fused sacral vertebrae. The central portion of the sacrum consists of the fused bodies of the five sacral segments. On its dorsal surface a series of tubercles is noted in the midline to form a sacral crest. On each side of this crest a series of tubercles form an intermediate crest, representing the vestigial articular processes. Dorsally there is a sacral hiatus at the lower portion of the sacral canal. The sacral foramina are typically located opposite each other, forming a communicating canal from the pelvic to the dorsal surface of the sacrum. This canal also communicates medially with the sacral portion of the vertebral canal. These foramina allow for the exit of the dorsal and ventral branches of the spinal nerves.

The superior articular processes arise from the dorsal aspect of the sacrum and face posteriorly for articulation with the inferior articular process of the fifth lumbar vertebra. Laterally the sacrum articulates with the ilium. The surface that forms the actual articulation resembles an external ear. These articular processes represent the small part of the sacroiliac articulation and have a synovial cavity. Dorsal to this articular surface are roughened areas or tuberosities that receive the strong sacroiliac ligaments.

The Coccyx

The coccyx, often referred to as the tailbone, consists of four tiny fused vertebrae. It is connected to the inferior end of the sacrum and is solid. There is no spinal canal in the coccyx.

THE INTERVERTEBRAL DISCS

The intervertebral discs form approximately 25 percent of the length of the vertebral column above the sacrum. However, this percentage varies in the different parts of the spinal column. In the cervical region the discs contribute 22 percent of the length of the column, in the thoracic region 20 percent, and in the lumbar area 33 percent. The discs are the chief structural units between adjacent vertebral bodies. They serve to allow greater motion between the vertebral bodies than would occur if the vertebrae were in direct apposition. More importantly, the discs distribute weight over a large surface of the vertebral body during bending motions—weight that would otherwise be concentrated eccentrically on the edge toward which the spine is bent.

Each intervertebral disc is made up of a gelatinous nucleus pulposus surrounded by a laminated, fibrous annulus fibrosus (Fig. 1–5). Each disc is situated between the cartilaginous end plates of two vertebrae.

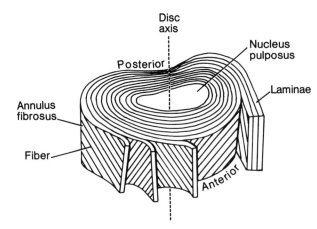

Figure 1–5. The intervertebral disc. The outer portion, the annulus fibrosus, is composed of 90 sheets of laminated collagen fibers that are oriented vertically in the peripheral layers and more obliquely in the central layers. Successive laminae run at angles to each other. (From Borenstein DG, Wiesel SW: Low Back Pain: Medical Diagnosis and Management. Philadelphia, W.B. Saunders, 1989.)

The annulus fibrosus forms the outer boundary of the disc. It is composed of fibrocartilaginous tissue and fibrous protein, which are arranged in concentric layers or lamellae and run obliquely from one vertebra to another. Successive layers of these fibers slant in alternate directions so that they cross each other at different angles depending upon the intradiscal pressure of the nucleus pulposus. Thus, the annulus fibrosus can absorb stress by expanding and contracting like a Japanese fingertrap. Its peripheral fibers pass over the edge of the cartilaginous end plate to unite with the bone of each vertebral body. The most superficial fibers blend with the anterior and posterior longitudinal ligaments. With age, these fibers of the annulus fibrosus deteriorate, become fissured, and lose their capacity to restrain the nucleus pulposus. If there is sufficient internal stress, the nucleus pulposus material can penetrate through the annulus, and the resulting injury is termed a herniated disc.

The nucleus pulposus is situated posteriorly and centrally within the disc and consists of collagen fibrils enmeshed in a mucoprotein gel. The nucleus pulposus occupies about 40 percent of the disc's cross-sectional area. It has a high water content at birth (88 percent), which mechanically allows it to absorb a significant amount of stress; however, with age, the percentage of water decreases, reflecting both an absolute decrease in available proteoglycans and a change in the ratio of the different proteoglycans present. This desiccation (loss of water) reduces the functional ability of the nucleus pulposus to withstand stress and will be discussed in more detail in Chapter 2.

The cartilaginous end plates limit the upper and lower borders of the discs and are composed of hyaline cartilage. They are at the region of the junction between the bone and the disc. This cartilage covers the perforated bony end plate but does not cover the compact peripheral epiphysis. Many of the collagen fibers that blend into the annulus fibrosus originate from these cartilaginous end plates.

In the cervical spine, the discs are thicker anteriorly than posteriorly and are entirely responsible for the normal cervical lordosis. They do not conform completely to the surfaces of the vertebral bodies with which they are connected, being slightly smaller in width than the vertebral bodies. The discs bulge anteriorly beyond the adjacent vertebrae. The nucleus pulposus in the cervical spine is located more anteriorly than in other portions of the spine.

The discs in the thoracic region are of equal height anteriorly and posteriorly, and thus the thoracic kyphosis is due primarily to the shape of the vertebral body rather than to that of the disc. The thoracic discs are thinner than those in the cervical or lumbar area. Accordingly, the mobility of the thoracic vertebral column is somewhat restricted as compared to that of the cervical and lumbar spine.

The lumbar intervertebral discs tend to be of greater height anteriorly than posteriorly, and this tendency is most marked in the fifth lumbar disc. In the upper portion of the lumbar spine, the lordosis is due almost entirely to the shape of the disc, but in the lower lumbar region, the shape of the vertebral body is also a contributory factor.

LIGAMENTS OF THE VERTEBRAL COLUMN

The anterior longitudinal ligament is a broad, strong ligament on the anterior and anterolateral aspects of the vertebral bodies from the atlas to the sacrum (Fig. 1–6). Its deepest fibers blend with the intervertebral disc and extend from the body of one vertebra, to the disc, to the body of the adjacent vertebra. These deep fibers bind the disc and the margins of the vertebra. Most of the superficial fibers extend over several vertebrae, occasionally spanning as many as five. This ligament is most firmly attached to the vertebral bodies at their periphery. The edges of the ligament are thinner than the centermost portion.

The posterior longitudinal ligament lies on the posterior surface of the bodies of the vertebrae from the axis to the sacrum (Fig. 1–7). The

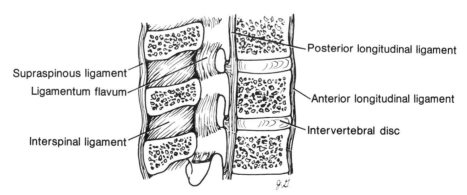

Figure 1–6. Lateral view of the lumbar spine demonstrating the ligaments that support the anterior (anterior longitudinal), middle (posterior longitudinal) and the posterior (supraspinous, intraspinous) elements of the vertebrae. Note the position of the ligamentum flavum forming a smooth posterior wall of the neural foramen. (From Borenstein DG, Wiesel SW: Low Back Pain: Medical Diagnosis and Management. Philadelphia, W.B. Saunders, 1989.)

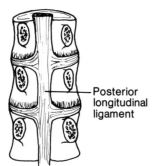

Posterior
longitudinal
ligament

Figure 1-7. Posterior view of the lumbar vertebrae. The posterior longitudinal ligament expands laterally to cover the intervertebral discs. The posterior longitudinal ligament is weakest in this location. (From Borenstein DG, Wiesel SW: Low Back Pain: Medical Diagnosis and Management. Philadelphia, W.B. Saunders, 1989.)

tectorial membrane is continuous, and the ligament passes onto the occiput. This ligament is attached most firmly to the ends of the vertebrae and most deeply to the intervening discs. The midportion of the body is only loosely attached to this ligament. In the thoracic and lumbar regions, the posterior longitudinal ligament narrows as it passes over the vertebral bodies and then expands over the discs, taking on the configuration of an hourglass. The lateral expansions over the intervertebral discs are rather weak and represent a more vulnerable area for disc herniation compared to the strong central band.

Capsular ligaments surround the synovial joints between the superior and inferior articular processes of adjacent vertebrae. Of necessity these ligaments are lax to allow gliding motion between these joints, and they therefore add little stability. The intertransverse ligaments, best developed in the lumbar region, join the transverse processes of adjacent vertebrae.

Posteriorly between adjacent laminae are found the highly elastic ligamenta flava. These yellow ligaments extend from the bases of the articular processes on one side to those on the opposite. They extend laterally into the intervertebral foramen, forming a portion of the roof of the foramen, and in certain areas, such as the thoracic spine, actually turn dorsally out of the foramen and fuse with the capsule of the apophyseal joint. The ligamenta flava are attached inferiorly to the superior edge of the posterosuperior surface of the lamina. Superiorly they are attached to the inferior and anterior inferior surfaces of the lamina. This unique attachment, combined with the anterior tilting of the lamina, has the effect of creating an extremely smooth posteroinferior wall of the spinal canal, which remains smooth in the various postural positions and serves to protect the neural elements.

Supraspinous and interspinous ligaments are found between adjacent spinous processes. The supraspinous ligament is thin, composed of a high percentage of elastic tissue, and runs over the tips of the spinous processes. In the cervical region it is continuous with the ligamentum nuchae. The infraspinous ligaments are thin and relatively weak, passing from one spinous process to the next. They are best developed in the lumbar area.

Atlanto-occipital and Atlantoaxial Joints and Ligaments

The occiput and the atlas articulate through two joints (Fig. 1–8). Each of these joints is formed by the deeply concave, oval, superior articular surface of the lateral mass of the atlas and the corresponding convex condyle of the occiput. These joints are condyloid in configuration, and the articular surfaces are reciprocally curved. In spite of the massive size of the atlanto-occipital joint, strong accessory ligaments are necessary to provide stability.

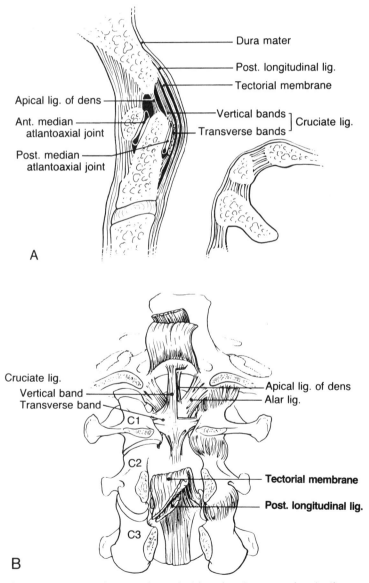

Figure 1–8. Soft tissue anatomy of the craniocervical junction demonstrating the ligaments and surrounding structures. *A,* Sagittal plane. *B,* Coronal plane. Posterior view of vertebrae. The laminae have been removed. (From Kricun ME: Imaging Modalities in Spinal Disorders. Philadelphia, W.B. Saunders, 1988.)

The anterior atlanto-occipital membrane is a strong, dense band composed of thick fibers that stretch across the anterior margin of the foramen magnum above, to the upper border of the anterior arch of the atlas below. In the midline there is a round tough band of fibers connecting the anterior tubercle of the atlas with the occiput. This structure may be considered a continuation of the anterior longitudinal ligament. The posterior atlanto-occipital membrane is thinner than its anterior counterpart and connects the posterior margin of the foramen magnum with the upper border of the posterior arch of the atlas. Inferiorly and laterally, there is an arched defect that permits the passage of the vertebral artery and the first cervical nerve. The articular capsules of the atlanto-occipital joints are loose, thin structures connecting the condyles of the occiput with the superior articular processes of the axis.

In addition to the ligaments between the occiput and the atlas, stability of the cranium on the vertebral column is further enhanced by a group of ligaments between the occiput and the axis. The alar ligaments are short, strong bundles of fibrous tissue directed obliquely upward and laterally from either side of the upper part of the odontoid process to the medial aspect of the condyles of the occiput. Because these ligaments restrict motion of the head on the atlas, they are often referred to as check ligaments. The apical odontoid ligament is a tough fibrous cord arising from the apex of the odontoid process between the alar ligaments. It inserts into the anterior margin of the foramen magnum.

The tectorial membrane, or occipitoaxial ligament, is a broad strong band in the vertebral column that lies immediately behind the body of the axis and its ligaments. Inferiorly, it is anchored to the posterior surface of the body of the axis and superiorly to the basilar groove of the occiput. The structure is essentially a continuation upward of the posterior longitudinal ligament.

There are three true synovial articulations between the atlas and the axis—the two lateral atlantoaxial joints and the median atlantoaxial joint. The lateral joints are formed by the inferior articular surfaces of the atlas and the superior articular surfaces of the axis. They are a large mass of arthrodial or gliding joints. Their broad surfaces are directed slightly downward and laterally. The median atlantoaxial joint is essentially a pivot joint with two synovial cavities, one anteriorly between the odontoid and the posterior surface of the anterior arch of the atlas, and the other between the posterior aspect of the odontoid and the front of the transverse ligament of the atlas.

The articular capsules and their accessory ligaments provide stability between the atlas and the axis. The capsular tissues are loose but are reinforced posteriorly and medially by stout fibrous bands termed accessory ligaments. These are anchored below to the body of the axis on either side of the odontoid process and above to the lateral mass of the atlas in relation to the transverse ligament. The anterior atlantoaxial ligament is a broad, dense membrane extending from the inferior border of the anterior arch of the atlas to the anterior aspect of the body of the axis. Anteriorly and in the midline, it is reinforced by a round cord that is a continuation of the anterior longitudinal ligament. It is attached above to the tubercle of the anterior arch of the atlas and below to the body of the axis.

The posterior atlantoaxial ligament is also a broad fibrous band, but it is thinner than its anterior counterpart. It stretches from the lower border of the posterior arch of the atlas to the upper margin of the lamina of the axis. In effect, it corresponds to the ligamentum flavum of the lower vertebra.

The transverse ligament of the atlas is undoubtedly the most important component of the ligamentous system in this region. It is a broad, strong, triangular ligament arching across the ring of the atlas and firmly anchored on each side to a tubercle in the medial surface of the lateral masses of the atlas. It divides the ring of the atlas into a small anterior and a large posterior compartment. In the anterior compartment lies the odontoid process, which is held firmly against the anterior arch of the atlas by the transverse ligament. There are two synovial cavities, one between the arch of the atlas and the odontoid anteriorly, and the other between the transverse ligament and the odontoid posteriorly. The posterior compartment is occupied by the spinal cord and its membranes; this compartment is equally divided between free space and the spinal cord. The transverse ligament gives off two strong fasciculi. The superior fascicle is elongated upward to the basal part of the occiput. Inferiorly, it is attached to the posterior surface of the body of the axis. This gives the transverse ligament a cruciate configuration.

INNERVATION OF THE SPINE

The question of the exact source of neck and back pain has not yet been answered. It is generally assumed that the sinuvertebral nerve carries many of the important sensory fibers from the organs concerned with the production of back pain. The sinuvertebral nerve arises from its spinal nerve near the ramus communicans (Fig 1–9). The nerve enters the spinal canal by way of the intervertebral foramen and curves upward around the base of the pedicle, proceeding toward the midline on the posterior longitudinal ligament (Fig 1–10). It innervates the posterior longitudinal ligament, the blood vessels of the epidural space, the dura mater, and the periosteum. The posterior rami of the spinal nerves supply branches to the skin, muscle, intertransverse ligaments, and apophyseal joints. The lumbodorsal fascia, supraspinous ligaments, and interspinous ligaments are innervated by fine, free nerve fibers and complex unencapsulated nerve endings. The intervertebral joint capsules exhibit the triad of nerve endings found in all other synovial joint capsules: fine, free fibers and both complex unencapsulated and small encapsulated nerve endings. The vertebral periosteum exhibits both fine, free fibers and complex unencapsulated nerve endings.

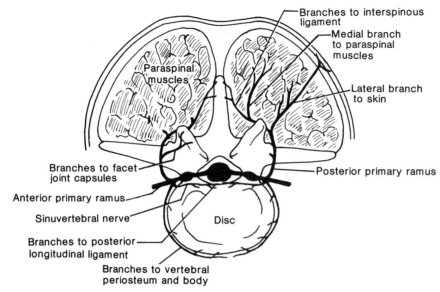

Figure 1–9. Cross-sectional view depicting nerve supply to the anterior (sinuvertebral) and posterior (posterior ramus) portions of the lumbar spine. (From Borenstein DG, Wiesel SW: Low Back Pain: Medical Diagnosis and Management. Philadelphia, W.B. Saunders, 1989.)

This nerve supply to the various structures has been anatomically delineated. It must be stressed that there is no definitive correlation between the structure and the function of these sensory elements. It would be nice to be able to associate a specific nerve supply with a descriptive type of pain, but unfortunately, this is not possible at present.

THE BLOOD SUPPLY OF THE INTERVERTEBRAL DISC

The intervertebral discs are without an active blood supply during the adult phase of life. The small vessels that supply the disc up to the age of 8 years are gradually obliterated during the first three decades of life. By the time growth has stopped, the nucleus pulposus and annulus

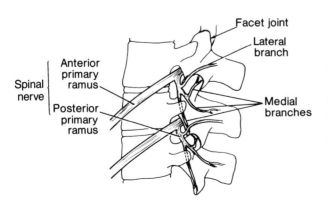

Figure 1–10. Lateral view of the posterior primary rami supplying facet joints at two vertebral levels. (From Borenstein DG, Wiesel SW: Low Back Pain: Medical Diagnosis and Management. Philadelphia, W.B. Saunders, 1989.)

fibrosus no longer have an active blood supply and receive only marginal sustenance from the transfer of tissue fluid across the cartilaginous end plate.

RELATIONAL ANATOMY

Relations of the Spinal Cord

The upper end of the spinal cord can be defined by the beginnings of the first rootlets of the first cervical nerve at the foramen magnum. The average length of the spinal cord is 45 cm in the male and 42 cm in the female. The cord usually terminates between the lower border of the first and the upper border of the second lumbar vertebra.

There is marked variation in the cross-sectional configuration of the cord. Its lateral dimension is usually greater than its anteroposterior one. The average width of the cord in the cervical area is 13.2 mm, in the thoracic region 8 mm, and in the lumbar area 9.6 mm. The average depth is 7.7 mm in the cervical area, 6.5 mm in the thoracic region, and 8.0 mm in the lumbar area.

In the cervical spine the relationship between the cord and vertebral canal is critical. In certain individuals the cervical cord fills a substantially larger percentage of the anteroposterior diameter of the canal. Should spondylosis develop in these persons, a significant myelopathy may occur. The disparity between the oval spinal cord and the triangular cervical canal allows the formation of a gutter anterolaterally between the cord and the walls of the canal. This recess permits some narrowing of the canal anterolaterally without compression of the spinal cord. The effect of disc herniations in relationship to the above-noted dimensions will determine the clinical significance of the herniation.

Relations of the Intervertebral Foramina

The intervertebral foramina are quite significant in the cervical spine (Fig. 1–11). They are essentially small canals approximately 4 mm

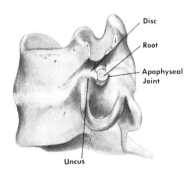

Figure 1–11. This figure illustrates the various components of the motor unit that can compress the nerve root as it courses through the intervertebral foramen. The disc and the uncinate process anteriorly, as well as the apophyseal joint posteriorly, can compromise the nerve root. The anteroposterior diameter is usually more critical than the superoinferior diameter. (From Rothman RH, Simeone FA: The Spine, 2nd ed. Philadelphia, W.B. Saunders, 1982.)

in length that are directed anteriorly and inferiorly. They are ovoid in shape with vertical diameters of approximately 10 mm in height; the anteroposterior diameter is approximately half of this. The roots and floors of the foramina fill the grooves in the bases of the adjacent vertebral arches. The posterolateral wall of each foramen is formed by the adjacent posterolateral articular processes. The superior process of the caudal vertebra contributes more to the formation of this boundary than the inferior process of the cephalad vertebra. The anterolateral wall of each foramen is formed by the lateral portion of the adjacent bodies, the uncovertebral (Luschka) joints, and the inferior portion of the superior vertebra.

All of the cervical spinal nerves except the first and second are contained within the intervertebral foramina. The first cervical nerve lies close to the superior articulation of the atlas and the vertebral artery, and the second in close proximity to the atlantoaxial articulation of the vertebral artery.

The nerve roots and mixed spinal nerve completely fill the anteroposterior diameter of the intervertebral foramen. The upper one quarter of the foramen is filled with areolar tissue and small veins. In addition to these structures, small arteries arising from the vertebral arteries and the sinovertebral nerves traverse the canals. Any space-occupying lesion that encroaches on the anteroposterior diameter of the intervertebral foramen can be expected to cause compression of the nervous tissue elements traversing this limited space. The close proximity of the contents of the intervertebral foramen to the uncovertebral joints anteromedially and to the apophyseal joints posterolaterally should be noted, since these are potential sites of hyperplastic processes that can constrict the canal. Flexion of the cervical spine increases the vertical diameter of the neural foramen, while extension decreases it.

In the lumbar region, the intervertebral foramen is limited in front by a portion of the adjacent vertebral body and the intervertebral disc. The pedicles of two adjacent vertebrae form the superior and inferior boundaries of the foramen. Posteriorly the superior and inferior articular processes, together with the ligamentum flavum, form the remainder of the borders of the foramen.

The lumbar intervertebral foramen is normally five to six times the diameter of the spinal nerve that traverses it (Fig. 1–12). This permits the spinal nerve relative freedom from any type of constriction in the intervertebral foramina. Extension and lateral flexion can decrease the diameter of this foramen significantly. In the lumbar area the foramina are sufficiently elongated that the spinal nerve exists at a level across the vertebral body above the disc space rather than across from the disc proper. Thus, a protruding lumbar disc will narrow the foramen below the level of the exit of the nerve. A disc will then produce its clinical effect by compressing through the dura the most laterally situated nerve of the cauda equina at that level; that is, the nerve that makes its exit at the foramen below the level of the disc. Thus, a herniated disc at the L5-S1 level will produce compression of the S1 nerve and an S1 radiculitis.

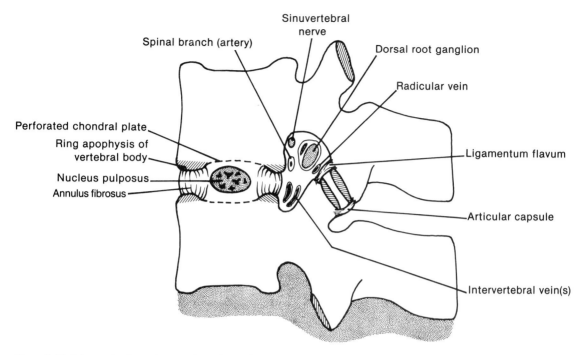

Figure 1-12. Schematic of a sagittal section of the spine showing contents of an intervertebral foramen in relation to a disc. The two vertebral bodies and intervertebral disc along with supporting structures constitute a motor unit, which includes all components of a somite present in an embryo. (From Borenstein DG, Wiesel SW: Low Back Pain: Medical Diagnosis and Management. Philadelphia, W.B. Saunders, 1989.)

Nerve-Disc Relationships

All spinal nerves below the cervical spine emerge from the intervertebral foramina below the corresponding numbered vertebra. Thus, the L5 spinal nerve exits in the intervertebral foramen between L5 and the sacrum. In the cervical region, however, the spinal nerves emerge above the similarly numbered vertebra. The fifth cervical nerve, for instance, emerges between the fourth and fifth cervical vertebrae.

In attempting to localize a disc lesion by the affected nerve root, many factors need to be considered. As noted earlier, the lumbar nerves are nestled sufficiently high in the intervertebral foramina that they will not be affected by a herniated disc at the same level unless the disc fragment migrates upward. The fifth lumbar nerve root, therefore, will be compressed not by a herniated L5-S1 disc but more often by a herniated L4-5 disc. In the cervical spine, disc protrusion will usually affect the nerve root exiting at the same level as the disc, but as mentioned, the numbering system is different. It should also be noted that the rootlets in the cervical spine may arise from a rather wide area one segment above or below the level of the nerve, and thus a disc one segment above or below may cause compression of a particular nerve root.

The Vertebral Artery

The vertebral artery ascends in the foramina of the transverse processes of the cervical vertebrae, in most instances beginning at the level of the sixth cervical vertebra. The artery lies anterior to the anterior primary rami of the third to sixth cervical nerves, inclusive. The second cervical nerve has no foramen and lies posterior to the vertebral artery. The first cervical nerve, after emerging from the dura, lies on the posterior arch of the atlas immediately beneath the vertebral artery. It has been demonstrated that flexion, extension, and rotation of the cervical spine may alter the blood flow in one or both vertebral arteries. It has also been suggested that muscle spasm in the posterior and superior cervical region can produce vascular impairment in a vertebral artery.

References

1. Bradford FK, Spurling RG: The Intervertebral Disc. Springfield, IL, Charles C Thomas, 1945.
2. Compere EL: Origin, anatomy, physiology, and pathology of the intervertebral disc. Instruc Lect Am Acad Orthop Surg 18:15–20, 1961.
3. Crock HV, Yoshizawa H: The Blood Supply of the Vertebral Column and Spinal Cord in Man. New York, Springer-Verlag, 1977.
4. Edgar MA, Ghadially JA: Innervation of the lumbar spine. Clin Orthop 115:35–41, 1976.
5. Galante JO: Tensile properties of the human lumbar annulus fibrosis. Acta Orthop Scand (Suppl) 100:1–91, 1967.
6. Hirsch C, Ingelmark B, Miller M: The anatomical basis for low back pain. Acta Orthop Scand 33:1–17, 1963.
7. Hollinshead WH: Anatomy for Surgeons. The Back and Limbs, Vol. 3, 3rd ed. New York, Harper & Row, 1982.
8. Parke WW: The vascular relations of the upper cervical vertebrae. Orthop Clin North Am 9(4):879–889, 1978.
9. Schmorl G, Junghanns H: The Human Spine in Health and Disease. New York, Grune & Stratton, 1959.
10. Siberstein CE: The evolution of degenerative changes in the cervical spine and an investigation into the "joints of Luschka." Clin Orthop 40:184–204, 1965.
11. Wiberg G: Back pain in relation to nerve supply of intervertebral disc. Acta Orthop Scand 19:211–221, 1949.

CHAPTER 2

Pathophysiology of the Aging Spine

THE AGING INTERVERTEBRAL DISC

It is difficult to differentiate the pathophysiology of intervertebral disc disease from the normal aging process. As clinicians, we deal with the clinical signs and symptoms of this aging process but often do not consider the pathophysiology involved. The changes seen in the normal aging spine grossly, radiographically, biochemically, and biomechanically are within the spectrum of changes seen in a pathologic and symptomatic spine. It is extremely difficult to predict at what point along the continuum of degenerative changes symptoms may arise. The purpose of this section is to describe the changes that occur in the normally aging spine as well as the abnormalities seen with the basic pathologic entities of disc protrusion, spinal stenosis, and instability.

Theories of Aging

The cause of age-related changes remains unknown; however, several theories should be considered. The developmental theory suggests that a failure occurs in the basic embryonic tissue and cellular developmental mechanism. The genetic theory maintains that a failure in maintenance of cellular steady-state energy is due to instability of certain cellular structures caused by faulty gene coding or transcription. Another theory holds that avascular tissues, such as the intervertebral disc, are subject to degeneration owing to the natural loss of cross-linking of macromolecules in the extracellular matrix over time. In reality, the aging process may involve one, all, or none of these concepts.

Morphologic Changes

In the first decades of life, the gross appearance of the spine and its components remains unchanged. The intervertebral disc is a hydrostatic load-bearing structure between vertebral bodies. The nucleus pulposus acts as a confined fluid within the annulus fibrosus and is able to convert axial loads into tensile strain on the annular fibers and the vertebral end plates. The discs maintain their full height, the vertebrae are nearly square in shape, and the facet joints are well defined with smooth capsules and healthy articular cartilage. The ligamentum flavum is only a few millimeters thick, and ample space is present for the neural elements within the canal (Fig. 2–1). In these first few decades, disc protrusions

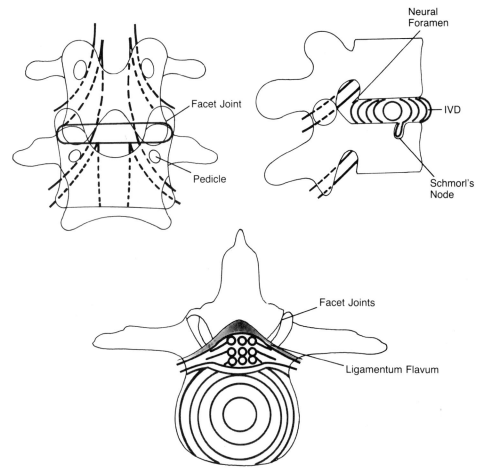

Figure 2–1. AP, lateral, and axial schematics of the spine in the first two decades of life. At this age, the neural structures can be compromised only by trauma, infection, neoplasm, and (relatively rarely) posterior or posterolateral disc herniation. (From Wiesel SW, Bernini P, Rothman RH: The Aging Lumbar Spine. Philadelphia, W.B. Saunders, 1982.)

through the cartilaginous end plate (Schmorl's node) and facet tropism (asymmetric facet configurations) may be seen but are not felt to be responsible for any well-defined symptoms. Trauma to the spine can frequently initiate or accelerate the natural aging process.

During the third through fifth decades of life, changes occur in the spine that may be quite pronounced (Fig. 2–2). In general, the first manifestations of aging are seen in the intervertebral disc, and subsequently changes in the bones and articular processes become evident.[36] Degeneration with diffuse bulging or focal extrusion of disc material will result in narrowing of the intervertebral disc space. The loss of disc height allows close approximation of adjacent vertebral bodies, which may lead to osteophyte formation, facet joint arthritis with hypertrophic changes, and encroachment on the neural elements in the foramina or within the spinal canal itself. These findings may also be manifest in the older spine as end-stage changes of the general aging process (Fig. 2–3). In addition, the facet joint capsule thickens and the ligamentum flavum hypertrophies.

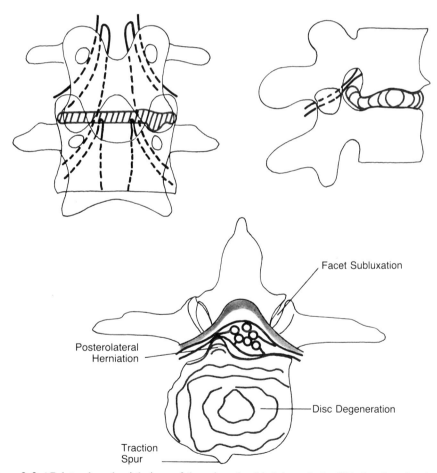

Figure 2–2. AP, lateral, and axial views of the spine, the third through the fifth decades, showing disc degeneration with herniation of the nuclear material. Facet joints in the axial view may show some subluxation, implying a hypermobile phase of motion segment instability. A typical traction spur is demonstrated on the lateral view. (From Wiesel SW, Bernini P, Rothman RH: The Aging Lumbar Spine. Philadelphia, W.B. Saunders, 1982.)

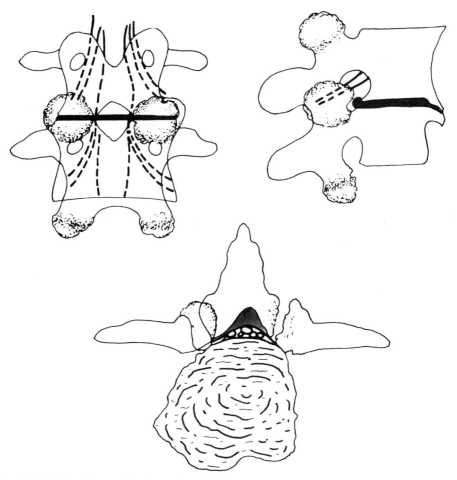

Figure 2–3. AP, lateral, and axial views of the fourth-decade-and-older spine show significant disc degeneration, a traction spur developing into a large osteophyte, and significant hypertrophic changes occurring within the facet joints compromising the neural elements both in the canal and in the neural foramina. Markedly thickened or redundant ligamentum flavum is also seen contributing to this neural compromise. (From Wiesel SW, Bernini P, Rothman RH: The Aging Lumbar Spine. Philadelphia, W.B. Saunders, 1982.)

Loss of disc space height is commonly felt to be part of the degenerative changes that occur in both the cervical and the lumbar spine. While reduction of stature in old age has been attributed to loss of disc height, measurements of average disc heights in cadaveric lumbar spines have shown that only a minority of lower lumbar discs show significant thinning.[34] Thus, loss of stature in the elderly spine is likely due to diminished vertebral body height rather than loss of disc height.[33]

The previously discussed changes in the intervertebral disc and facet joint are generally associated with decreased movement in each motion segment. An olisthesis, or slip (forward or backward), of one vertebra on another may occur as a result of disc incompetence followed by facet subluxation (Fig. 2–4). Such slips are noteworthy but rarely show significant motion on flexion-extension films. Anterior osteophytes, sometimes

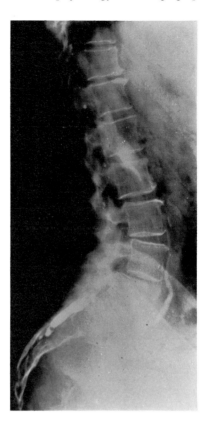

Figure 2–4. Spondylolisthesis resulting from degeneration occurring at L5-S1 with retrolisthesis occurring at L3-4. The direction of slip depends upon the location within the lumbar spine, but the slip itself is subsequent to both disc space degeneration and facet incompetence. (From Wiesel SW, Bernini P, Rothman RH: The Aging Lumbar Spine. Philadelphia, W.B. Saunders, 1982.)

called traction spurs, are frequently indicative of abnormal motion at a spinal segment.

Disc degeneration in adults can occasionally result in disc space calcification (Fig. 2–5); in children, this process is generally asymptomatic and only of minor clinical significance. The etiology of this hydroxyapatite deposition is unclear.

As the spine ages, postural alterations are also common. In the lumbar spine, a reduction in lordosis can be seen as an attempt to unload the degenerating articular facets by maintaining a more flexed rather than extended posture. A flexed position can also provide more room for the susceptible neural elements within the canal and foramina, which are dynamically compromised in extension.

Intervertebral disc degeneration is closely associated with aging, as shown in many cadaveric and radiologic surveys. In the cervical region, the majority of spines after the fourth decade show implications of degeneration in one or more discs, and after the fifth decade, there is a sharp rise in the severity of the degenerative process. DePalma and Rothman found that in specimens from patients over the age of 70, 72 percent showed severe cervical abnormalities,[8] with the C5-6 and C6-7 levels most frequently involved. In the lumbar spine, degenerative changes are almost universal after age 60, and the most frequently involved levels are L4-5, L3-4, and L5-S1.[20]

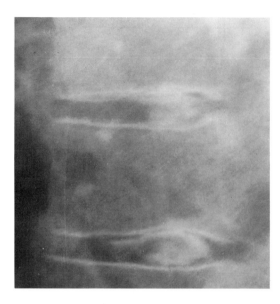

Figure 2–5. Calcification of nucleus pulposus. (From Kricun ME: Imaging Modalities in Spinal Disorders. Philadelphia, W.B. Saunders, 1988.)

Biochemical Changes

Perhaps the major consequence of disc degeneration is the loss of hydrostatic properties. In a young adult disc, the nucleus pulposus is 85 percent water and the annulus, 78 percent water. With aging, the water content in both tissues falls to about 70 percent.[19] There is a gradual decrease in the osmotic swelling pressure of the intervertebral disc and a twofold increase in creep under compression from age 30 to 80.[16] The ability of the disc to imbibe water and evenly distribute load deteriorates with aging, largely owing to changes in the molecular meshwork of proteoglycans and collagen.[21]

The major structural components of the intervertebral disc, aside from water, are collagen and proteoglycans. The nucleus pulposus is able to hold its fluid pressure largely because of the presence of negatively charged groups of glycosaminoglycan chains (Fig. 2–6). The crossing collagen fibril arrangement in the layers of the annulus is ideally suited to accommodate the complex stresses caused by compression of the nucleus.[13] The collagen in the nucleus is largely type II, that seen in hyaline cartilage, while the collagen in the annulus is mostly type I, providing increased tensile strength as in tendons.

The biochemical changes in the aging disc can be summarized as follows: (1) loss of clear distinction between nucleus and annulus; (2) gradual increase in collagen content within the disc; (3) loss of negatively charged proteoglycan side chains, decreasing the imbibing capability of the nucleus; and (4) greatly reduced numbers of proteoglycan aggregates.[6,10,27] Similar changes have been seen in herniated intervertebral discs.[7,36] The initiating event, if one exists, remains unknown. Evidence has demonstrated that normal discs do contain collagenase enzymes capable of degrading their extracellular macromolecular matrix.[31]

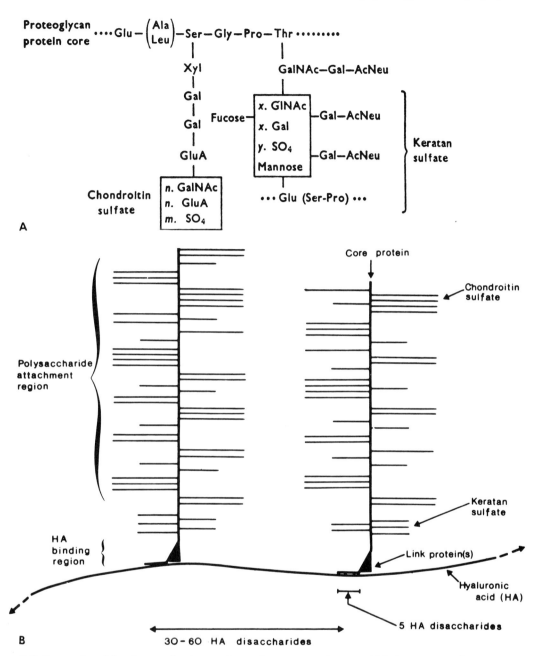

Figure 2-6. Composite of the glycosaminoglycans that make up proteoglycans, which, in turn, contribute to the much larger proteoglycan aggregates. *A,* Proposed structure for chondroitin sulfate–keratan sulfate protein unit. (From Hopwood JJ, Robinson HC: The structure and composition of cartilage keratan sulfate. Biochem J 111: 517, 1971.) *B,* Model of proteoglycan aggregation. (*A,* From Hopwood JJ, Robinson HC: structural studies on keratan sulphate from cartilage. Biochem J Molec Aspects 141:524, 1974).

Changes in the annulus fibrosus have also been noted with aging. The number of cells per unit of tissue surface decreases progressively, along with a gradual reduction in cellular metabolic activity.[28] The major biochemical change in the aging annulus seems to be a decrease in the total content of proteoglycans. Larger collagen fibrils also appear, which may increase the likelihood of failure of an overstressed region of annulus.[14] Localized biochemical changes may predispose certain areas of the annulus to tearing. Focal decrease in collagen content and increase in type III collagen have been associated with annular tears.[1,3,29,32] Unfortunately, significant healing of the torn annulus does not appear to occur.[11]

In addition to changes in the nucleus and annulus with aging, there are also associated changes in the vertebral end plates and adjacent bone marrow.[22,35] Such changes can affect the nutrition of the avascular disc, which is dependent on diffusion of nutrients through the cartilaginous vertebral end plates. Calcification of the end-plate cartilage and vascular changes seen in older vertebrae probably impede the delivery of disc nutrients from the blood.[2] It is possible that these adverse alterations in the nutrient delivery system to the intervertebral disc initiate or at least potentiate the undesirable biochemical changes in the degenerating disc.

In summary, a series of biochemical events can be postulated in which there is a rapid breakdown of proteoglycan aggregates in the disc. During this breakdown of glycosaminoglycans, there is a disproportionate loss of chondroitin sulfate as compared with keratan sulfate. At the same time, there is a rise in the collagen content and decreased delivery of disc nutrients. These changes ultimately result in a reduction in the imbibing capacity of the disc and a loss of its ability to function as a perfect gel. Subsequently, biomechanical compensation by other structures results in further degenerative changes.

Biomechanical Changes

Although the final pathway of the biochemical changes described is altered biomechanics, the initiating event may be mechanical rather than biochemical. There is evidence to suggest that disc degeneration begins with a loss of confined fluid in the nucleus pulposus in an abortive repair attempt, rather than with biochemical changes in proteoglycans.[19] In addition, local mechanical forces may influence the type and distribution of collagen and other macromolecules.[5] Certainly, biochemical and biomechanical changes are closely interwoven.

With degeneration of the disc, a variety of aberrant mechanics occur.[24] As the disc loses its turgor, its capacity to convert vertical load to tangential load for distribution to the annulus diminishes. In addition, the degenerated discs display altered centers of motion that can lead to segmental instability.[17]

Autoimmune Changes

Autoimmune processes may contribute to or accelerate biomechanical failure and biochemical alterations in the degenerating intervertebral disc. An autoimmune etiology for disc degeneration was proposed by Naylor, and Bobechko and Hirsch demonstrated that disc material could act as an antigen.[17, 23] After an annular rupture, previously avascular disc material is exposed to the blood stream and can cause a cellular immune response. Such a theory remains to be validated in vivo.

CLINICAL SEQUELAE OF DISC AGING

In the majority of patients, many of these structural, biochemical, and biomechanical changes occur gradually over time without resulting symptoms. In others, perhaps those with smaller (less tolerant) canals or faster rates of degeneration, symptoms may become severe. In evaluating the various clinical syndromes that result, individual differences in the susceptibility of the anatomic pathways involved and cortical perception of the painful stimuli must be kept in mind. One should consider the pathophysiology of disc disease not only in terms of anatomic, biochemical, and biomechanical factors but also with an appreciation for the complex cortical modulations in a given patient. The remainder of this chapter will discuss the etiology of some of the clinical problems of intervertebral disc aging as they result from disc protrusions, spinal stenosis, and segmental instability. Clinical diagnosis and management of these entities are discussed in subsequent chapters.

Disc Protrusion

With aging, the annulus fibrosus fibrillates and weakens. Radial cracks develop centrally and extend outward toward the periphery. These radiating clefts in the annulus reduce its resistance, and nuclear herniation or annular protrusion ensues. With nuclear herniation, the nuclear material is forced through a tear in the annulus and forms a well-circumscribed mass. This acute form of the pathologic process more commonly affects younger people. In the cervical spine, frank herniation, or a "soft disc," is frequently but not always associated with trauma.

If herniation does not occur early in the process, disc degeneration continues with a subsequent decrease in proteoglycans and increase in collagen. The results are disc fibrosis, loss of disc height, and annular weakening, which produce the second type of disc protrusion, namely annular protrusion or bulging. In the cervical spine, secondary osteophytes forming a "hard disc" can result in the gradual onset of symptoms.[18] Bony hypertrophy can occur at the uncovertebral joints in addition to the facet joints as in the lumbar spine.

Herniation through the annulus is a much greater threat in the younger individual. Between the ages of 30 and 50, the nuclear material still has good turgor and can generate a focal herniation. In the elderly, the disc is desiccated and fibrotic, making herniation less likely. This may explain the predominance of acute disc syndromes in the middle-aged population and their rarity in the elderly.

Nuclear disc material can herniate anterior, posterior, or lateral to the disc space. The weakest portion of the posterior annulus is on either side of the midline where it lacks reinforcement by the strong central fibers of the posterior longitudinal ligament (PLL). Thus it is not surprising that posterolateral protrusions are the most common. Posterior disc herniations can be further distinguished by the structures through which the nuclear material has herniated. If the nuclear material herniates through the annulus but not the PLL, it is called a contained herniation. If the nuclear material also violates the PLL, the herniation is not contained, and free or sequestered fragments may be present in the canal or neural foramen (Fig. 2–7). A true midline posterior protrusion is usually contained within the PLL but may dissect cephalad or caudad, shift laterally, or even stretch the PLL to the point of rupture.

The origin of a disc protrusion, as well as its direction, will determine the clinical signs and symptoms (Fig. 2–8). In the lumbar spine, the posterolateral protrusion is most common; however, in the cervical spine, intraforaminal herniations are more frequent (Fig. 2–9). Unlike a

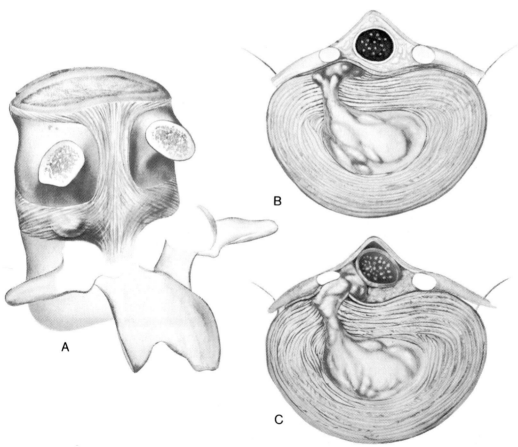

Figure 2–7. *A,* Posterolateral protrusion. The protrusion lies lateral to the midline and lateral to the strong central fibers of the posterior longitudinal ligament. This is the weakest portion of the annulus. *B,* The nuclear material is still contained by the posterior longitudinal ligament. *C,* The nuclear material has penetrated the posterior longitudinal ligament and now lies in the spinal canal. (From DePalma AF, Rothman RH: The Intervetebral Disc. W.B. Saunders, 1970.)

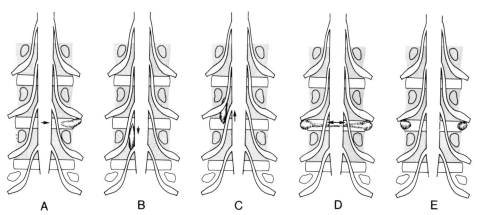

Figure 2–8. Different pathways extruded disc material may take. *A,* If a protrusion arises from the L4-5 disc and migrates directly laterally, it may impinge on the fourth lumbar root. This is a rare situation. *B,* Generally the protrusion migrates downward and laterally and involves the fifth root before it reaches the foramen at the L5-S1 level or it may proceed into the foramen. *C,* The protrusion may travel upward and involve the fourth root before it enters the L4-5 foramen. *D,* Posterolateral protrusions usually involve the root crossing the disc from which the protrusion originated. *E,* Large or double protrusions may involve both roots at this level. (Redrawn from DePalma AF, Rothman RH: The Intervertebral Disc. W.B. Saunders, 1970.)

lumbar disc protrusion, a cervical protrusion may cause myelopathy in addition to radicular pain owing to the presence of the spinal cord in the cervical region. Many cervical protrusions present with some element of upper motor neuron signs.[4,25] In the lumbar spine, clinically significant herniations generally produce radicular symptoms, resulting from compression of individual nerve roots or occasionally the entire cauda equina.

The clinical symptoms of disc protrusions are likely the result of more than just mechanical forces acting on the neural elements. Large protrusions, in addition to generating tension on the neural roots, may also compress the nerve against bone or hypertrophied ligamentum flavum. Because of the lack of elasticity of the roots, minimal tension may generate secondary local inflammatory changes and eventually fibrosis around the nerve root. The root responds to the abnormal situation by becoming injected, edematous, and cordlike. The neurologic deficits from this process may be permanent.

The entity of anterior disc herniation has been infrequently discussed in the literature. However, it is being diagnosed more often with the advent of magnetic resonance imaging, and the incidence of anterior protrusions may be as high as 30 percent in the lumbar spine.[15] Although anterior protrusions do not result in nerve root or cord compression, they may play a role in discogenic and autonomic mediated pain syndromes.

Spinal Stenosis

The secondary alterations that occur in the wake of intervertebral disc degeneration involve all the elements comprising the spinal motion segment. With the loss of the hydrostatic mechanism between the vertebrae, the anterior portions of the vertebral bodies are in closer prox-

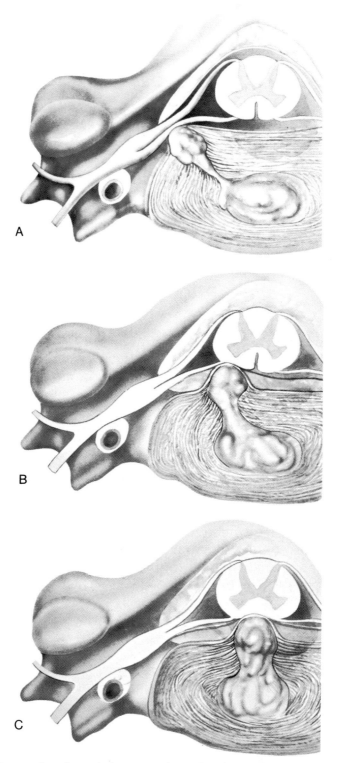

Figure 2–9. *A,* Compression of a cervical nerve root by nuclear tissue at its site of exit from the spinal canal. *B,* Posterolateral lesion encroaching upon the nerve root and lateral aspect of the cord. *C,* Midline lesion encroaching on the central anterior portion of the cord. (Redrawn from DePalma AF, Rothman RH: The Intervertebral Disc. W.B. Saunders, 1970.)

imity and may be subjected to direct compressive forces. As a result, beak-shaped osteophytes may form along the vertebral body rims (Fig. 2–10). There is telescoping of the articular facets of the posterior joints (and the uncovertebral joints in the cervical spine) and stretching of their capsules. Continuous stretch of the posterior joint capsule and ligaments results in a profound thickening of these structures. Compression of the intervertebral joints results in hypertrophic osteophyte formation, which may encroach on the neural foramen or the canal itself (Fig. 2–11).

Ultimately, these degenerative changes result in a narrowing of the spinal canal diameter and a decrease in the size of the neural foramina. The decrease in disc height results in foraminal encroachment from facet hypertrophy posteriorly, the relative descent of the pedicle superiorly, and disc bulging anterior to the foramen. These changes occur gradually, and the patient may remain asymptomatic until late in the degenerative process.

The most common clinical finding associated with early spinal stenosis is nondisabling chronic neck or back pain. Over a few years a radicular pain develops because the neural elements become progressively entrapped within a smaller space. Patients with acquired or congenital canal stenosis are more likely to have severe symptoms with acute disc protrusion.

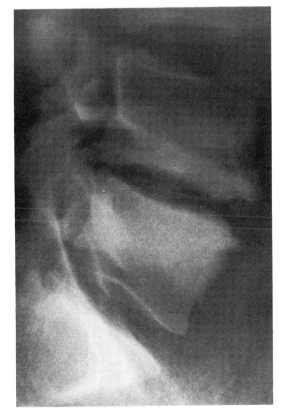

Figure 2–10. Radiograph illustrates a traction osteophyte at the L4-5 level associated with disc degeneration. Note sclerosis at the adjacent vertebral bodies and narrowing of the disc space. (From Rothman RH, Simeone FA: The Spine, 2nd ed. Philadelphia, W.B. Saunders, 1982.)

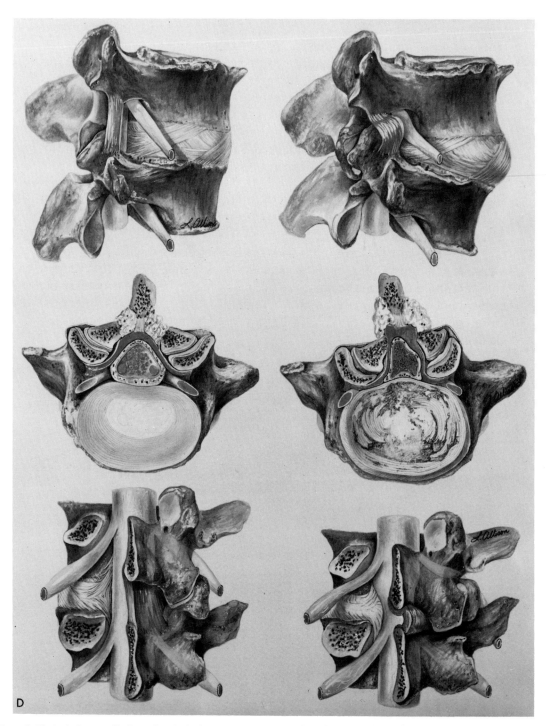

Figure 2–11. Artist's compilation of pathologic changes that result in spinal stenosis (*right*) compared with three normal views of the L4-5 intervertebral joint (*left*). (From Rothman RH, Simeone FA: The Spine, 2nd ed. Philadelphia, W.B. Saunders, 1982.)

In the cervical spine, stenosis may result in radicular symptoms or myelopathy. Although fewer than 5 percent of patients with cervical spondylosis develop myelopathy, these patients are likely to require surgical treatment. The changes of myelopathy are most often gradual and associated with posterior osteophyte formation with secondary spinal canal narrowing. Acute myelopathy is most often the result of a central soft disc herniation producing a high-grade block on a myelogram. Edward and LaRocca have categorized symptomatic spinal stenosis as almost certain with midcervical canal diameters less than 10 mm, at risk (premyelopathic) with diameters of 10 to 13 mm, myelopathy-prone with diameters of 13 to 17 mm, and rarely seen with diameters greater than 17 mm.[9] Hayashi and colleagues have shown that other factors such as vascular changes in the cord, repeated trauma, soft tissue entrapment from disc protrusion, and invagination of the ligamentum flavum are also important in predicting cervical myelopathy.[12]

In the lumbar spine, a claudication-type pain related to ambulation frequently develops secondary to spinal stenosis. During ambulation, there are mechanical irritation and poor excursion of the spinal nerves secondary to entrapment, edema, and ischemia from vasonervosum compromise in the cauda equina. This pseudoclaudication (neurogenic claudication) must be distinguished from true vascular claudication.

Spinal Instability

Spinal instability, or abnormal motion beyond physiologic constraints at a spinal segment, can have many etiologies. Although ligaments can be injured in acute trauma, instability in the older population is more commonly due to chronic disc degeneration, with associated arthritis of the intervertebral joints and laxity of the spinal supporting structures. Slippage of one vertebra on another (olisthesis) is called spondylolisthesis when the superior body is displaced anteriorly or retrolisthesis when the superior body slips posteriorly. Degenerative spondylolisthesis is most common in the older population. Pathologic spondylolisthesis due to a structural weakness secondary to tumor, infection, or metabolic disease may also be seen.

In the cervical spine, instability can occur at a single level, but with chronic disc degeneration multiple level involvement may be seen. Radiographically, anteroposterior subluxation of more than 3.5 mm in flexion or extension is generally considered significant (Fig. 2–12). Cervical instability can result in nerve root irritation and symptoms or frank cord impingement.

Degenerative spondylolisthesis in the lumbar spine occurs most often in the latter half of life. It is most common in black females and occurs six times more often at L4-5 than at L3-4.[30] Unlike isthmic spondylolisthesis, which occurs in younger patients, usually at L5-S1, degenerative spondylolisthesis does not involve a pars interarticularis defect and slip-

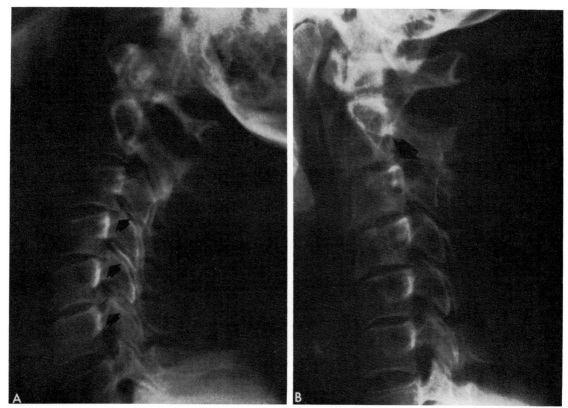

Figure 2–12. Neck and suboccipital pain secondary to multiple level subluxation in flexion and extension. *A,* At the C3-4, C4-5, and C5-6 levels, there was posterior overriding of the vertebral bodies in extension. At this time the patient experienced neck and shoulder pain. *B,* In flexion, there was good alignment of these vertebrae, but C2 subluxed anteriorly on C1, at which time the patient noted marked suboccipital pain. Stabilization in a cervical collar alleviated her symptoms. (From Rothman RH, Simeone FA: The Spine, 2nd ed. Philadelphia, W.B. Saunders, 1982.)

page is never greater than 30 percent (Fig. 2–13). Patients with spondylolisthesis are frequently asymptomatic and often do not demonstrate radiographic instability. In general, normal lumbar horizontal translation is considered to be less than 3.0 mm, but this remains an area of continued uncertainty owing to a large range in normal values.[26]

References

1. Adam M, Deyl Z: Degenerated annulus fibrosus of the intervertebral disc contains collagen type II. Ann Rheum Dis 43:258–263, 1984.
2. Bernick S, Cailliet R: Vertebral end-plate changes with aging of human vertebrae. Spine 7:97–102, 1982.
3. Blumenkrantz N, Sylvest J, Asboe-Hansen G: Local low-collagen content may allow herniation of intervertebral disc: Biochemical studies. Biochem Med 18:283–290, 1977.
4. Bohlman HH, Emery SE: The pathophysiology of cervical spondylosis and myelopathy. Spine 13:843–846, 1988.
5. Brickley-Parsons D, Glimcher MJ: Is the chemistry of collagen in intervertebral discs an expression of Wolff's law? A study of the human lumbar spine. Spine 9:148–163, 1984.
6. Brown MD: The pathophysiology of disc disease. Orthop Clin North Am 2:359–370, 1971.
7. Davidson EA, Woodhall B: Biochemical alterations in herniated intervertebral disks. J Biol Chem 234:2951–2954, 1959.

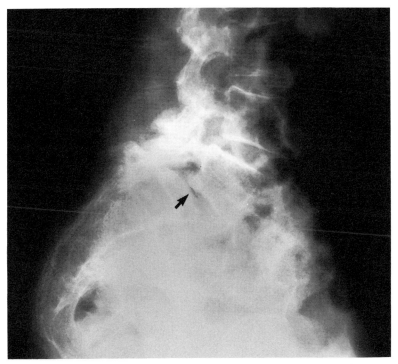

Figure 2–13. An 82-year-old woman was evaluated for low-back pain of 2 months' duration. The pain was constant, exacerbated by anterior flexion and relieved by lying supine. Lateral view of the lumbosacral spine reveals a grade II degenerative spondylolisthesis at the L5-S1 interspace. A vacuum phenomenon is also present at the same interspace (*arrow*). (From Borenstein DG, Wiesel SW: Low Back Pain: Medical Diagnosis and Management. Philadelphia, W.B. Saunders, 1989.)

8. DePalma AF, Rothman RH: The Intervertebral Disc. Philadelphia, W.B. Saunders, 1970, pp. 37–38.
9. Edward WC, LaRocca SH: The developmental segmental sagittal diameter in combined cervical and lumbar spinal spondylosis. Spine 10:43–49, 1985.
10. Gower WE, Pedrini V: Age-related variations in protein polysaccharides from human nucleus pulposus, annulus fibrosus, and costal cartilage. J Bone Joint Surg 51A:1154–1162, 1969.
11. Hampton D, Laros G, McCarron R, et al: Healing potential of the annulus fibrosus. Spine 14:398–401, 1989.
12. Hayashi H, Okada K, Hamada M, et al: Etiologic factors of myelopathy. A radiographic evaluation of the aging changes in the cervical spine. Clin Orthop 214:200–209, 1987.
13. Hickey DS, Hukins DWL: Relation between the structure of the annulus fibrosus and the function and failure of the intervertebral disc. Spine 5:106–115, 1980.
14. Hickey DS, Hukins DWL: Aging changes in the macromolecular organization of the intervertebral disc. An X-ray diffraction and electron microscopic study. Spine 7:234–242, 1982.
15. Jinkins JR, Whittenmore AR, Bradley WG: The anatomic basis of vertebrogenic pain and the autonomic syndrome associated with lumbar disk extrusion. Am J Neuroradiol 10:219–231, 1989.
16. Koeller W, Muehlhaus S, Meier W, et al: Biomechanical properties of human intervertebral discs subjected to axial dynamic compression: Influence of age and degeneration. J Biomech 19:807–816, 1986.
17. LaRocca H: New horizons in research on disc disease. Orthop Clin North Am 2:521–531, 1971.
18. Lestini WF, Wiesel SW: The pathogenesis of cervical spondylosis. Clin Orthop 239:69–93, 1989.
19. Lipson SJ, Muir H: Proteoglycans in experimental intervertebral disc degeneration. Spine 6:194–210, 1981.
20. Miller JAA, Schmatz C, Schultz AB: Lumbar disc degeneration: Correlation with age, sex and spine level in 600 autopsy specimens. Spine 13:173–178, 1988.
21. Mitchell PEG, Hendry NGC, Billewicz WZ: The chemical background of intervertebral disc prolapse. J Bone Joint Surg 43B:141–151, 1961.
22. Modic MT, Steinberg PM, Ross JS, et al: Degenerative disk disease: Assessment of changes in vertebral body marrow with MR imaging. Radiology 166:193–199, 1988.
23. Naylor A: The biochemical changes in the human intervertebral disc in degeneration and nuclear prolapse. Orthop Clin North Am 2:343–358, 1971.

24. Panjabi MM, Krag MH, Chung TQ: Effects of disc injury on mechanical behavior of the human spine. Spine 9:707–713, 1984.
25. Parke WW: Correlative anatomy of cervical spondylotic myelopathy. Spine 13:831–837, 1988.
26. Pearcy MJ: Stereoradiography of lumbar spine motion. Acta Orthop Scand (Suppl) 56 (212):1–41, 1985.
27. Pedrini-Mille A, Pedrini VA, Tudisco C, et al: Proteoglycans of human scoliotic intervertebral disc. J Bone Joint Surg 65A:815–823, 1983.
28. Postacchini F, Bellocci M, Massobrio M: Morphologic changes in annulus fibrosus during aging. An ultrastructural study in rats. Spine 9:596–603, 1984.
29. Roberts S, Beard HK, O'Brien JP: Biochemical changes of intervertebral discs in patients with spondylolisthesis or with tears of the posterior annulus fibrosus. Ann Rheum Dis 41:78–85, 1982.
30. Rosenberg NJ: Degenerative spondylolisthesis. Surgical treatment. Clin Orthop 117:112–120, 1976.
31. Sedowofia KA, Tomlinson IW, Weiss JB, et al: Collagenolytic enzyme systems in human intervertebral disc. Their control, mechanism, and their possible role in the initiation of biomechanical failure. Spine 7:213–222, 1982.
32. Stevens RL, Ryvar R, Robertson WR, et al: Biological changes in the annulus fibrosus in patients with low-back pain. Spine 7:223–233, 1982.
33. Twomey LT, Taylor JR: Age changes in lumbar intervertebral discs. Acta Orthop Scand 56:496–499, 1985.
34. Twomey LT, Taylor JR: Age changes in lumbar vertebrae and intervertebral discs. Clin Orthop 224:97–104, 1987.
35. Twomey LT, Taylor JR, Furniss B: Age changes in the bone density and structure of the lumbar vertebral column. J Anat 136:15–25, 1983.
36. Vernon-Roberts B, Pirie CJ: Degenerative changes in the intervertebral discs of the lumbar spine and their sequelae. Rheumatol Rehabil 16:13–21, 1977.

The Cervical Spine

CHAPTER 3

Clinical Syndromes and Physical Examination of the Cervical Spine*

CERVICAL SPONDYLOSIS

As humans have achieved erect posture, the cervical spine has evolved to obtain a remarkable degree of mobility and flexibility. Although subjected to loads of less magnitude than the lumbar spine, it manifests degenerative changes of aging with exceptional regularity.[52] It may be because of this remarkable mobility that degenerative changes are so consistently seen during the process of aging.

The radiographic and pathologic consequences of the aging process begin to manifest themselves in the third decade of life. Cervical spondylosis is a term used to describe the sequence of degenerative changes that occurs in the vertebral body, intervertebral disc, uncovertebral joints, zygoapophyseal joints, ligamentum flavum, dura, and soft tissues with increasing age. Intervertebral disc degeneration, disc space collapse, spinal canal and foraminal osteophyte formation, and hypertrophy of the facet, lamina, ligamentum flavum, and dura are morphologic changes seen in cervical spondylosis and, to a lesser degree, in asymptomatic elderly patients. Because the natural history of cervical spondylosis parallels the aging process, it is often difficult to determine whether these morphologic changes are due to the aging process or to disease states. Indeed, the anatomic and radiographic expressions of cervical spondylosis become significant only when etiologically related to distinct clinical syndromes. Three clinical syndromes arise from cervical spondylosis: neck pain, cervical spondylotic radiculopathy, and cervical spondylotic myelopathy.

Pathogenesis

In 1989, Lestini and Wiesel published a comprehensive review on the pathogenesis of degenerative processes in the cervical spine.[39] In 1555, Vesalius gave the first description of the intervertebral disc.[66] The original description of spinal cord compression from a spondylotic bar was not reported until 1838.[34] Von Luschka gave an accurate description of the disc and postulated its embryology in 1858.[68]

During the first half of this century, radicular symptoms and spinal cord compression were attributed to the consequences of arthritic changes of the spine.[5,19] Research has continued in the embryology, physiology, and pathology of the intervertebral disc and in the anatomy and pathology of disc protrusion.[35,54,55,59] Others have focused on the consequences of joint degeneration,[13,45] disc protrusion,[22,45,60] vascular changes,[10,42] ligamentum flavum compression,[63] and spinal cord dimension[4,48] in the cervical spine. More recently, researchers have studied the impact of dynamic as well as static reduction of spinal canal diameter[1–3,12,28,49,50,62] and have examined premorbid spinal canal dimensions, developmental cervical spinal stenosis, and the factors that trigger symptoms.[8,20,70]

HISTORY

The mildest form of neck injury, and the most common, is cervical strain. This soft tissue injury results from stretching of the tissues beyond their elastic limit. The vast majority of patients presenting with complaints of neck pain following minimal or no trauma and with normal neurologic findings have this injury.

In the elderly, however, comparatively less force is needed to create significant injury. The head and neck should be regarded as a unit, and any evidence of blunt trauma to the head (altered mental status, scalp laceration, facial laceration) justifies radiographic evaluation of the cervical spine.[9] Elderly patients with spondylotic changes may demonstrate acute traumatic cervical myelopathy (central cord syndrome) following seemingly mild trauma. In this clinical setting, radiographs may not demonstrate any evidence of fracture or instability attributable to the trauma. Individuals with developmental stenosis and degenerative spondylosis are predisposed to develop myelopathy after minor trauma.

After determining the timing of the onset of complaints, the frequency, quality, and precise distribution of symptoms become important points. Careful questioning about subtle long tract symptoms (clumsy gait, bowel and/or bladder changes) is also essential to avoid missing an early myelopathy. A history of previous malignancies, metabolic disorders, and arthritis in other joints is also relevant.

CLINICAL SYNDROMES

Neck Pain

Referred neck pain is a common clinical syndrome that may be seen in the presence or absence of trauma or radiographic findings. It is prevalent in industrial employees.[69] The pathogenesis of neck pain is attributed to structures innervated by the sinovertebral nerve or the nerves innervating the paravertebral soft tissues. In contradistinction to radicular pain, which is characterized by deep aching, burning, or shooting arm pain following a radicular distribution, referred pain is more vague, diffuse, axial, nondermatomal, and poorly localized. Stimulation of sinovertebral nerve fibers to the annulus fibrosus, facet joints, and anterior and posterior longitudinal ligaments can elicit this pain. Variable success with the localization and diagnosis of the origin of referred neck pain by infiltration of local anesthetic into the disc, nerve root, or facet joint has been reported.[36,53,56]

The natural history of conservative treatment of neck pain was outlined by Rothman and Simeone.[52] The literature has consistently reported a guarded prognosis for referred neck pain.[24–26,32,38,41,52] Ten-year follow-up of patients with neck pain[24] continues to underscore these findings: (1) approximately one third of the patients remain in moderate or severe pain; (2) clinical and radiographic data are of little value in directing treatment or predicting outcome; (3) patients reporting severe initial pain are more likely to have an unsatisfactory outcome; and (4) patients in litigation report severe initial pain more frequently.

A standardized approach to the evaluation and treatment of industrial patients with cervical spine problems has had encouraging initial results and is discussed in Chapter 5.[69] Using this approach, appropriate and reasonable medical care resulted in a decrease in the number of injuries, in the number of lost work days, and in costs.

Radicular Symptoms

Nerve root irritation may vary in anatomic location and degree of involvement. Single or multiple, unilateral or bilateral, symmetric or asymmetric root involvement can occur. The degree of root involvement can vary from monoradiculopathy to multilevel radiculopathy and associated cord compression. Stookey as well as Rothman and Marvel have described the types of soft disc protrusion.[51,60] Intraforaminal herniations are the most common and produce dermatomal radiculopathy. Posterolateral lesions present with a preponderance of motor signs, while central herniations may demonstrate myelopathy (Fig. 3–1). Although it is theoretically possible for cervical radiculopathy to manifest on either side of the spine and at any number of levels, a more confined distribution is usually encountered. The extensive experience of Henderson and associates has shown cervical radiculopathy to be localized to the C5-6 or C6-7 interspace in the vast majority of cases.[31]

The clinical manifestations of radiculopathy vary.[17] Acute radiculopathy, in the absence of cervical spondylosis or disc degeneration, can occur in the young patient. This may be seen in blunt trauma involving vertebral dislocation or end-plate disruption. Acute disc herniation is seen in individuals with varying degrees of spondylotic changes. Often a history of prior neck symptoms or minor trauma can be elicited. The more acute forms of radiculopathy are more likely to be associated with a soft disc herniation[51,52] (Fig. 3–2). Patients with long-standing radiographic evidence of cervical spondylosis may present with mono- or polyradiculopathy without a history of trauma. The majority of these patients respond to conservative treatment.

Chronic radiculopathy typically presents in elderly patients as the insidious onset of symptoms referable to root involvement. Chronic radiculopathy can result in persistence of signs and symptoms of acute or subacute radiculopathy following conservative treatment.[39] The diagnosis of cervical radiculopathy is established by the clear identification of the signs and symptoms of nerve root irritation (see Table 3–1). Diagnostic confirmation is provided by imaging studies demonstrating compression of the clinically suspected nerve root (Fig. 3–3).

Sensory symptoms are present in nearly all patients. Curiously, nondermatomal, diffuse pain and/or paresthesias are quite common, occurring in 45 percent of 841 cases reviewed by Henderson and co-workers.[31] Pain and/or paresthesia followed a dermatomal pattern in 54 percent of cases, and a demonstrable deficit in pinprick sensation was observed in 85 percent.

In summary, cervical radiculopathy is diagnosed when a symptom complex specific for an affected root or roots is observed. Commonly, patients will describe relief of monoradicular pain with abduction of the shoulder.[6,16,57,58,67] The diagnosis is confirmed when imaging studies demonstrate nerve root compression.

Cervical Myelopathy

The progressive degenerative process of cervical spondylosis can culminate in myelopathy. Patients with developmental cervical stenosis are predisposed to manifest myelopathy at a younger age.[8,20,21,65] The degenerative changes implicated in the development of cervical

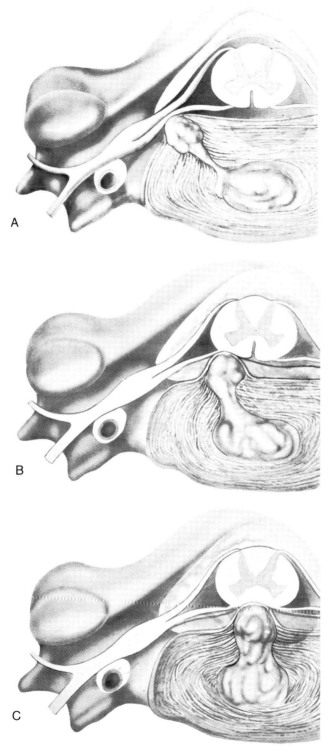

Figure 3–1. Types of soft disc protrusion. *A,* Intraforaminal, most common. *B,* Posterolateral, produces mostly motor signs. *C,* Midline, may manifest as myelopathy. (Modified from DePalma AF, Rothman RH: The Intervertebral Disc. Philadelphia, W.B. Saunders, 1970.)

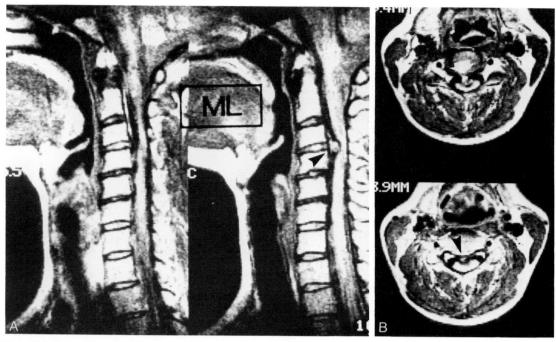

Figure 3–2. This 32-year-old female presented with acute radiculopathy and myelopathy. *A,* Midsagittal MRI demonstrates midline soft disc herniation at C3-4 *(arrow)* with cord compression. *B,* Axial MRI confirms midline soft disc herniation and cord compression *(arrows).*

Table 3–1. CERVICAL RADICULOPATHY SYMPTOMS AND FINDINGS

Disc Level	Nerve Root	Symptoms and Findings
C2-3	C3	*Pain:* Back of neck, mastoid process, pinna of ear *Sensory Change:* Back of neck, mastoid process, pinna of ear *Motor Deficit:* None readily detectable except by EMG *Reflex Change:* None
C3-4	C4	*Pain:* Back of neck, levator scapula, anterior chest *Sensory Change:* Back of neck, levator scapulae, anterior chest *Motor Deficit:* None readily detectable except by EMG *Reflex Change:* None
C4-5	C5	*Pain:* Neck, tip of shoulder, anterior arm *Sensory Change:* Deltoid area *Motor Deficit:* Deltoid, biceps *Reflex Change:* Biceps
C5-6	C6	*Pain:* Neck, shoulder, medial border of scapula, lateral arm, dorsal forearm *Sensory Change:* Thumb and index finger *Motor Deficit:* Biceps *Reflex Change:* Biceps
C6-7	C7	*Pain:* Neck, shoulder, medial border of scapula, lateral arm, dorsal forearm *Sensory Change:* Index and middle fingers *Motor Deficit:* Triceps *Reflex Change:* Triceps
C7-T1	C8	*Pain:* Neck, medial border of scapula, medial aspect of arm and forearm *Sensory Change:* Ring and little fingers *Motor Deficit:* Intrinsic muscles of hand *Reflex Change:* None

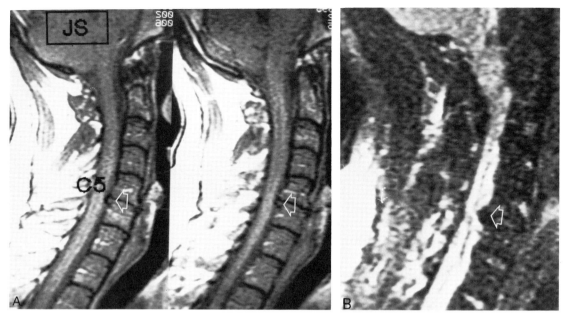

Figure 3–3. This 45-year-old male presented with unilateral C6 radiculopathy. *A,* Midsagittal MRI shows more pathologic anatomy than the parasagittal view of the unaffected side *(arrows).* *B,* Parasagittal MRI of the affected side shows hard disc pathology *(arrow).*

spondylotic myelopathy include hypertrophy of the lamina, facets, ligamentum flavum, and dura, redundant annulus fibrosus, compression of radicular vessels by foraminal osteophytes, spinal cord compression by vertebral osteophytes, tethering of the spinal cord by dentate ligaments, and ossification of the ligamentum flavum or posterior longitudinal ligament.* Reduction of the functional volume of the spinal canal can result in direct compression and can cause intrinsic or extrinsic ischemia.† A decrease in the anteroposterior canal diameter is a necessary[18,30,70] but not sufficient cause of myelopathy.[4,5,30]

Dynamic stenosis further reduces osseous canal dimensions.[1–3,28,30,49,62] Spinal cord compression by the pincer mechanism was described by Penning and van der Zwaag in 1966. The spinal cord is pinched between the posteroinferior osteophyte of the rostral vertebra and the anterosuperior margin of the lamina of the caudal vertebra.[49] Flexion stretches the cord over vertebral body osteophytes, and extension may cause retrolisthesis of a vertebral body or buckling of the ligamentum flavum.[12,50] In the aging cervical spine, dynamic and static canal stenosis are essential for the development of myelopathy. Retrolisthesis of the upper cervical spine (C3-4 and C4-5) can combine with disc protrusion and osteophytosis at C5-6 and C6-7 to produce multilevel canal stenosis.

The clinical picture of cervical spondylotic myelopathy varies considerably. The onset of symptoms is usually after 50 years of age and

*Refs. 1–3,8,15,20,22,37,43,44,47,48,61,62,65,70.
†Refs. 7,11,23,27,33,46,61,62,64.

males are more often affected. Onset is usually insidious, although there is occasionally a history of trauma. The natural history is that of initial deterioration followed by a plateau period lasting several months. The resulting clinical picture is often one of an incomplete spinal lesion with a patchy distribution of deficits. Disability varies with the number of vertebrae involved and the degree of involvement at each level.[38,44,71]

Common presenting symptoms of cervical myelopathy include numbness and paresthesias in the hands, clumsiness of the fingers, weakness (greatest in the lower extremities), and gait disturbances. Abnormalities of micturition are seen in about one third of cases and indicate more severe cord involvement. Symptoms of radiculopathy can coexist with myelopathy and confuse the clinical picture. Sensory disturbances may show patchy distribution. Spinothalamic tract (pain and temperature) deficits may be seen in the upper extremities, thorax, or lumbar region and may be in a stocking or glove distribution. Posterior column deficits (vibration and proprioception) are more commonly seen in the feet than hands. Usually there is no gross sensory impairment but a diminished sense of appreciation of light touch and pinprick.[39,71]

In summary, the diagnosis of cervical spondylotic myelopathy is suspected in a patient with a clinical presentation typical of myelopathy, with or without radiculopathy, and imaging studies demonstrating single or multilevel cervical spinal cord compression. The diagnosis is confirmed when the many disorders with a similar clinical presentation have been excluded. Since cervical spondylosis is so prevalent in elderly patients, the diagnosis of cervical spondylotic myelopathy must be carefully considered.[11,14,52,71]

PHYSICAL EXAMINATION

For the clinician treating patients with cervical spondylosis, the most critical problem is identification of the level (or levels) responsible for symptomatology. The physical examination is vitally important for the demonstration or exclusion of alternative sources of symptomatology.[29] Compressive neuropathies, thoracic outlet syndrome, and chest and shoulder pathology are differential diagnoses for cervical radiculopathy.[9,29] Chest, shoulder, and abdominal pathology must be excluded for the diagnosis of referred neck pain. Cervical spondylotic myelopathy must be carefully diagnosed.[11] In one study, as many as 17 percent of patients initially diagnosed with cervical spondylotic myelopathy were later shown to have other disease.[14]

Observations should be made of the patient's general health, mental status, facial expressions, and head and body posture. Gait abnormalities and micturition disturbances should be sought. Patients with spondylosis or cervical radiculopathy are often awakened with severe neck pain. The pain results from stimulation of the sinuvertebral nerve fibers and may be referred to the head, neck, shoulders, or scapulae. There may be no motor, sensory, gait, or reflex abnormalities. Patients with referred neck pain secondary to cervical spondylosis may demonstrate limitation of cervical range of motion.

Radicular Signs

Patients with radiculopathy complain of pain distributed along a clearly defined dermatome. Unfortunately, diffuse nondermatomal pain is as commonly noted in patients with abnormal myelograms.[31] The Valsalva maneuver, or any maneuver that stretches the involved nerve root, may increase the pain. Attacks of sharp acute pain that radiates into the fingers may be associated with paresthesias. Shoulder abduction, neck hyperextension, and neck compression tests are often positive in patients with compressive radiculopathy.[6,16,67] Wasting, focal weakness, and diminished reflexes of the involved nerve root may be revealed on examination.

Henderson and colleagues and Lunsford and co-workers found a demonstrable motor deficit in about 65 percent of patients with cervical radiculopathy.[31,40] The incidence of a specific motor deficit was 37 percent for the triceps, 28 percent for the biceps, 1.9 percent for the deltoid, and 0.6 percent for those muscles involved in grip. Thirty-two percent of patients showed no motor deficit.[31]

Diminished deep tendon reflexes are observed in the majority of patients. In Henderson's series, a specific decrease in a deep tendon reflex was seen in 71 percent of 846 patients. Thirty-six percent had a diminished triceps jerk, 35 percent had a diminished biceps jerk, and 29 percent showed no deep tendon reflex change.[31]

In addition to motor, sensory, and reflex examination, manual tests and maneuvers that increase or decrease radicular symptoms may also be useful. In the neck compression test, the patient's head is flexed laterally, slightly rotated, and then compressed to elicit aggravation of radicular symptoms. The axial manual traction test is performed in the presence of radicular symptoms in the supine position. With 20 to 30 lb of axial traction, a positive finding is the decrease or disappearance of radicular symptoms. The shoulder abduction test is performed in the sitting position. A positive result is the decrease or disappearance of radicular symptoms when the patient lifts a hand above the head. All of these tests are highly specific for the diagnosis of root compression, but the sensitivity is less than 50 percent.[67]

Myelopathic Signs

Patients affected with spondylotic myelopathy may complain of micturition and gait disturbances. The patient's gait should be observed, and the extent of motor disability, which may vary from mild to severe, should be ascertained. Pyramidal tract weakness and atrophy are more commonly seen in the lower extremities and are the most common abnormal signs. The usual clinical findings in the lower extremities are spasticity and weakness. Weakness and wasting of the upper extremities and hands may also be due to combined spondylotic myelopathy and radiculopathy. The patient usually complains of hand clumsiness. A diminished or absent upper extremity deep tendon reflex, often the triceps jerk, can indicate compressive radiculopathy superimposed on spondylotic myelopathy.

Sensory deficits in spinothalamic (pain and temperature) and posterior column (vibration and proprioception) function should be documented. Usually there is no gross impairment of sensation; rather, a patchy decrease in light touch and pinprick is seen. Hyper-reflexia, clonus, and upgoing Babinski's signs are seen in the lower extremities. Hoffmann's sign and hyper-reflexia may be observed in the upper extremeties.

After a complete history and physical examination, a working diagnosis is formulated, which can be confirmed or refined with the appropriate diagnostic studies. Chapter 4 discusses imaging and electrodiagnostic studies of the cervical spine.

References

1. Adams CBT, Logue V: Studies in cervical spondylotic myelopathy. I. Movement of the cervical roots, dura and cord, and their relation to the course of the extrathecal roots. Brain 94:557–568, 1971.
2. Adams CBT, Logue V: Studies in cervical spondylotic myelopathy. II. The movement and contour of the spine in relation to the neural complications of cervical spondylosis. Brain 94:569–586, 1971.
3. Adams CBT, Logue V: Studies in cervical spondylotic myelopathy. III. Some functional effects of operations for cervical spondylotic myelopathy. Brain 94:587–594, 1971.
4. Arnold JG: The clinical manifestations of spondylochondrosis (spondylosis) of the cervical spine. Ann Surg 141:872–889, 1955.
5. Bailey P, Casamajor L: Osteoarthritis of the spine as a cause of compression of the spinal cord and its roots. J Nerv Ment Dis 38:588, 1911.
6. Beatty RM, Fowler FD, Hanson EJ: The abducted arm as a sign of ruptured cervical disc. Neurosurg 21(5):731–732, 1987.
7. Bedford PD, Bosanquet FD, Russell WR: Degeneration of the spinal cord associated with cervical spondylosis. Lancet 2:55–59, 1952.
8. Bohlman HH: Cervical spondylosis with moderate to severe myelopathy: A report of 17 cases treated by Robinson anterior cervical discectomy and fusion. Spine 2:151–162, 1977.
9. Bohlman HH: The neck. In D'Ambrosia RD (ed): Musculoskeletal Disorders: Examination of Differential Diagnosis, 2nd ed. Philadelphia, J.B. Lippincott, 1986.
10. Brain WR, Knight GC, Bull JWD: Rupture of the intervertebral disk in the cervical region. Proc R Soc Med 41:509–516, 1948.
11. Brain WR, Northfield D, Wilkenson M: Neurological manifestations of cervical spondylosis. Brain 75:187–225, 1952.
12. Breig A, Turnbull I, Hassler O: Effects of mechanical stresses on the spinal cord in cervical spondylosis. J Neurosurg 25:45–56, 1966.
13. Bull J: Review of cerebral angiography. Proc R Soc Med 42:880, 1949.
14. Campbell AMG, Phillips DG: Cervical disk lesions with neurological disorder. Differential diagnosis, treatment, and prognosis. Br Med J 2:481–485, 1960.
15. Clarke E, Robison PV: Cervical myelopathy: A complication of cervical spondylosis. Brain 79:483–510, 1956.
16. Davidson RI, Dunn EJ, Metzmaker JN: The shoulder abduction test in the diagnosis of radicular pain in the cervical extradural compressive monoradiculopathies. Spine 6:441–446, 1981.
17. Dillin W, Booth R, Cuckler J, et al: Cervical radiculopathy. Spine 11(10):988–991, 1986.
18. Edwards WC, LaRocca H: The developmental segmental sagittal diameter of the cervical spinal canal in patients with cervical spondylosis. Spine 8:20–27, 1983.
19. Elliot GR: A contribution to spinal osteoarthritis involving the cervical region. J Bone Joint Surg 8:42, 1926.

20. Epstein J, Carras R, Epstein BS, et al: Myelopathy in cervical spondylosis with vertebral subluxation and hyperlordosis. J Neurosurg 32:421–426, 1970.
21. Epstein J, Janin Y, Carras R, et al: A comparative study of the treatment of cervical spondylotic myeloradiculopathy: Experience with 50 cases treated by means of extensive laminectomy, foraminotomy, and excision of osteophytes during the past 10 years. Acta Neurochir 61:89–104, 1982.
22. Frykholm R: Cervical nerve root compression resulting from disk degeneration and root sleeve fibrosis. Acta Chir Scand 160:1–149, 1951.
23. Gooding M, Wilson CB, Hoff JT: Experimental cervical myelopathy effects of ischemia and compression of the canine cervical spinal cord. J Neurosurg 43:9–17, 1975.
24. Gore DR, Sepic SB, Gardner GM, et al: Neck pain: A long-term follow-up of 205 patients. Spine 12(1):1–5, 1987.
25. Gotten N: Survey of one hundred cases of whiplash injury after settlement of litigation. JAMA 162:865–867, 1956.
26. Greenfield J, Ilfeld FW: Acute cervical strain: Evaluation and short-term prognostic factors. Clin Orthop 122:196–200, 1977.
27. Griffiths I: Some aspects of the pathology and pathogenesis of the myelopathy caused by disc protrusions in the dog. J Neurol Neurosurg Psychiatr 35:403–413, 1972.
28. Guidetti B, Fortuna A: Long-term results of surgical treatment of myelopathy due to cervical spondylosis. J Neurosurg 30:714–721, 1969.
29. Hawkins RJ: Cervical spine and the shoulder. AAOS Instructional Lectures 14:191–195, 1985.
30. Hayashi H, Okada K, Hashimoto J, et al: Cervical spondylotic myelopathy in the aged patient: A radiographic evaluation of the aging changes in the cervical spine and etiologic factors of myelopathy. Spine 13(6):618–625, 1988.
31. Henderson CM, Hennessy R, Shuey H, et al: Posterior-lateral foraminotomy as an exclusive operative technique for cervical radiculopathy: A review of 846 consecutively operated cases. Neurosurgery 13(5):504–512, 1983.
32. Hohl M: Soft tissue injuries of the neck in automobile accidents: Factors influencing prognosis. J Bone Joint Surg 56A:1675–1682, 1974.
33. Hukuda S, Wilson C: Experimental cervical myelopathy: Effects of compression and ischemia on the canine cervical cord. J Neurosurg 37:631–652, 1972.
34. Key CA: On paraplegia depending on the ligaments of the spine. Guys Hosp Rep 3:17, 1838.
35. Keyes DC, Compere EL: The normal and pathological physiology of the nucleus pulposus of the intervertebral disk. J Bone Joint Surg 14:897, 1932.
36. Kikuchi S, MacNab I, Moreau P: Localization of the level of symptomatic cervical disc degeneration. J Bone Joint Surg 63B:272–277, 1981.
37. Kubota M, Baba I, Sumida T: Myelopathy due to ossification of the ligamentum flavum of the cervical spine: A report of two cases. Spine 6:553–559, 1981.
38. Lees F, Turner JWA: Natural history and prognosis of cervical spondylosis. Br Med J 2:1607–1610, 1963.
39. Lestini WF, Wiesel SW: The pathogenesis of cervical spondylosis. Clin Orthop 239:69–93, 1989.
40. Lunsford L, Bissonette DJ, Jannetta PJ, et al: Anterior surgery for cervical disc disease. J Neurosurg 53:1–11, 1980.
41. MacNab I: The "whiplash syndrome." Orthop Clin North Am 2:389–403, 1971.
42. Mair WG, Druckman R: The pathology of spinal cord lesions and their relations to the clinical features in protrusion of cervical intervertebral disks. Brain 76:70–91, 1953.
43. Nugent G: Clinicopathologic correlations in cervical spondylosis. Neurology 9:272–281, 1959.
44. Nurick S: The natural history and the results of surgical treatment of the spinal cord disorder associated with cervical spondylosis. Brain 95:101–108, 1972.
45. O'Connell JE: Involvement of the spinal cord by intervertebral disk protrusions. Br J Surg 43:225–247, 1955.
46. Olsson SE: The dynamic factor in spinal cord compression: A study on dogs with special reference to intervertebral disc protrusion. J Neurosurg 15:308–321, 1958.
47. Ono K, Ota H, Tada K, et al: Ossified posterior longitudinal ligament. Spine 2:126–138, 1977.
48. Payne EE, Spillane JD: The cervical spine. An anatomicropathological study of 70 specimens (using a special technique) with particular reference to the problem of cervical spondylosis. Brain 80:571–596, 1957.
49. Penning L, van der Zwaag P: Biomechanical aspects of spondylotic myelopathy. Acta Radiol (Diagn) 5:1090–1103, 1966.
50. Reid J: Effects of flexion-extension movements of the head and spine upon the spinal cord and nerve roots. J Neurol Neurosurg Psychiatr 23:214–221, 1960.
51. Rothman RH, Marvel JP: The acute cervical disk. Clin Orthop 109:59–68, 1975.
52. Rothman RH, Simeone FA: The Spine, 2nd ed. Philadelphia, W.B. Saunders, 1982, p. 477.
53. Roy DF, Fleury J, Fontaine SB, et al: Clinical evaluation of cervical facet joint infiltration. J Can Assoc Radiol 39:118–120, 1988.
54. Schmorl G: Ueber NorpelKnoten an der Hinterflache der Wirbeldandscheiden. Fortscher Rontgenstr 40:629, 1929.
55. Schmorl G, Yunghans H: The Human Spine in Health and Disease. New York, Grune & Stratton, 1959.

56. Simmons E, Bhalla SK, Butt WP: Anterior cervical discectomy and fusion. J Bone Joint Surg 51B:225–237, 1969.

57. Simmons JCH: Rupture of cervical intervertebral disc and cervical spondylosis, sections in miscellaneous affections of joints. In Crenshaw AH, ed: Campbell's operative orthopaedics, 5th ed. St. Louis, C.V. Mosby, 1971, pp. 1044–1053.

58. Spurling RG: Lesions of the Cervical Intervertebral Disc. Springfield, IL, Charles C Thomas, 1956.

59. Stookey B: Compression of the spinal cord due to ventral extradural cervical chondromas. Arch Neurol Psychiatr 20:275–291, 1928.

60. Stookey B: Compression of spinal cord and nerve roots by herniation of nucleus pulposus in cervical region. Arch Surg 40:417–432, 1940.

61. Tarlov I, Klinger H: Spinal cord compression studies. II. Time limits for recovery after acute compression in dogs. Arch Neurol Psychiatr 71:271–290, 1954.

62. Tarlov I, Klinger H, Vitale S: Spinal cord compression studies. I. Experimental techniques to produce acute and gradual compression. Arch Neurol Psychiatr 70:813–819, 1953.

63. Taylor AR: Mechanism and treatment of spinal cord disorders associated with cervical spondylosis. Lancet 1:717–720, 1953.

64. Taylor A: Vascular factors in the myelopathy associated with cervical spondylosis. Neurology (Minneapolis) 14:62–68, 1964.

65. Tsuyama M: The ossification of the posterior longitudinal ligament of the spine (OPLL). J Jpn Orthop Assoc 55:425, 1981.

66. Vesalius A: Die Humani Corporis Fabrica Libri Septem. Basileae, per J Ororinum, 1555, pp. 71–73.

67. Viikari-Juntura E, Porras M, Laasonen EM: Validity of clinical tests in the diagnosis of root compression in cervical disc disease. Spine 14(3):253–257, 1989.

68. Von Luschka H: Die Halbgelenke des Menschlichen Korpers. Berlin, G Reimer, 1858.

69. Wiesel SW, Feffer HL, Rothman RH: The development of a cervical spine algorithm and its prospective application to industrial patients. J Occup Med 27(4):272–276, 1985.

70. Wolf BS, Khilnani M, Malis L: The sagittal diameter of the bony cervical spinal canal and its significance in cervical spondylosis. J Mt Sinai Hosp 23:283–292, 1956.

71. Yu YL, Woo E, Huang CY: Cervical spondylotic myelopathy and radiculopathy. Acta Neurol Scand 75:367–373, 1987.

CHAPTER 4

Confirmatory Diagnostic Studies in the Cervical Spine*

PLAIN RADIOGRAPHS

Degenerative changes develop in the cervical spine and surrounding tissues as part of the aging process. In the elderly, the radiographic manifestations of cervical spondylosis occur with such regularity that they may not be related to symptoms. In many instances, it is difficult to verify the clinical symptoms or the sequelae of the degenerative changes of cervical spondylosis. There is often no direct relationship between symptoms and the radiographic changes of degenerative disc disease in the cervical spine.

While radiographic evidence of chronic disc degeneration is common in middle age, it is almost universal in the elderly (Fig. 4–1). Degenerative disc disease of the cervical spine is not seen as an isolated finding; rather, it is part of a process that affects the structure of the entire cervical spine. DePalma and Rothman reported gross, microscopic, and radiographic studies of aging cervical spine specimens.[11] Severe disc degeneration was seen in 72 percent of the specimens over 70 years of age. The most commonly affected level was C5-6, with 86 percent of specimens having observable abnormalities. The C6-7 level was the next most frequently affected, and the C2-3 disc was the least often involved in chronic disc degeneration.[11,16]

---

*Written with Neil Shonnard, M.D.

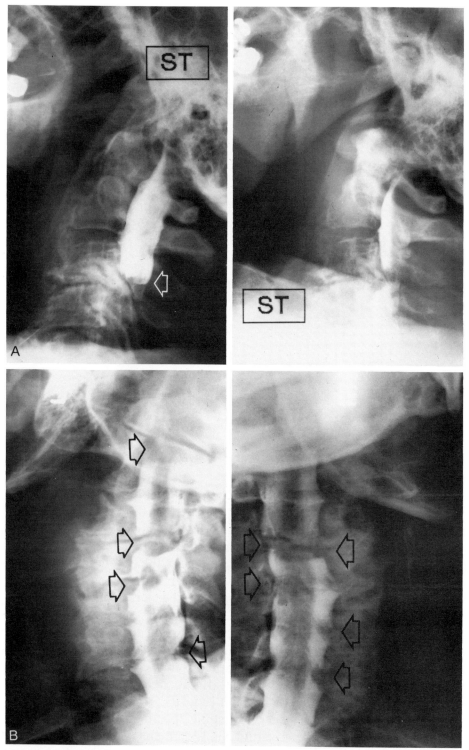

Figure 4–1. This 73-year-old male presented with progressive bilateral upper extremity poly-radiculopathy, atrophy, and hand ataxia associated with gait disturbance. *A,* Lateral myelograms show a complete C3 block *(arrow)* and multilevel blocks. *B,* Left and right oblique views show multilevel blocks and multiple bilateral root sleeve cut-offs *(arrows).*

The radiographic and morphologic findings of cervical spondylosis are as readily observed in asymptomatic patients. Gore and co-workers reported that by age 65, 95 percent of men and 70 percent of women had at least one degenerative change on their radiographs.[18] Anterior osteophyte formation and disc space narrowing were common findings. Anterior osteophyte formation was the only component of cervical spondylosis that occurred as an isolated finding. DePalma and Rothman stated that anterior osteophyte formation, in contrast to posterior osteophyte formation, was more likely related to ligamentous stress than to disc degeneration.[11] A similar study comparing groups of symptomatic and asymptomatic individuals found no difference between the two groups in the incidence of degenerative changes at the joints of Luschka, the intervertebral foramen, or the posterior articular processes.[17]

It is well known that patients with all the radiographic changes of cervical spondylosis may be asymptomatic, while other patients with minimal radiographic findings may manifest advanced symptoms of cervical myelopathy. This discrepancy may be attributable to the differences in the premorbid cervical spinal canal diameter. Wolf and colleagues found that the normal adult cervical spinal canal had an average diameter of 17 mm.[49] Patients who manifest cervical spondylotic myelopathy, however, were found to have an average canal diameter of 14 mm. When the cervical spinal canal is decreased by the presence of osteophytes, the smallest anteroposterior (AP) measurement observed is seen between the posterior osteophyte at the inferior edge of the rostral vertebral body and the superior margin of the lamina of the caudal vertebra.[37,49] Recently, Hayashi and associates demonstrated that the dynamic AP canal diameter (flexion-extension measurements) became much narrower than the static canal as aging progressed.[19]

Plain roentgenography is a rapid, inexpensive way to screen for unsuspected bony pathology. Congenital anomalies, the destructive effects of infection or tumor, cervical canal dimensions, and vertebral disc heights as well as degenerative changes are readily discernible. Plain films, however, have limited use for planning therapeutic intervention because of the difficulty in correlating them with a patient's symptoms. Canal encroachment and neural compression from soft tissues cannot be visualized on plain films. Roentgenograms must be interpreted with an awareness of the wide variations among normal patients as well as the frequent findings of degenerative changes in asymptomatic patients. In a study of asymptomatic patients ranging in age from 30 to 70 years, Friedenberg and Miller found that 35 percent had radiographic evidence of spondylosis.[17]

MYELOGRAPHY

The major advantage of water-soluble contrast myelography is its capacity to demonstrate spinal cord dimensions and nerve root sleeve configurations throughout the cervical region (see Fig. 4–1). Extradural disease manifests as defects in the contrast column. The goal of myelography is to establish conclusive evidence of compressive pathology impinging on nerve roots or the spinal cord. Because myelographic contrast extends only a relatively short distance along the nerve root sleeve, large laterally placed lesions may produce only slight indentations in the visible portion of the nerve root sleeve. Myelographic evidence of extradural compression, however subtle or obvious, is significant only when there is clinical correlation.

Myelography has been the standard for the evaluation of cervical radiculopathy.[12,40] Complications are rare, and if necessary the examination can be done on an outpatient basis. The major disadvantages of myelography are its invasive nature and lack of diagnostic specificity.[15] Retrospective studies correlating clinical symptoms with myelographic findings have shown the inability of myelography to unequivocally and accurately localize cord or nerve root compression.[9,15] Water-soluble myelography, however, provides excellent contrast for subsequent computed tomographic (CT) examination, and plain film myelography is often necessary to tailor adjunctive CT studies (Fig. 4–2).

COMPUTED TOMOGRAPHY

The advantages of contrast CT include excellent differentiation of bone and soft tissue (disc or ligament) lesions, direct demonstration of

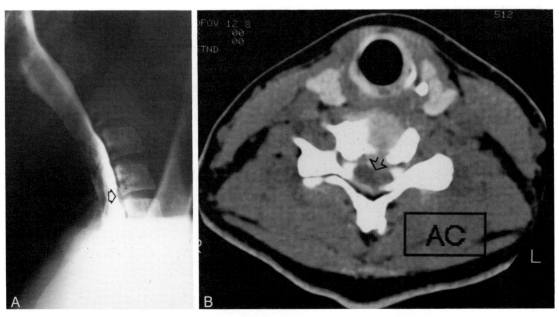

Figure 4–2. This 23-year-old female presented with bilateral hand clumsiness and myelopathy. *A,* Lateral myelogram shows loss of C5-6 disc space height and distortion of the contrast column *(arrow). B,* Axial CT myelogram confirms cord compression *(arrow).*

spinal cord and spinal canal dimensions, assessment of foraminal encroachment, and visualization of regions distal to myelographic blockade (Fig. 4–3). Contrast CT can be performed at a reduced cost and can be done safely on an outpatient basis, often following plain film myelography.[1,7,10,13,26,36,41] In addition, CT has been used for functional diagnosis of rotatory instability in the cervical spine.[14]

The clinical significance of CT myelographic findings in cervical spondylosis was studied by Penning and associates.[38] A 100 percent correlation was found between the side of disc herniation with an occlusion of the intervertebral foramen and the side of nerve root symptoms. Long track signs were noted after the cross-sectional area of the spinal cord had been reduced by 30 percent, to a value of about 60 mm^2 or less. Penning also noted that in the presence of a normal conventional plain film myelogram, postmyelographic CT studies were superfluous. CT investigation in these cases may lead to false-positive interpretation of clinically irrelevant findings.

MAGNETIC RESONANCE IMAGING

Teresi and colleagues and Boden and co-workers have documented the degenerative changes in asymptomatic patients studied with magnetic resonance imaging (MRI).[2,47] A wide variety of abnormalities were displayed in over 20 percent of asymptomatic subjects. Disc protrusion was seen in about 10 to 15 percent of subjects and may have an increased frequency in older individuals. The prevalence of disc narrowing, disc degeneration, and spurs increased from 25 percent in subjects under age 40 to 60 percent in those over 40.[2] Foraminal stenosis was present in 7 percent of subjects under age 40 and in 23 percent of those over age 40. Spinal cord impingement was seen in 10 to 15 percent of younger subjects and in 20 to 25 percent of older asymptomatic subjects. Spinal cord compression was seen in fewer than 5 percent and was due solely to disc protrusion. Cord area reduction averaged 7 percent and never exceeded 16 percent.[47] Thus, the cord appears to tolerate a certain amount of volume loss without demonstrating symptoms (Fig. 4–4).

An early report compared surgically confirmed predictions of myelography, CT myelography, and MRI.[31] In this study, myelography was the least specific modality and MRI was as sensitive as CT myelography for localization of the diseased level. However, MRI was not as sensitive as CT myelography for identification of the cause of neural encroachment (soft tissue vs. bone). Excellent sensitivity and specificity for inflammatory processes were noted with MRI. Marrow changes associated with degenerative disc disease or neoplastic involvement were also well depicted.[31]

Several technical modifications have improved the accuracy of MRI.[30,32–35] The distinction between disc and bone and the relationship of

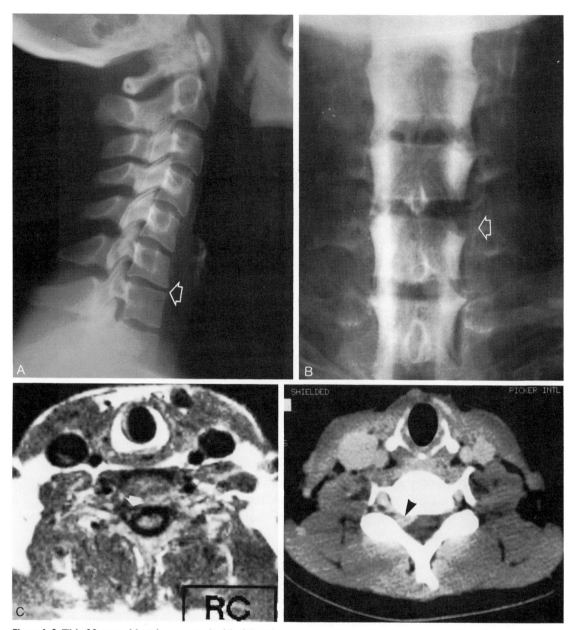

Figure 4–3. This 33-year-old male presented with right triceps weakness, C7 radicular pain, and absent triceps reflex. *A,* Lateral radiograph of C6-7 shows loss of disc height *(arrow). B,* AP myelogram confirms right C7 root sleeve cut-off. *C,* Axial MRI *(left)* and CT *(right)* show occlusion of the right C6-7 foramen *(arrows).*

both to the neural foramen are clearer. Pulse sequence techniques may enhance cerebrospinal fluid signal intensity relative to extradural structures. Gadolinium, a paramagnetic contrast agent, may enhance the dural-extradural interface and parenchymal lesions on T1-weighted images. Intramedullary abnormalities (e.g., syringomyelia, myelomalacia, intramedullary neoplasms, demyelinating disease) are better appreciated with MRI than with CT myelography. Several operator-dependent parameters can influence the clarity of MR images. Many options exist (e.g., car-

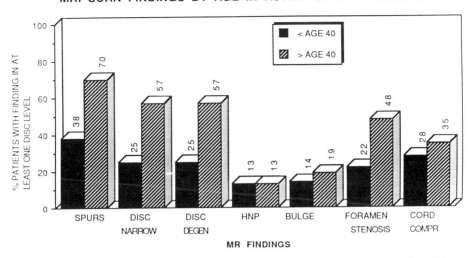

Figure 4–4. Graph of abnormal findings seen in at least on disc level on cervical spine MR1 scans from 74 asymptomatic volunteers.[2]

diac gating of T2-weighted sequences, fast low flip-angle scans) to reduce examination time, ghosting artifacts, and motion between views and to sharpen margins.[20,32,33]

Myelography and CT myelography are currently the studies with which surgeons are most comfortable. CT myelography is less operator-dependent than MRI and remains superior for detecting lateral encroachment. As familiarity with MRI increases and reproducible accuracy improves, this modality is likely to become the initial study of choice for the cervical spine. Quality MR images, combined with plain films, permit an accurate, noninvasive initial radiographic evaluation of cervical radiculopathy and myelopathy, while CT myelography is the preferred follow-up examination.[4]

DISCOGRAPHY

Since its introduction by Smith in 1957, cervical discography has remained controversial.[44] Many authors believe that the procedure has diagnostic value,[5,6,28,39,43,48] while others maintain that it is useless and misleading and should be discontinued altogether.[8,21–23,25,29,42,45,46] Advocates of the procedure have stated that a normal disc will accept no contrast material or at most 0.1 to 0.2 cc. Injection of a normal disc infrequently produces pain at the base of the neck. Injection of an abnormal disc, however, generally reproduces the type of pain and discomfort from which the patient is suffering. Injection of a local anesthetic promptly relieves this pain and is confirmatory for the level of involvement. More than one disc is generally studied. Cervical discography may be useful in patients who present with chronic neck, shoulder, and upper extremity pain after noninvasive imaging has been inconclusive.[48]

ELECTRODIAGNOSTIC TESTING

The particular value of electromyography (EMG) in the investigation of patients with compressive radiculopathy or myelopathy from cervical spondylosis is that it may help to accurately localize the level of the lesion.[3,27] Secondarily, EMG may demonstrate the presence of other more peripheral compressive neuropathies (e.g., carpal or cubital tunnel syndrome, anterior interosseous syndrome).[24] It is important to exclude or identify the various compressive neuropathies of the upper extremity when investigating the origin of symptoms in patients with cervical spondylosis. A combination of EMG and nerve conduction studies is occasionally necessary to make the correct diagnosis in these cases.

As a valuable adjunct in the diagnosis of the different syndromes of cervical spondylosis, the EMG can detect motor unit dysfunction. Radiculopathy may show fibrillation and fasciculation potentials. These potentials are seen with the muscle at rest and indicate nerve root irritation or injury. Abnormal insertional activity (positive waves and fibrillations) is more easily seen in acute radiculopathies. Chronic radiculopathies usually show motor unit action potentials with longer duration, higher amplitude, and more polyphasic activity.

The EMG is useful in the evaluation of suspected spondylotic myelopathy. There may be anterior horn cell degeneration secondary to compression or ischemia. The EMG changes in the affected segments may be indistinguishable from those of motor neuron disease. In cervical spondylotic myelopathy, the EMG abnormalities are generally confined to a few adjacent cervical segments, while in motor neuron disease they may be widespread and involve both upper and lower extremities. The EMG is useful in differentiating cervical spondylotic myelopathy and amyotrophic lateral sclerosis.

The EMG is an electronic extension of the physical examination. Although it is 80 to 90 percent accurate in establishing cervical radiculopathy as the cause of pain, false-negative results do occur. If cervical radiculopathy affects only the sensory root, the EMG will be unable to demonstrate an abnormality. A false-negative examination can occur if the patient with acute symptoms is examined early (4 to 28 days from onset of symptoms). A negative study should be repeated in two to three weeks if symptoms persist. The accuracy of the EMG increases if both the paraspinal and extremity muscles innervated by the suspected root demonstrate abnormalities.

Somatosensory evoked potentials (SSEPs) may also be useful in the assessment of cervical spondylosis. This modality involves electric stimulation of peripheral nerves (e.g., peroneal, radial) and measurement of the amplitude and latency of the electric potential transmitted to the sensory cortex of the brain. Although this modality may be of limited benefit in evaluating cervical radiculopathy, some feel it is more useful than EMG in assessing cervical myelopathy.[50]

Summary

The problem in cervical spondylosis is the identification of the level or levels that are productive of symptomatology. The accuracy of the diagnostic tools that are employed is commonly compared to surgical findings. Although the surgeon can confirm or disprove the radiologic assessment of the anatomic status within the spinal canal, he is no more able than the radiologist to unequivocally ascertain that the patient's symptoms are etiologically related to the morphologic status of the canal. In other words, both the radiologist and the surgeon are capable of describing the morphologic features of cervical spondylosis but neither can tell with certainty whether these features are responsible for the patient's symptoms. The results of an operation can provide an indication of the accuracy of these imaging modalities but they are by no means conclusive. The importance of strict correlation of positive diagnostic studies with a patient's signs and symptoms cannot be overstressed. Imaging studies are useful to confirm a clinical diagnosis, but should never be interpreted in isolation from the overall clinical picture.

References

1. Badami JP, Norman D, Barbaro NM, et al: Metrizamide CT myelography in cervical myelopathy and radiculopathy: Correlation with conventional myelography and surgical findings. Am J Roentgenol 144:675–680, 1985.
2. Boden SD, McCowin PR, Davis DO, et al: Abnormal cervical spine MR scans in asymptomatic individuals: A prospective and blinded investigation. J Bone Joint Surg, 72A:1178–1184, 1990.
3. Braddom RL: Role of Electromyography in Cervical Spondylosis, Vol. XXVII. St. Louis, CV Mosby, 1978.
4. Brown BM, Schwartz RH, Frank E, et al: Preoperative evaluation of cervical radiculopathy and myelopathy by surface-coil MR imaging. Am J Roentgenol 151:1205–1212, 1988.
5. Cloward RB: Cervical discography. Technique, indications and use in diagnosis of ruptured cervical disks. Am J Roentgenol 79:563–574, 1958.
6. Cloward RB: Cervical discography. A contribution to the etiology and mechanism of neck, shoulder, and arm pain. Ann Surg 150:1052–1064, 1959.
7. Coin CG, Coin JT: Computed tomography of cervical disk disease: Technical considerations with representative case reports. J Comput Assist Tomogr 5:275–280, 1981.
8. Collins HR: An evaluation of cervical and lumber discography. Clin Orthop 107:133–138, 1975.
9. Crandall PH, Batzdorf U: Cervical Spondylitic Myelopathy. J Neurosurg 25:57–66, 1966.
10. Daniels DL, Grogan JP, Johansen JB, et al: Computed tomography and myelography compared. Radiology 151:109–113, 1984.
11. DePalma AF, Rothman RH: The Intervertebral Disc. Philadelphia, W.B. Saunders, 1970.
12. Dillin W, Booth R, Cuckler J, et al: Cervical radiculopathy. Spine 11(10):988–991, 1986.
13. Dublin AB, McGahan JP, Reid MH: The value of computed tomographic metrizamide myelography in the neuroradiological evaluation of the spine. Radiology 146:79–86, 1983.
14. Dvorak J, Penning L, Hayek J, et al: Functional diagnostics of the cervical spine using computed tomography. Neuroradiology 30:132–137, 1988.
15. Fox AJ, Lin JP, Pinto RS, et al: Myelographic cervical nerve root deformities. Radiology 116:355–361, 1975.
16. Friedenberg ZB, Ediken J, Spenser N, et al: Degenerative changes in the cervical spine. J Bone Joint Surg 41A:61–72, 1959.

17. Friedenberg ZB, Miller WT: Degenerative disk disease of the cervical spine. J Bone Joint Surg 45A:1171–1178, 1963.
18. Gore DR, Sepie SB, Gardner GM: Roentgenographic findings of the cervical spine in asymptomatic people. Spine 11(6):521–524, 1986.
19. Hayashi H, Okada K, Hamoda M, et al: Etiologic factors of myelopathy. A radiographic evaluation of the aging changes in the cervical spine. Clin Orthop 214:200–209, 1987.
20. Hedberg MC, Drayer BP, Flom RA, et al: Gradient echo (GRASS) MR imaging in cervical radiculopathy. Am J Roentgenol 150:683–689, 1988.
21. Hirsch C, Schajowicz F, Galante J: Structural changes in the cervical spine. Acta Orthop Scand (Suppl) 109:1–77, 1967.
22. Holt EP: Fallacy of cervical discography. JAMA 188:799–801, 1964.
23. Holt EP: Further reflections on cervical discography. JAMA 231:613–614, 1975.
24. Kimura J: Electrodiagnosis in diseases of nerve and muscle: Principles and practice. Philadelphia, F.A. Davis, 1983.
25. Klafta LA: The diagnostic inaccuracy of the pain response in cervical discography. Cleve Clin Q 36:35–39, 1969.
26. Landman JA, Hoffman JC, Brawn IF, et al: Tomographic myelography in the recognition of cervical herniated disk. Am J Neuroradiol 5:391–394, 1984.
27. Lenman JAR, Ritchie AE: Clinical Electromyography, 4th ed. New York, Churchill Livingstone, 1987.
28. Massare C, Bard M, Tristant H: Cervical discography. Speculation on technique and indications from our own experience. J Radiol Electrol Med Nucl 55:395–399, 1974.
29. Meyer RR: Cervical discography. A help or hindrance in evaluating neck, shoulder, arm pain? Am J Roentgenol 90:1208–1215, 1963.
30. Modic MR, Hardy RW, Weinstein MA, et al: Nuclear magnetic resonance imaging of the spine: Clinical potential and limitations. Neurosurgery 15:583–592, 1984.
31. Modic MR, Masaryk TJ, Mulopulos GP, et al: Cervical radiculopathy: Prospective evaluation with surface coil MR imaging, CT with metrizamide, and metrizamide myelography. Radiology 161:753–759, 1986.
32. Modic MT, Masaryk TJ, Ross JS, et al: Cervical radiculopathy: Value of oblique MR imaging. Radiology 163:227–231, 1987.
33. Modic MT, Ross JS, Masaryk TJ: Imaging of degenerative disease of the cervical spine. Clin Orthop 239:109–120, 1989.
34. Modic MT, Weinstein MA, Pavlicek W, et al: Imaging of the spine. Radiology 148:757–762, 1983.
35. Modic MT, Weinstein MA, Pavlicek W, et al: Magnetic resonance imaging of the cervical spine: Technical and clinical observations. AJR 141:1129–1136, 1983.
36. Nakagawa H, Okumura T, Sugiyama T, et al: Discrepancy between metrizamide CT and myelography in diagnosis of cervical disk protrusions. Am J Neuroradiol 4:604–606, 1983.
37. Ogino H, Tada K, Okada K, et al: Canal diameter, anteroposterior compression ratio, and spondylotic myelopathy of the cervical spine. Spine 8:1–15, 1983.
38. Penning L, Wilmink JT, van Woerden HH, et al: CT myelographic findings in degenerative disorders of the cervical spine: Clinical significance. Am J Neuroradiol 7:119–127, 1986.
39. Roth DA: Cervical analgesic discography. A new test for the definitive diagnosis of the painful-disk syndrome. JAMA 235:1713–1714, 1976.
40. Rothman RH, Simeone FA: The Spine, 2nd ed. Philadelphia, W.B. Saunders, 1982, p. 477.
41. Scotti G, Scialfa G, Pieralli S, et al: Myelopathy and radiculopathy due to cervical spondylosis: Myelographic CT correlations. Am J Neuroradiol 4:601–603, 1983.
42. Shapiro R: Myelography, 4th ed. Chicago, Year Book Medical Publishers, 1984.
43. Simmons EH: An evaluation of discography in the localization of symptomatic levels in discogenic diseases of the spine. Clin Orthop 108:57–59, 1975.
44. Smith GW, Nichols P Jr: The technic of cervical discography. Radiology 68:163–165, 1963.
45. Sneider SE, Winslow OP, Pryor TH: Cervical discography: Is it relevant? JAMA 185:163–165, 1963.
46. Taveras J: Is discography a useful diagnostic procedure? J Can Assoc Radiol 18:294–295, 1967.
47. Teresi LM, Lufkin RB, Reicher MA: Asymptomatic degenerative disk disease and spondylosis of the cervical spine: MR imaging. Radiology 164:83–88, 1987.
48. Whitecloud TS, Seago RA: Cervical discogenic syndrome: Results of operative intervention in patients with positive discography. Spine 12(4):313–316, 1987.
49. Wolf BS, Khilnani M, Malis L: The sagittal diameter of the bony cervical spinal canal and its significance in cervical spondylosis. J Mt Sinai Hosp 23:283–292, 1956.
50. Yiannikas C, Shahani BT, Young RR: Short-latency somatosensory-evoked potentials from radial, median, ulnar, and peroneal nerve stimulation in the assessment of cervical spondylosis. Arch Neurol 43:1264–1271, 1986.

Standardized Approach to the Diagnosis and Treatment of Neck Pain and Brachialgia

GOALS OF TREATMENT

The task of the physician, when confronted with the cervical spine patient, is to integrate the complaints and physical findings into an accurate diagnosis and to prescribe appropriate therapy. The primary objective for the physician is to return the patient to a normal level of function as quickly as possible. In the process, there must be concern for the efficient and precise use of the diagnostic studies described in the previous chapter, minimization of ineffectual surgery or other treatments, and cost effectiveness. Achievement of these goals depends on the accuracy of the physician's decision-making process. Although specific information is not available for every aspect of neck pain, there is a large body of data to guide the handling of these patients.

Using the available knowledge, an algorithm for the diagnosis and treatment of neck pain has been designed (Fig. 5–1). The algorithm is, in effect, an organized sequence of clinical decisions and thought processes found to be useful in approaching the universe of aging patients with cervical spine problems. The algorithm follows well-delineated rules, es-

Cervical Spine Algorithm

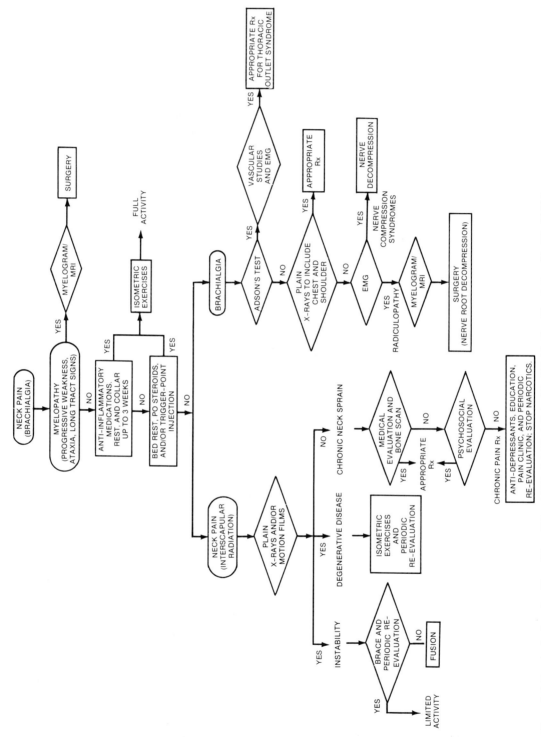

Figure 5–1. Cervical spine algorithm. (From Wiesel SW, et al: Neck Pain. The Michie Co, Charlottesville, VA, 1988.)

tablished from the consensus of a broad segment of qualified spine surgeons. It should be noted that the protocol is not inclusive of all cervical spine diagnoses but provides a useful framework for the most commonly encountered entities.

CERVICAL SPINE PROTOCOL

The protocol begins with the evaluation of patients who are initially seen for neck pain with or without arm or shoulder pain. Patients with major trauma including fractures and dislocations are not included. After an initial medical history and physical examination, and with the assumption that the patient's symptoms are originating from the cervical spine, the first major decision is to rule in or out the presence of a cervical myelopathy.

Cervical myelopathy is compression of the neural elements in the cervical spine. It can lead to a progressive and profound neurologic deficit. As discussed in Chapter 3, the etiology of the compression is usually a combination of osteoarthritis and degenerative disc disease, which leads to a decrease in the volume of the spinal canal. If the canal becomes too small, the spinal cord may be compromised.

The character and severity of the problem depend on the size, location, and duration of the lesion. Posterolateral lesions encroach on the nerve roots and ventral aspect of the spinal cord, producing all the manifestations of nerve root compression. The main radicular signs are weakness with loss of tone and volume of the muscles in the upper extremity. Pressure on the spinal cord can produce pyramidal tract signs and spasticity in the lower extremities.

Midline lesions intrude on the central aspect of the anterior spinal cord and generally do not produce signs of nerve root compression. Both lower extremities are usually involved, and the most common initial problem is gait disturbance.[1] As the process progresses, bowel and bladder control may be affected.

Although the natural history of cervical spondylotic myelopathy is one of gradual progression, severe myelopathy rarely develops in patients who do not show it when they first present.[7] Once the diagnosis of a cervical myelopathy is made, surgical intervention should be considered quickly. The best results are attained when only one or two motor units are involved and myelopathy is of relatively short duration. Cervical myelography or magnetic resonance imaging (MRI) should be performed to precisely define the neural compression, and an adequate surgical decompression should be undertaken as soon as possible to achieve the best results.

After cervical myelopathy has been ruled out, the remainder of neck pain patients (i.e., the overwhelming majority) should be started on a course of conservative (nonoperative) management. Initially, a specific diagnosis, whether it be a herniated disc, cervical spondylosis, or neck strain, is not required, as all these patients are treated in the same fashion.

Immobilization is the mainstay of therapy for both acute episodes and exacerbations in patients with chronic cervical disc disease.[2] A well-fitted soft felt collar will usually provide comfort for the patient. The collar should initially be worn continuously, day and night. The patient must understand that because the neck is especially unprotected from awkward positions and movements during sleep, nighttime use of the collar is very important. The other major component of the initial treatment program is drug therapy. Anti-inflammatory drugs, analgesics, and muscle relaxants will usually improve patient comfort and should supplement immobilization. However, medication is not a substitute for proper immobilization.

Most patients will respond to this approach of immobilization and pharmacotherapy in the first 10 days. Patients who do improve should be encouraged to gradually increase their activities and begin a program of exercises directed at strengthening the paravertebral musculature, rather than at increasing the range of motion. The patient is then weaned from the soft collar over the next 2 to 3 weeks. The unimproved group of patients should continue with full-time collar immobilization and anti-inflammatory medication.

If there is no significant improvement in symptoms at 3 to 4 weeks, a local injection into the area of maximum tenderness in the paravertebral musculature and trapezii should be considered. Marked relief of symptoms is often achieved by infiltration of these trigger points with a combination of 3 to 5 ml of lidocaine (Xylocaine) and 10 mg of a corticosteroid preparation. If the trigger-point injection is not successful at 4 to 5 weeks after the onset of symptoms, a trial of cervical traction may be instituted. A home traction device with minimal weights is preferred.

The patient should be treated conservatively for up to 6 weeks. The majority of cervical spine patients will get better and should return to a normal life pattern within 2 months. If the initial conservative treatment regimen fails, symptomatic patients may be separated into two groups. The first group comprises patients with neck pain as a predominant complaint, with or without interscapular radiation. The second group consists of those who complain primarily of arm pain (brachialgia).

NECK PAIN

If no symptomatic improvement is achieved after 6 weeks of conservative therapy in the neck-pain–predominant group, plain radiographs, including lateral flexion-extension bending films, should be carefully examined. Radiography before this point is not usually helpful because of the lack of significant differences between symptomatic and asymptomatic patients.[5,6] Nonspecific radiographic degenerative changes in the cervical spine are almost universal by age 60. Radiographs may be indicated earlier in the treatment course of older patients in whom infection or metastatic disease is suspected from the history or physical findings.

Some patients may have objective evidence of instability on the bending films. In the lower cervical spine (C3-7), instability has been defined as horizontal translation of one vertebra on another of more than 3.5 mm, or as an angulatory difference between adjacent vertebrae of more than 11°.[10] The majority of patients with degenerative (i.e., nontraumatic) instability will respond to further nonoperative measures, including a thorough explanation of the problem and some type of bracing. In some cases, segmental spinal fusion may be necessary.

Another group of patients complaining mainly of neck pain will be found on radiography to have degenerative disease. The roentgenographic signs include loss of height of the intervertebral disc space, osteophyte formation, secondary encroachment of the intervertebral foramina, and osteoarthritic changes in the zygoapophyseal joints. The diagnostic difficulty is not in identifying these abnormalities but in determining their clinical significance.

As discussed earlier, degeneration in the cervical spine can be a normal part of the aging process. Large numbers of asymptomatic patients show radiographic, myelographic, and MR evidence of abnormal degenerative disease. The most significant finding relevant to symptomatology is narrowing of the intervertebral disc space, particularly at C5-6 and C6-7.[5] Changes at the zygoapophyseal joints, foramina, and posterior articular processes do not correlate well with clinical symptoms.

These patients should be treated symptomatically with anti-inflammatory medications, cervical support, and trigger-point injections as required. In the quiescent stages, they should be placed on isometric exercises. Finally, they should be re-examined periodically because some may develop myelopathy.

The majority of patients with neck pain will have essentially normal roentgenograms. The preliminary diagnosis for this group is neck strain. However, with no objective findings and with failure to improve after appropriate conservative management, other pathology must be considered. These patients should undergo a bone scan and a complete medical evaluation to assess the cervical spine for infection, tumor, or inflammatory arthritis. A thorough medical examination may also reveal problems missed in the early stages of neck pain evaluation. If this work-up is negative, the patient should have a complete psychosocial evaluation and receive treatment when appropriate for depression or substance dependence, both of which are frequently seen in association with neck pain.

If the psychosocial evaluation proves normal, the patient is considered to have chronic neck pain. These patients require encouragement, patience, and education. They especially need to be detoxified from narcotic drugs and placed on an exercise regimen. Many will respond to antidepressant drugs such as amitriptyline (Elavil). Regardless, these patients need to be periodically re-evaluated to avoid missing any new problems.

Occasionally, it is difficult to distinguish patients who have a true neck problem from those individuals using neck pain as an excuse to stay out of work and collect compensation or because of pending litigation. The outcome of treatment of cervical disc disease has been shown to be adversely affected by litigation.[4] Frequently with hyperextension neck injuries, there are no objective findings to substantiate the subjective complaints. The best solution to this dilemma in the compensation setting is to recommend an independent medical examination early in the treatment course.

BRACHIALGIA

Patients in whom arm pain (brachialgia) predominates may have symptoms due to mechanical pressure from a herniated disc or hypertrophic bone and secondary inflammation of the involved nerve roots.[9] Extrinsic pressure on the vascular structures or peripheral nerves is the most likely imitator of brachialgia and must be excluded. Pathology in the chest and shoulder must also be considered. A careful physical examination including Adson's test, shoulder evaluation, and Tinel's test at the ulnar and carpal tunnels should be conducted. If these tests are equivocal, appropriate radiographs and an electromyogram (EMG) should be obtained.

In addition to spinal nerve root encroachment, disease processes that directly affect the brachial plexus can result in a variety of upper extremity symptoms that must be distinguished from cervical root syndromes. Although trauma is the most common cause of brachial plexus injury, compression by vascular structure, cervical ribs, muscular or fibrous bands, or tumors may result in a plexus neuropathy. Apical carcinoma of the lung may encroach upon the brachial plexus and may be seen with Horner's syndrome.

Peripheral nerve compression occasionally manifests by patterns of arm pain that exceed the expected regional involvement of the specific peripheral nerve. Although peripheral nerve entrapment can usually be identified by the motor and sensory loss pattern and by EMG studies, these peripheral lesions may coexist with cervical root compression. The double-crush hypothesis maintains that axons compressed in one region may become more susceptible to impairment at a distant site.

If there is unequivocal evidence of nerve root compression (neurologic deficit, positive EMG, and positive myelogram or MRI) consistent with the physical findings, surgical decompression should be considered. Some studies suggest that patients with radicular symptoms seem to do better with surgery.[4] Although conservative management of patients with radicular symptoms has shown that isolated nerve root compression rarely progresses to cervical myelopathy, persistent symptoms are common.[8]

Summary

The authors maintain that all patients with an exacerbation of cervical disc disease should have up to 6 weeks of conservative therapy in the absence of myelopathy. The specific temporal sequence for use of the various conservative modalities is variable. A program of a soft cervical collar and anti-inflammatory medications is recommended, occasionally followed by trigger-point injections or home traction if necessary. This regimen has been effective empirically in treating the vast majority of patients with exacerbations of cervical disc disease.

References

1. Clark CR: Cervical spondylotic myelopathy: History and physical findings. Spine 13:847–849, 1988.
2. DePalma AF, Rothman RH: The Intervertebral Disc. Philadelphia, W.B. Saunders, 1970.
3. DePalma AF, Rothman RH, Levitt RL, et al: The natural history of severe cervical disc degeneration. Acta Orthop Scand 43:392–396, 1972.
4. Dillin W, Booth R, Cuckler J, et al: Cervical radiculopathy: A review. Spine 11:988–991, 1986.
5. Friedenberg ZB, Miller WT: Degenerative disease of the cervical spine. J Bone Joint Surg 45A:1171–1178, 1963.
6. Gore DR, Sepic SB, Gardner GM: Roentgenographic findings of the cervical spine in asymptomatic people. Spine 11:521–524, 1986.
7. LaRocca H: Cervical spondylotic myelopathy: Natural history. Spine 13:854–855, 1988.
8. Lees F, Turner JW: Natural history and prognosis of cervical spondylosis. Br Med J 2:1607–1610, 1963.
9. Rothman RH, Marvel JP: The acute cervical disc. Clin Orthop 129:59–68, 1975.
10. White AA, Panjabi MM, Posner I, et al: Spinal stability: Evaluation and treatment. American Academy of Orthopaedic Surgeons Instructional Course Lectures 30:457–483, 1981.

CHAPTER **6**

Nonoperative
Treatment Modalities
for the Cervical Spine

All patients with neck pain, excluding those with fractures, dislocations, or cervical myelopathy, should be given an initial period of conservative therapy. There are many noninvasive treatment modalities
available; unfortunately, most are based on empiricism and tradition.
While there are few prospective, randomized, double-blind studies for
conservative treatment of lumbar disc disease, even less scientifically
valid data exist for cervical disc disease.[1] Each treatment in popular use
today is surrounded by conflicting claims for its indication and efficacy.
Therefore, treatments prescribed should at least be safe, inexpensive, and
have a reasonable chance of success.

The goals of noninvasive treatment of cervical disc disease are
to return the patient to normal activity rapidly with the least diagnostic
and therapeutic expense and, most of all, to do no harm. This chapter presents several of the more common therapeutic modalities along with the
available scientific evidence for and against their use. In addition, a strategy for initial conservative management of cervical disc disease is outlined (Fig. 6–1). This treatment protocol has been empirically developed
by the authors; other temporal sequences for the various treatment modalities may also be effective.

NECK PAIN TREATMENT FLOW CHART

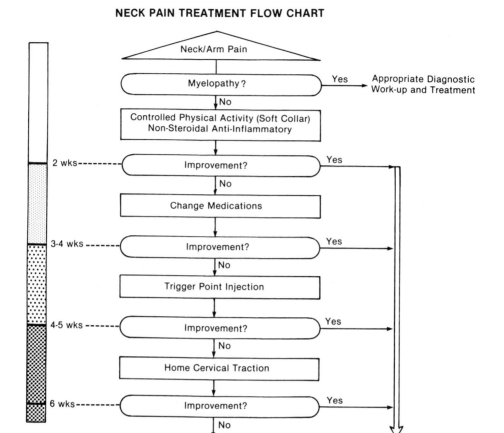

Figure 6–1. Algorithm for conservative treatment of neck pain.

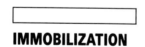

IMMOBILIZATION

The cornerstone of conservative therapy is immobilization of the cervical spine.[13] The goal of immobilization is to rest the neck to facilitate healing of torn and/or attenuated soft tissues and to reduce mechanical irritation or stretching of affected nerve roots. In patients with an exacerbation of chronic symptoms, the purpose of immobilization is to reduce any inflammation in the supporting soft tissues and around the nerve roots.

Immobilization can be best achieved by use of a soft cervical collar that holds the head in a neutral or slightly flexed position. The collar must fit properly; if the neck is held in hyperextension the patient is often uncomfortable and will derive no benefit from its use. Acutely, the collar should be worn 24 hours a day, until the pain begins to subside.

Then, gradual weaning from the collar is begun. The amount of immobilization required varies for each patient and should be guided by improvement of symptoms. Once acute symptoms have improved, long-term immobilization ideally comes from strong paracervical musculature. Therefore, excessive external immobilization that will cause atrophy of the muscles should be avoided.

In addition to the soft collar, other devices such as plastic collars and metal braces are available to achieve more rigid immobilization.[9] In the author's experience, these are more burdensome to the patient than soft collars and are less effective in the relief of pain. Furthermore, use of the rigid devices for a prolonged period of time may lead to marked soft tissue atrophy and stiffness, which are not generally found with use of the soft collar. Ultimately, stabilization of the cervical motion segments is best achieved by increasing the resting tone of the paraspinal muscles, providing a functional "internal splint."

Another component of immobilization is bedrest. Not only are the axial compressive forces on the cervical spine relieved, but confinement to bed also limits other daily activities that might exacerbate the problem. Bedrest with cervical support is a viable option acutely for extremely severe pain or for patients who would not otherwise comply with limitation of physical activities.

DRUG THERAPY

Inflammation in the soft tissues is believed to be a major contributor to pain production in the cervical spine. This is especially true for those patients with symptoms secondary to cervical disc herniation. The resulting arm pain is due not only to mechanical pressure from the ruptured disc but also to inflammation around the involved nerve roots.

None of the vast spectrum of anti-inflammatory drugs has been proven superior. Accordingly, the usual treatment plan is to begin the patient on adequate doses of aspirin, which is effective and inexpensive. If the response is not satisfactory, other agents such as naproxen, ibuprofen, or indomethacin are tried. Patients with peptic ulcer disease should not be treated with conventional anti-inflammatory agents. Some salicylates are now available with a pH-sensitive coating that prevents digestion in the stomach and duodenum. It should be stressed that anti-inflammatory agents are utilized in conjunction with immobilization; they do not replace adequate rest.

Analgesic medication is also important during the acute phase of an episode of neck pain. Most patients respond to the equivalent of 30 to 60 mg of codeine every 4 to 6 hours. If stronger analgesia is required, the patient should be monitored very closely and admitted to the hospital for observation.

Muscle relaxants are another class of medication useful in the conservative treatment of cervical disc disease. Muscle spasm may frequently be a significant contributor to the overall pain problem following acute injury to any of the tissues in the cervical spine. Severe headaches are a common sequela of cervical strain as a result of paracervical muscle spasm. Theoretically, muscle spasm leads to ischemia, which causes a further increase in pain. A muscle relaxant can frequently break the muscle spasm–pain cycle and allow an increased range of motion in the cervical spine. Methocarbanol and carisoprodol in adequate doses are the drugs commonly utilized. Valium is not recommended as a muscle relaxant because it is also a psychologic depressant, and many neck pain patients may already have some degree of clinical depression. A common side effect of the muscle relaxants is drowsiness, and patients must be cautioned about driving automobiles.

TRACTION

Although cervical traction has been used for many years, current opinions regarding its effectiveness vary. In theory, axial traction opens the neural foramina and tends to flatten a bulging disc by stretching the posterior longitudinal ligament. While some studies have suggested that traction is a valuable clinical therapy,[8,14] others have concluded that it is either ineffective or potentially harmful in an acutely injured cervical spine.[2,7] Certainly, traction should never be prescribed unless roentgenograms have been reviewed for fracture, tumor, and infection. Traction is an empirical form of therapy that should be employed only when more conservative treatment is not effective.

Cervical traction is contraindicated in malignancy, cord compression, infection, osteoporosis, and rheumatoid arthritis. It is also commonly believed that when there is a frank disc herniation either in the midline or laterally, traction should not be considered.

Cervical traction can be administered in several ways: mechanical or manual, continuous or intermittent, and sitting or supine. Many feel that manual traction is preferable due to the interaction between the therapist and patient and the potential for individually varying the traction. We prefer a home traction device with minimal weights (5 to 10 lb) pulling in slight flexion. Since there is evidence that at least 25 lbs are necessary to actually distract the cervical vertebrae, the major benefit of low-weight traction is probably from the immobilization.[12] There is no uniform theory as to how traction actually works, and there is no valid scientific evidence that traction in and of itself is effective.

TRIGGER POINT INJECTION

Myofacial pain syndrome involving the trapezius muscle or due to irritation of deeper structures is a common cause of cervical pain.

Many patients complain of very localized tender points in the paravertebral area. The object of a trigger point injection is to decrease the inflammation in a specific anatomic area. This therapy is most effective with well-localized trigger points. Injections can be repeated at intervals of 1 to 3 weeks. There have been no true randomized clinical trials to study the efficacy of this modality in the cervical spine, but the injections empirically seem to work quite well for both neck pain and brachalgia in some patients.

EPIDURAL STEROIDS

A large component of cervical radiculopathy is often due to secondary inflammation of the involved nerve root. Reduction of the edema and the local inflammatory response should theoretically help to relieve symptoms. Cervical epidural injections of a local anesthetic and steroid may provide some pain relief. This procedure, however, requires experience and technical competence and is not without complications.[10] While some have had limited success with this technique, we do not routinely utilize cervical epidural injections.

EXERCISES

After a patient's acute symptoms have resolved and there is no significant pain or spasm, an exercise regimen is recommended. The exercises should be directed at strengthening the paravertebral musculature rather than increasing the range of motion. Motion will generally return with the disappearance of pain.

The authors suggest isometric exercises be performed once each day with increasing repetitions. It should be appreciated that there are no scientific studies that demonstrate that isometric or any other type of exercises will reduce the frequency or duration of recurrent neck pain. Empirically, exercise regimens do appear to have a positive psychological effect and allow the patient to actively participate in the treatment program.

PHYSICAL THERAPY MODALITIES

Other unproven modalities are safe and may achieve relief in some patients. Moist heat, transcutaneous electrical nerve stimulation (TENS),[5] and ultrasound may be effective. Scientific data supporting these modalities are scant; however, they are safe, relatively inexpensive, and worthy of a brief trial in refractory patients. In addition, patient education about sleeping with the neck in a neutral position, avoiding automobile travel during the acute injury phase, and customizing work areas to avoid extreme neck flexion, extension, or rotation is worthwhile.

MANIPULATION

Manipulation of the cervical spine should be approached carefully. There is no scientific evidence that manipulation is effective in the treatment of acute or chronic neck problems, and there have been a number of tragic complications associated with its use.[11] It is the authors' feeling that the hazards are too great and that manipulation has no place in the treatment of cervical spine disorders.

Summary

While acute lumbar disc disease is usually self-limiting, at least one third of cervical disc disease patients have persistent pain.[6] Over time, most patients with degenerative problems in the cervical spine will improve with the nonoperative treatment program outlined. The role of conservative therapy in this disease is strengthened by studies that suggest that operative intervention may not provide any long-term advantages over nonoperative management.[3,4] However, much of the evidence for the conservative treatment modalities is empiric and there are no data to suggest that any of the conservative modalities influence the natural history of cervical disc disease other than by alleviating acute symptoms.[6] It is important to provide symptomatic relief, however, to avoid the development of a chronic pain syndrome.

References

1. Bloch R: Methodology in clinical back pain trials. Spine 12:430–432, 1987.
2. British Association of Physical Medicine: Pain in the neck and arm: A multicentre trial of the effects of physiotherapy. Br Med J 1:253, 1966.
3. DePalma AF, Rothman RH, Levitt RL, et al: The natural history of severe cervical disc degeneration. Acta Orthop Scand 43:392–396, 1972.
4. Dillin W, Booth R, Cuckler J, et al: Cervical radiculopathy: A review. Spine 11:988–991, 1986.
5. Eriksson M, Sjolund B, Nielzen S: Long-term results of peripheral conditioning stimulation as an analgesic measure of chronic pain. Pain 6:335–347, 1979.
6. Gore DR, Sepic SB, Gardner GM, et al: Neck pain: A long-term follow-up of 205 patients. Spine 12:1–5, 1987.
7. Greenfield J, Ilfeld FW: Acute cervical strain. Clin Orthop 122:196–200, 1977.
8. Harris W: Cervical traction: Review of the literature and treatment guidelines. Phys Ther 57:8, 1977.
9. Johnson RM, Hart DL, Simmons EF, et al: Cervical orthosis: A study in normal subjects comparing the effectiveness in restricting cervical motion. J Bone Joint Surg 59A:332–339, 1977.
10. Lilley JP, Fromme GA, Wang JK: Management of acute pain. Adv Anesthesiol 4:347–364, 1987.
11. Livingston MCP: Spinal manipulation causing injury (a three year study). Clin Orthop 81:82–86, 1971.
12. Rath WW: Cervical traction. A clinical perspective. Orthop Rev 13:430–449, 1984.
13. Rothman RH, Simeone F: The Spine, 2nd ed. Philadelphia, W. B. Saunders, 1982.
14. Zhongda L: A study of the effect of manipulative treatment on 158 cases of cervical syndrome. J Tradit Chin Med 7:205–208, 1987.

CHAPTER 7

Operative Management of the Aging Cervical Spine

While operations for cervical spine disease continue to be frequently utilized, this is an area of active research interest, and many questions and controversies remain. Whether a given problem should be approached anteriorly or posteriorly, whether a degenerated disc should be removed or replaced with a bone graft or prosthesis, whether instrumentation, wiring, or acrylic should be used are all matters of continuing concern. The purpose of this chapter is not to provide all the technical details of cervical spine surgery, but rather to afford the reader a general appreciation for the role of surgery in specific diagnoses with its attendant risks, benefits, and complications.

From a historical standpoint, the earliest cervical spine procedures were posterior laminectomies. Subsequently, the anterior approach with discectomy and interbody fusion was devised, and more recently numerous variations have appeared. Ingenious forms of instrumentation have been developed and continue to be improved.

The pathophysiology of the cervical spine includes structural, biomechanical and neurologic aspects, all of which are pertinent to the aging spine. The cervical spine is required to support the relatively heavy and poorly balanced weight of the head against gravity and also to provide for appropriate, rapid, and accurate movement of the head. The normal anatomy of the atlas on the axis and the normal cervical curvature provide the basis for both support and flexibility. The spinal elements depend upon the cervical ligaments and musculature to perform this task, and disease processes affecting ligaments, intervertebral joints, intervertebral discs, cervical muscles, cervical nerves, and the bones themselves can all produce pathologic malfunction. The effects of gravity and normal "wear and tear" over the years can result in degenerative disease of the spine, which may be accelerated by minor trauma and by constitutional disorders such as osteoporosis and rheumatoid disease.

INDICATIONS

Trauma can affect the cervical spine at any age. Cervical fractures and dislocations can have grave implications for spinal cord function and must be stabilized and reduced, often surgically. In the elderly, trauma without actual fracture or dislocation can injure the spinal cord, as the spondylotic changes that occur with aging can narrow the anteroposterior dimension of the spinal canal. Trauma, usually with hyperextension of the spine, can contuse the spinal cord and produce the characteristic central spinal cord syndrome with profound loss of function in the upper extremities and relative sparing of function and sensation in the lower extremities.

Congenital problems that can affect the structure and function of the cervical spine include congenital diseases of bone and vertebral anomalies such as occipitalization of the atlas, underdevelopment of the odontoid, and variations of the Klippel-Feil syndrome with congenital vertebral fusions and hemivertebrae. Congenital diseases can also affect the cervical muscles, and secondary postural abnormalities may lead to degenerative changes. A congenitally small cervical spinal canal can produce spinal cord abnormalities and aggravate other pathologic conditions.

Neoplasms can affect the spine itself, the spinal cord and its meninges, and the nerve roots and nerve trunks of the brachial plexus. Disc space and vertebral infections are the most common types of infectious processes, and surgical management is often indicated. Degenerative and metabolic disease processes can have direct or indirect effects. Rheumatoid disease, because of its effects on ligaments, can produce cervical instability and subluxation, most often at C1-2. Degenerative disc disease and spondylosis are the most common disorders treated by surgery.

These categories of disease are important to consider during the differential diagnosis of patients with signs and symptoms suggestive of problems with the cervical spine.

SURGICAL APPROACHES

The choice of surgical approach for exposure of the cervical spine depends upon a thorough knowledge of anatomy and upon the level or levels to be exposed, from C1 rostrally to T1 caudally.

Anterior exposure of the odontoid may be necessary, particularly for processes that produce ventral compression at the cervicomedullary junction. Approaches for this level include transoral, submandibular, transcervical, and mandible-splitting transoral routes.

For the cervical spine from C3 to C7, an anterolateral approach is quite satisfactory and may be accomplished through either a transverse or a longitudinal incision, depending upon the extent of exposure desired. More lateral approaches to the lower cervical spine are sometimes indicated, and a sympathectomy type exposure through a supraclavicular incision permits access to the proximal brachial plexus.

On rare occasions an anterior approach to C7-T1 may be an indication for splitting of the sternum.

Posterior approaches to the cervical spine can also be tailored to the amount of exposure needed.[6] Midline exposures are standard for decompressive laminectomies, spinal cord tumors, most posterolateral disc herniations, foraminotomies, and fusions for instability. Paramedian approaches are occasionally used for foraminotomy.

Fixation and immobilization of the cervical spine are essential for achieving successful fusions in the management of spinal instability secondary to trauma, degenerative disease, or surgery. A number of methods, internal and external, are available. Rapid control of the unstable cervical spine is achieved with halo fixation or Gardner-Wells tongs. Depending on the mechanism of instability, anterior or posterior fixation may be chosen (sometimes both). Anteriorly, one may utilize interbody fusion with bone or one of a number of instrumentation concepts using plates and screws (e.g., Caspar's). Posteriorly, the spinal elements may be wired, fused with bone, or subjected to instrumentation with clamps, rods, or more complex devices. The use of methylmethacrylate to supplement fixation has been advocated in some cases. Experimental work involves the development of prostheses to replace intervertebral discs or entire vertebral bodies. External fixation is an important interim measure for many patients with cervical spine disorders. Simple cervical collars such as the Philadelphia collar are useful for some patients but provide poor immobilization; rigid two-poster or four-poster cervical braces are more effective. Halo-vest fixation provides good stabilization, particularly for C1-2 fractures.

CERVICAL RADICULOPATHY

The most common condition for which cervical spine surgery is ultimately recommended is cervical radiculopathy. This clinical syndrome is the result of nerve root compression in the neural foramen[2,8]. The anterior aspect of the neural foramen consists of the cervicovertebral joints and the annulus fibrosus of the intervertebral disc at each level from C2-3 down. For this reason, both osteophytes associated with the uncovertebral joint and posterolateral disc herniations can compress a cervical nerve root in the foramen proper. The former situation is usually the result of chronic changes related to disc degeneration and spondylosis and is theoretically aggravated by motion at the disc space, which promotes osteophyte development. The latter situation can occur whenever a combination of physical stress affecting the disc and weakening of the annulus allow disc herniation to occur.

Most patients will complain of posterior neck pain as an initial part of the radiculopathy syndrome. If the space affected is C5-6 or lower, aching radiating interscapular pain may be present and is probably related to nociceptors in the disc space itself. Depending upon the level, pain will radiate to the proximal shoulder and arm, ultimately reflecting the anatomic distribution of the nerve root involved, and will be accompanied by numbness or paresthesias in the same distribution. With severe or prolonged nerve root compression, motor weakness and reflex loss occur, again in the appropriate distribution for the root involved (Fig. 7–1). Long-standing root compression can lead to atrophy of the muscles innervated by the affected root.

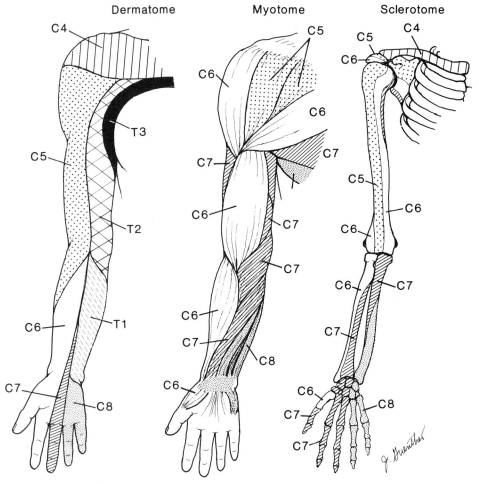

Figure 7–1. Pattern of referred pain associated with cervical radiculopathy based on embryologic origin of structures.

Important features to consider in the differential diagnosis of cervical radiculopathy are shoulder joint disease, muscle strain, or inflammation, nerve root entrapment syndromes in the upper extremities, and neoplasms affecting the spinal cord, meninges, or nerve roots.

The diagnosis can be confirmed by a combination of physical and neurologic findings along with appropriate imaging studies. Plain radiographic studies should include flexion, extension, and oblique views that show the foramina. Computed tomographic (CT) studies can detect cervical spondylosis and many disc herniations. Magnetic resonance imaging studies are excellent for evaluating the discs and the spinal cord in relation to the spinal canal (Fig. 7–2). Myelography with CT can also provide definitive anatomic information (Fig. 7–3). Discography and venography play no major role in modern diagnosis. Conservative management is successful in resolving symptoms and signs in 60 to 70 percent of patients. When conservative management fails to relieve disabling symptoms or when significant or progressive motor weakness is present, surgical management is recommended.

Operative Technique

Posterior Approach

The posterior approach to cervical foraminotomy has been traditional and provides excellent results in the classical patient operated upon by an experienced surgeon. The goals of the procedure are to perform a decompressive foraminotomy, to expose the compressed nerve root with great care, and to remove any accessible free fragments of disc. The patient's position is either upright or prone, with the head carefully fixed, and the neck in neutral or slightly flexed position. Radiographic control assures surgery at the appropriate level. The incision is usually midline, but some surgeons use a paramedian, muscle-splitting (McBurney) approach. Subperiosteal dissection is employed to expose the appropriate lamina, facet joint, and lateral mass. A burr or high-speed drill is used to perform partial hemilaminectomy and foraminotomy, and the exposure of the nerve root is completed with curettes and Kerrison-type punches when possible. Magnification of vision with loupes or microscope is a most helpful adjunct for this portion of the procedure and throughout the rest of the operation.

Once the bony decompression is complete, the ligamentum flavum is carefully dissected, placed under tension with a hook or pointed clamp, and incised with a scalpel, unroofing the epidural space from medial to lateral. Bleeding from the epidural venous plexus is controlled by bipolar cautery, and careful exposure of the nerve root is accomplished, again working from medial to lateral with great care. It is important to realize that at the axilla of the nerve root where it emerges from the common dural sac, the motor and sensory roots may be separate. It is critical to avoid misinterpreting the ventrally placed motor root as a disc herniation

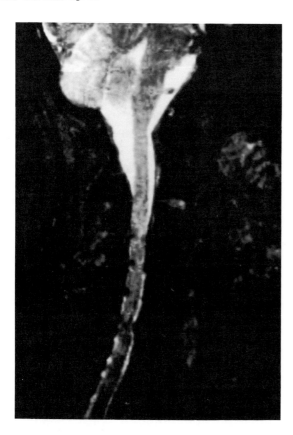

Figure 7–2. Lateral MRI study showing multiple level cervical spondylosis in an elderly patient. The spinal canal is compromised anteriorly by osteophytes and bulging discs and posteriorly by buckling of the ligamentum flavum.

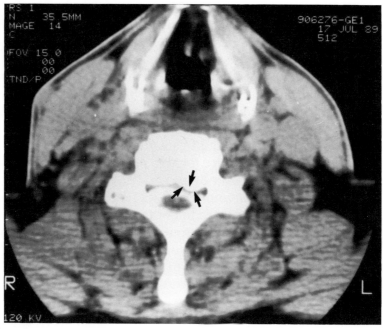

Figure 7–3. Myelogram-CT study of the cervical spine; axial view at C5-6. There is left-sided spondylosis deforming the thecal sac and compromising the left C6 nerve root (*arrows*).

under the posterior longitudinal ligament. Once complete decompression of the nerve root is accomplished, the root itself is gently mobilized with a blunt hook working toward the axilla. Palpation ventral to the common dural sac and the nerve root usually reveals a herniated disc or a hard bony ridge at the uncovertebral joint. With the nerve root gently retracted, the disc capsule is incised with the scalpel and disc fragments are "milked" out and removed with a small punch. Occasionally, portions of a bony ridge may be removed, but this can be hazardous to the root and the spinal cord. With complete decompression achieved, hemostasis is assured with bipolar cautery and Gelfoam, and the wound is closed. Ordinarily, no form of immobilization is necessary and most patients can resume full activity within 7 to 10 days after surgery.

Anterior Approach

The anterior approach for treatment of cervical radiculopathy also has its advocates and is highly effective in experienced hands.[3,9-11,13-15] The patient is placed in the supine position and the head is immobilized in 5 lbs of halter or Gardner-Wells traction with the neck slightly extended by a sandbag placed at the cervicothoracic junction. The hip from which the bone graft is to be taken is also elevated by a sandbag, and the shoulders are carefully taped down so that a satisfactory lateral radiograph can be taken. For the same reason, towel clips are avoided in draping the neck.

Using preoperative plain films as a guide, an appropriately placed transverse incision is made in a skin fold from the midline laterally just past the leading border of the sternomastoid. The platysma is isolated and divided sharply, taking care to preserve the external jugular vein. The fascial plane anterior to the sternomastoid is dissected and sharply divided, and the remainder of the exposure can usually proceed with blunt dissection using the fingertips and a Kitner dissector ("peanut") to expose the prevertebral fascia at the midline. Blunt dissection serves to avoid damage to the carotid artery (lateral), the esophagus and trachea (medial), and the recurrent laryngeal nerve. The prevertebral fascia is opened with sharp dissection, exposing the anterior longitudinal ligament bordered on either side by the longus colli.

With exposure secured, the level is checked by a lateral radiograph with a discogram needle carefully placed into the assumed proper disc space. A saline injection into the disc using a tuberculin syringe confirms the disc degeneration: a normal disc will not accept the injection. The ligament anterior to the degenerated disc is resected after rectangular incision with a scalpel. A small square periosteal elevator defines the borders of the cartilaginous end plates of the disc against the bodies above and below. The disc is entered with curettes and rongeurs and is removed piecemeal. Magnification of vision with loupes or microscope is ordinarily employed. The offending herniated disc fragment is frequently attached to the nucleus pulposus and is readily excised along with the remainder of the disc. Alternatively, a rent in the posterior longitudinal ligament can be seen. This can be enlarged and the extruded fragments then removed. A thorough disc removal is accomplished, aided by increasing the cervical traction or by using intervertebral body spreading devices. Some surgeons use a high-speed drill or curettes to remove offending osteophytes. This must be done with great care and control if damage to the nerve root and spinal cord is to be avoided.

With the disc removed and decompression accomplished, the disc space is carefully measured. An appropriately sized bone graft is obtained from the iliac crest. Ideally, it will have three cortical surfaces and will be high enough to provide some distraction of the interspace once it is in place. The graft is carefully impacted within the interspace after a few perforations have been made through the end plates above and below. An increase in the cervical traction assists this maneuver. Hemostasis is assured and the wounds are closed, often with a closed drain in the hip, which remains for 24 hours.

Patients are up and about the following day. A Philadelphia collar is utilized for 6 weeks, at which time the progress of the fusion is checked radiographically. Most patients can resume full activity within a week, and the success rate is high, often with immediate relief of preoperative pain.

Both the posterior and the anterior approach are effective, with similar success and complication rates. Selection of the appropriate patient and skillfully performed surgery remain the keys to a satisfactory outcome.

CERVICAL SPONDYLOSIS AND MYELOPATHY

Degenerative changes in the aging spine can lead to diffuse cervical spondylosis. When coupled with a congenitally narrow spinal canal or with buckling of a thickened posterior ligamentum flavum, this can produce spinal cord compression and resultant myelopathy.[2,8,12,16] The usual presentation is that of painless gradual loss of control of the lower extremities, ultimately resulting in spastic paraparesis with long tract signs and spastic bladder dysfunction. Occasionally, the spondylotic process also affects the cervical nerve roots, with associated weakness and atrophy in the upper extremities. Rarely, a painless lower motor neuron type syndrome can affect one arm, and even more rarely, multiple level spondylosis can present a picture similar to amyotrophic lateral sclerosis.

Diagnosis can be clarified by electromyographic and nerve conduction studies. Plain radiographs are helpful but may not be diagnostic. Myelography with CT and, more recently, MRI have greatly aided in establishing an accurate diagnosis.

Operative Technique

Surgical management of cervical spondylosis has been less than ideal. The standard operation has been a decompressive laminectomy extending at least one segment above and below the involved levels as seen on imaging studies. Debate has occurred about whether to open the dura, but this is not recommended unless an associated disc herniation is anticipated. It is no longer thought necessary or desirable to section the dentate ligaments in order to allow the spinal cord to move posteriorly. When nerve root compression is present in addition to the myelopathy, foraminotomies are performed as well, taking care not to produce instability of the spine.

The patient is placed either upright or prone with the head fixed and the neck in strict neutral position. Through a midline incision the spinous processes and laminae are exposed in a subperiosteal plane. The laminectomy may be performed as an osteoplastic laminectomy by using a high-speed drill to divide the laminae laterally, lifting off the posterior elements as one structure after sectioning the ligamentum flavum. More commonly, the spinous processes and laminae are simply resected using ronguers. In either case, great care must be utilized, as there is no room for technical error and the already compromised cervical spinal cord is unforgiving. The initial decompression is completed with fine Kerrison-type ronguers or the drill, and nerve root decompression is accomplished where necessary. Although some surgeons attempt to reconstruct the spinal canal by wiring back the removed intact elements in such a fashion as to widen the canal, more commonly, no bony reconstruction is attempted and the wound is simply closed in layers, with or without closed drainage.

Results of decompressive laminectomy for cervical spondylosis are variable. The goal is mainly prophylactic—to prevent progressive neurologic deficit. Often improvement to the clinical state present 6 months prior to surgery can be achieved, and occasionally more dramatic recovery will occur. The procedure has yielded between 70 and 85 percent satisfactory (good to excellent) results.[1,5]

Cervical spondylotic myelopathy may be successfully treated by anterior surgical approaches as well, particularly in the case of focal disease at one or two levels. Bohlman has shown that the posterior osteophytes or spurs resorb once solid bony fusion occurs and may not need to be removed at the time of anterior disc excision and fusion (Fig. 7–4).[1] DePalma and associates reported only 63 percent good or excellent results in a large retrospective series.[4] More recent results and overall complication rates tend to be similar to those of the posterior approach.

COMPLICATIONS

Even with meticulous surgical exposure and intimate knowledge of anatomy, complications will occur during cervical spine surgery. Some complications are unique to the anterior or posterior approach, while others are common to both. The overall complication rate is estimated to

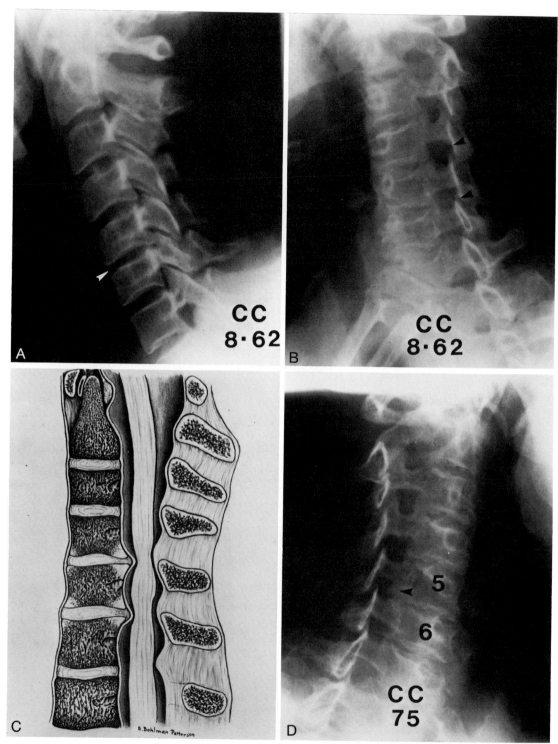

Figure 7–4. *A,* Lateral roentgenogram of a 52-year-old female presenting with neck and left shoulder pain in August 1962. There is minimal disc space narrowing at C5-6 (*arrow*). *B,* Note that there is very little foraminal encroachment in the oblique roentgenogram (*arrows*). *C,* A diagrammatic illustration of a cervical spondylotic spine showing a narrow canal, decreased height of the disc spaces, posterior osteophytes, and disc protrusions with a buckled posterior longitudinal ligament and ligamentum flavum. (From Bohlman HH: Cervical spondylosis with moderate to severe myelopathy: A report of seventeen cases treated by Robinson anterior cervical discectomy and fusion. Spine 2:151–162, 1977.) *D,* Oblique roentgenogram revealing a large osteophyte and osteochondrophyte spur formation in the foramen between the fifth and sixth cervical vertebrae (*arrow*).

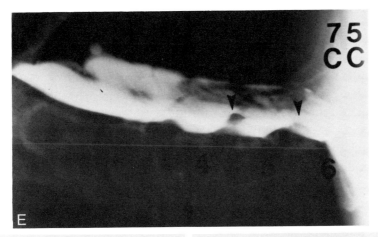

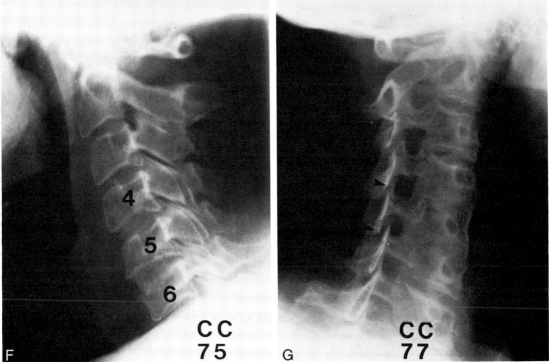

Figure 7–4 *Continued E,* Lateral view of the myelogram revealing disc and osteophyte protrusions at C4-5 and C5-6 (*arrows*) *F,* Lateral roentgenogram taken 2 months after Robinson anterior cervical discectomy and fusions at C4-5 and C5-6. Note the distracting bone blocks and the intentional lack of removal of posterior osteophytes. The patient was relieved of her neck and shoulder pain at this time. *G,* Oblique roentgenogram 2 years after surgery revealing total resorption of osteophytes in the foramina of C4-5 and C5-6 secondary to the normal process of bone remodeling (*arrows*).

be 3 to 4 percent, with the frequency of neurologic complications at 1 to 2 percent. While the anterior approach has a lower rate of neurologic complications (less than 1 percent) than the posterior approach (1 to 2 percent), it is associated with a higher rate of complications related to the bone graft used for fusion (1 to 5 percent).[7]

Intraoperative complications unique to the anterior approach include perforation of the pharynx, trachea, and esophagus, which can be devastating if unrecognized during surgery. Vascular injury to the carotid artery, jugular vein, and vertebral artery must be avoided, as well as injury to the thoracic duct. The most frequent neurologic complication is injury to the recurrent laryngeal nerve, but injury to the spinal cord, nerve roots, and sympathetic chain may also occur. Complications associated with the autogenous iliac crest bone graft include improper positioning with cervical canal compromise, anterior extrusion of the graft, and graft donor site problems such as injury to the cutaneous femoral nerve or hematoma.

Intraoperative complications associated with the posterior approach include injury to the spinal cord or nerve roots, most frequently C5. Also late instability due to aggressive decompression without fusion may occur. The most common complications of posterior cervical fusion include wire pull-out and pseudarthrosis.

Postoperative complications are similar with both approaches and include hematoma, infection, and failure of fusion with subsequent kyphosis. The anterior approach also may rarely be complicated by discitis. Pulmonary atelectasis, deep venous thrombosis, and intestinal ileus may occur. Most of these complications can be prevented or at least minimized if recognized and treated early.

Summary

The aging cervical spine represents a continuing surgical challenge and is an area in which much remains to be done in research, in diagnosis, and in clinical practice.

References

1. Bohlman HH: Cervical spondylosis with moderate to severe myelopathy. Spine 2:151–162, 1977.
2. Brain WR, Northfield D, Wilkinson M: The neurological manifestations of cervical spondylosis. Brain 75:187–225, 1952.
3. Cloward RB: The anterior approach for removal of ruptured cervical disks. J Neurosurg 15:602–614, 1958.
4. DePalma AF, Rothman R, Lewinnek G, et al: Anterior interbody fusion for severe cervical disc degeneration. Surg Gynecol Obstet 134:755–758, 1972.
5. Epstein JA, Janin Y: Management of cervical spondylotic myeloradiculopathy by the posterior approach. In Bailey RW, et al: The Cervical Spine, 1st ed. Philadelphia, J.B. Lippincott, 1983, pp. 402–410.
6. Fager CA: Results of adequate posterior decompression in the relief of spondylotic cervical myelopathy. J Neurosurg 38:684–692, 1973.
7. Graham JJ: Complications of cervical spine surgery. In Sherk HH, et al: The Cervical Spine, 2nd ed. Philadelphia, J.B. Lippincott, 1989, pp. 831–837.
8. Hoff JT, Wilson CB: The pathophysiology of cervical spondylotic radiculopathy and myelopathy. Clin Neurosurg 24:474–487, 1977.

9. Lunsford LD, Bissonette DJ, Jannetta PJ, et al: Anterior surgery for cervical disc disease. I. Treatment of lateral cervical disc herniation in 253 cases. J Neurosurg 53:1–11, 1980.
10. Lunsford LD, Bissonette DJ, Zorub DS: Anterior surgery for cervical disc disease. II. Treatment of cervical spondylotic myelopathy in 32 cases. J Neurosurg. 53:12–19, 1980.
11. Martins AN: Anterior cervical discectomy with and without interbody bone graft. J Neurosurg 44:290–295, 1976.
12. Mayfield FH: Cervical spondylosis: Observations based on surgical treatment of 400 patients. Postgrad Med 38:345–357, 1965.
13. Robinson RA, Walker AE, Ferlich DE: The results of anterior interbody fusion of the cervical spine. J Bone Joint Surg 44A:1569–1586, 1962.
14. Smith GW, Robinson RA: The treatment of certain cervical spine disorders by anterior removal of the intervertebral disc and interbody fusion. J Bone Joint Surg 40A:607–624, 1958.
15. Southwick WO, Robinson RA: Surgical approaches to the vertebral bodies in the cervical and lumbar regions. J Bone Joint Surg 39A:631–644, 1957.
16. Stoltman HF, Blackwood W: The role of the ligamenta flava in the pathogenesis of myelopathy in cervical spondylosis. Brain 87:45–50, 1964.

The Thoracic Spine

CHAPTER 8

Thoracic Disc Disease

The thoracic spine is uniquely protected from many of the pathophysiological mechanisms that affect the cervical and lumbar spine. The rib cage effectively splints the thoracic spine and prevents many of the degenerative stresses that accompany bending and twisting movements. The lack of a normal curvature of the thoracic spine also helps to avoid some of the unbalanced forces that affect other areas when one assumes an upright posture and otherwise opposes the force of gravity. These same features tend to protect the thoracic spine from physical trauma, with most traumatic fracture-dislocations occurring at the thoracolumbar junction.

An extremely important feature of the thoracic spine, and one that differentiates it from the lumbar spine, is the presence of the spinal cord and the conus medullaris within the spinal canal. The cord fits more tightly within the canal in the thoracic region than in the cervical, and, therefore, small anatomic or pathologic disturbances can produce profound neurologic consequences.

Thoracic disc herniations, although much less common than those in the cervical or lumbar regions, occur for the same basic reasons.[1,5,6,7] Increase in intradiscal pressure and weakening of the restraining annulus fibrosus are the major factors. They may occur with trauma, in association with other conditions such as scoliosis, or as part of the effects of age and "wear and tear" on the spinal elements, ligaments, and other soft tissues.

Historically, operations on the thoracic spine, especially for disc pathology, have been associated with significant risk of intraoperative and postoperative complications. However, great progress has been made in diagnosis, surgical techniques, and most importantly, surgical philosophy, permitting safer and more effective management of disorders affecting the thoracic spine.

ETIOLOGY

Each basic category of disease can contribute to pathology in the thoracic spine. Congenital anomalies can affect the bone, nerves, and soft tissues. Spina bifida and meningoceles in the thoracic area are rare. Neurenteric cysts are also rare congenital lesions but most commonly affect the thoracic spine. Scoliosis is the most frequently seen congenital anomaly of the thoracic spine and may be idiopathic or associated with other conditions such as neurofibromatosis. The stresses associated with scoliosis can lead to progressive degeneration of thoracic discs.

Trauma to the thoracic spine can result in fractures, dislocations, and traumatic disc herniations. These most commonly occur at either end of the thoracic spine, but axial trauma can result in disc herniations at any level.

Neoplasms affecting the thoracic spine can involve the vertebral bodies, meninges, nerve roots, or the spinal cord itself. Chordomas arise from notochordal remnants and may affect the vertebral body or the disc itself. Tumors metastatic to the vertebral bodies seldom affect the discs but may narrow the spinal canal. The most common primary tumor in this region is the meningioma, which usually appears as an intradural extramedullary lesion in middle-aged women.

Infectious processes have a predilection for the disc in the thoracic region as elsewhere. Tuberculosis, although now uncommon, classically results in pathologic changes in the thoracic spine, with paravertebral infectious abscesses and vertebral collapse with the typical deformity of Pott's disease.

Metabolic diseases such as osteoporosis can affect the thoracic spine, resulting in vertebral collapse at one or more levels. Acromegaly may be associated with hypertrophic changes that can affect any part of the spinal canal.

Most pertinent to the aging thoracic spine are degenerative changes, which may occur in the discs themselves or in any of the vertebral elements or intervertebral joint structures.

CLINICAL MANIFESTATIONS

Thoracic disc disease usually presents either with pain because of thoracic nerve root compression or with progressive myelopathy due to spinal cord compression. The latter usually is painless, and when subacute or chronic can be confused with multiple sclerosis or other spinal cord degenerative processes. Root compression usually causes typical bandlike thoracic radicular pain, but visceral type pain may also occur, particularly when lower segments are involved.

The neurologic examination ordinarily reveals a spastic paraparesis, with upper motor neuron signs in the lower extremities, increased deep tendon reflexes, and Babinski signs. Sensory findings are frequently present and may help to identify the level of the lesion.

DIAGNOSTIC PROCEDURES

Magnetic resonance imaging has revolutionized diagnosis of diseases affecting the thoracic spine and its discs.[2,4] The vertebral bodies, discs, and spinal canal can be seen clearly and distortions of the spinal cord are readily visualized (Fig. 8–1). Computed tomographic scanning and myelography are often helpful (Fig. 8–2). Myelography and spinal angiography are utilized when an arteriovenous malformation of the thoracic spinal cord is a consideration. Electrophysiologic diagnosis can often confirm or clarify clinical findings. Electromyography and spinal cord evoked potential studies may be useful in diagnosis and also as an adjunct in monitoring spinal cord function during surgery. Plain films are used to evaluate scoliosis. Disc space narrowing, vertebral body collapse, and pathologic calcification within a degenerated disc are also visible on plain radiographs.

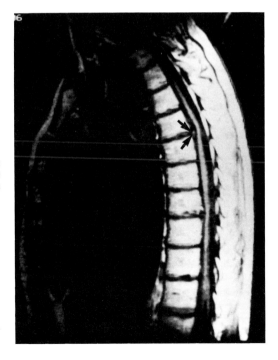

Figure 8–1. Lateral MRI scan of patient with T5-6 disc herniation (*arrows*) displacing the spinal cord. Ventral discogenic disease is also present at T8-9.

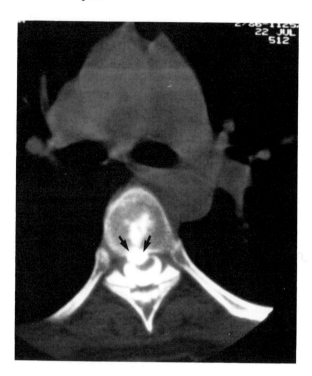

Figure 8–2. Axial view of myelogram-CT scan showing a calcified thoracic disc herniation (*arrows*) displacing the spinal cord (*gray*) from right to left within the thecal space (*white*).

DIFFERENTIAL DIAGNOSIS

Pain in the thoracic spine with or without radiation into the chest and abdomen can be caused by a plethora of entities other than thoracic disc disease. Rheumatoid or ankylosing spondylitis affecting the thoracic spine can give rise to sensations of pain and stiffness. Radiographs and a history of arthritis in other joints can help make this distinction; however, radiographs are frequently negative early in the course of the spondyloarthropathies.

Malignant or benign tumors, either intraspinal or extraspinal, can give rise to dorsal spine pain mimicking a thoracic disc. The advent of magnetic resonance imaging has made this diagnosis much easier than in the days of myelography alone.

Disc space infections are usually found in a younger age group than disc herniations and present a unique radiographic appearance, which is outlined in Chapter 15. Nevertheless, spinal tuberculosis, as well as other infections, is still seen in immunocompromised hosts. These disc infections may present in older patients without significant elevation in temperature or white cell count.

Herpes zoster produces a typical vesicular rash and pain along a radicular cutaneous distribution. The midline component of the radicular pain can be absent initially, but may appear within a relatively short time.

[   ]

SURGICAL APPROACHES

Symptomatic thoracic discs, unlike cervical and lumbar discs, are treated only by surgical intervention. When the diagnosis is suspected on the basis of clinical signs and symptoms and confirmed with an imaging study, surgery should be performed as soon as possible to prevent irreversible spinal cord changes.

Although the midline approach with a standard laminectomy or laminotomy is quite satisfactory for many kinds of pathologic processes affecting the thoracic spine, most notably benign tumors such as dorsally situated meningiomas, ventrally located midline lesions such as thoracic disc herniations are frequently inaccessible.[8] The spinal cord occupies nearly all of the space within the spinal canal, and it cannot safely be displaced. For that reason, and because many thoracic disc herniations are calcified and not easily removed, posterolateral and anterior approaches have been developed and are used with great success.[9,10] The posterior laminectomy is performed in a manner similar to that described for the cervical spine. Its limitations have been noted, and it will not be considered further.

The most widely employed posterior approach to thoracic disc pathology is accomplished through a costotransversectomy. The initial exposure can be achieved through either a midline or a paramedian incision. Subperiosteal dissection exposes the lamina and transverse process at the desired level, usually confirmed by an intraoperative radiograph. Dissection is carried out laterally to the head of the rib, which is resected, exposing the nerve root. A hemilaminectomy exposes the dural sac over the spinal cord. The pedicle is then drilled down, and this provides excellent visualization of the disc without retraction of the spinal dura. A posterolateral entry is made into the disc space, and the offending fragments are removed or drilled away. Ordinarily, no reconstruction or fixation is necessary and the wound can be closed in standard fashion, with or without drainage. The surgeon must keep in mind the possibility of damage to the pleura, and the wound must be evaluated for an air leak prior to closure.

In some cases of thoracic disc disease, the posterolateral route may not provide a safe or effective angle of approach, and a more anterior trajectory may be desirable.[3] Anterior approaches to the thoracic spine are of necessity transthoracic or, in the case of the lowest discs, thoracoabdominal. These approaches are carried out with the patient in the lateral position, through a standard thoracotomy, respecting the anatomy and position of the great vessels. These procedures are performed in conjunction with a thoracic surgeon and are a team effort.

References

1. Benjamin J: Diagnosis and management of thoracic disc disease. Clin Neurosurg 30:577–605, 1983.

2. Blumenkopf B: Thoracic intervertebral disc herniations: diagnostic value of magnetic resonance imaging. Neurosurgery 23:36–40, 1988.
3. Bohlman HH, Zdeblick TA: Anterior excision of herniated thoracic discs. J Bone Joint Surg 70A:1038–1047, 1988.
4. Francavilla TL, Powers A, Dina T, et al: MR imaging of thoracic disk herniations. J Comput Assist Tomogr 11:1062–1065, 1987.
5. Hedge S, Staas WE Jr: Thoracic disc herniation and spinal cord injury. Am J Phys Med Rehabil 67:228–229, 1988.
6. Krag MH, Seroussi RE, Wilder DG, et al: Internal displacement distribution from in vitro loading of human thoracic and lumbar spinal motion segments: experimental results and theoretical predictions. Spine 12:1001–1007, 1987.
7. Lehman LB: Paraparesis during myelography associated with a ruptured thoracic intervertebral disc. Neurosurgery 24:909–912, 1989.
8. Lesoin F, Rosseaux M, Autricque A, et al: Thoracic disc herniations: evolution in the approach and indications. Acta Neurochir 80:30–34, 1986.
9. Otani K, Yoshida M, Fujii E, et al: Thoracic disc herniation. Surgical treatment in 23 patients. Spine 13:1262–1267, 1988.
10. Sekhar LN, Jannetta PJ: Thoracic disc herniation: operative approaches and results. Neurosurgery 12:303–305, 1983.

The Lumbar Spine

CHAPTER 9

Clinical Syndromes and Physical Examination of the Lumbar Spine

The lifetime incidence of low back pain is frequently reported to be about 65 percent, but it may be somewhat lower in the United States.[4,40] Degeneration of the lumbar disc, associated degenerative arthritis of the facet joints, and spinal stenosis are the most common causes of low back and leg pain in the aging population. The clinical presentation ranges from backache with or without referred pain, to radicular pain, to neurogenic claudication. These symptoms are a reflection of the totality of degeneration of the intervertebral discs and facet joints. The clinical features in the early phases are related directly to derangement of the intervertebral disc and its effect on the adjacent nerve roots. During the later phases of the pathologic process, the clinical picture may be clouded by secondary changes that occur in the spinal segment and motor unit as a whole.

It is important to recognize that the clinical syndromes to be discussed represent manifestations of the sequential spectrum of degeneration that affects the aging spine. Accordingly, the clinical syndromes that evolve are multifaceted and must be recognized as such if diagnosis is to be correct and treatment effective. It is disturbing to see missed diagnoses of herniated lumbar discs that present in an atypical fashion. It is equally precarious, however, to attribute all cases of back and leg pain to abnormalities of the intervertebral disc or "arthritis of the spine," especially in the aging spine. A spectrum of neoplastic, infectious, and vascular disorders can mimic lumbar disc herniation or spinal stenosis. This chapter will first outline the etiology of pain in the lumbar spine and describe the classical clinical presentations of lumbar disc degeneration, as well as the more common variants. Then, the most important aspects of the physical examination will be discussed.

ETIOLOGY OF PAIN IN THE LUMBAR SPINE

Back Pain

The majority of patients with degenerative disease in the lumbar spine have back pain as the earliest symptom, often preceding leg pain or other radicular symptoms by 2 to 10 years.[39,43] Pain in the early stages of disc disease is probably caused by early degeneration of the annulus fibrosus and dessication of the nucleus pulposus. Since the nucleus no longer functions as a perfect gel with viscoelastic properties, it transmits forces in a nonlinear and asymmetric fashion (Fig. 9–1).[23] The intermittent episodes of mechanical low back pain are nonspecific and cannot be differentiated from the syndromes commonly labeled as "low back

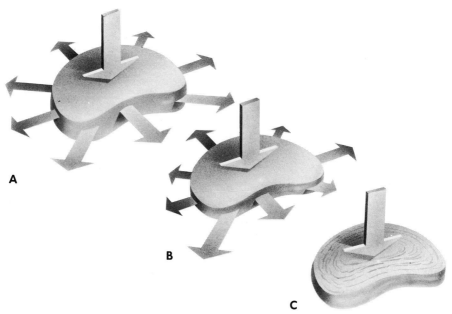

Figure 9–1. Distribution of forces in the normal and abnormal disc. *A,* When the disc functions normally, as in the early decades of life, the nucleus distributes the forces of compression and tension equally to all parts of the annulus. *B,* With degeneration, the nucleus no longer functions as a perfect gel and the forces transmitted to the annulus are unequal. *C,* With advanced degeneration of the nucleus, the distribution of forces to the annulus from within is completely lost since the nucleus now acts as a solid rather than a liquid. For this reason, disc herniation is unusual in the elderly. (From Rothman RH, Simeone FA: The Spine. 2nd ed. Philadelphia, W.B. Saunders, 1982.)

strain" or "acute lumbago." Because this clinical situation frequently progresses to the more typical disc herniation with unequivocal findings, the pathologic basis for this episodic low back pain is likely to be disc degeneration.

Since the intervertebral disc is innervated by dorsally situated sinovertebral sensory nerves, degeneration can reasonably be implicated in this low back pain syndrome. The age-related defective diffusion mechanism at the vertebral endplate–annular interface provides a basis for the loss of structural integrity of the disc early in the aging process of the axial skeleton.[3] The mechanical intensification and relief seen in this syndrome can be understood in light of Nachemson's in vivo determination of disc pressures in various postural positions (Fig. 9–2).[27] Accordingly, it is not surprising that many low back pain episodes begin in the morning hours after the patient has been in an extended supine position during sleep and when the hydration (turgor) of the nucleus pulposus is at its maximum (Fig. 9–3).[28]

Referred Pain

Pain in the lumbar region alone or associated with pain in the lower extremities is the result of stimuli applied to the mesodermal structures of the spine or to the nerve roots, either within the dural sac or after they emerge from the dura. Based on the site of origin, pain can be classified as sclerotogenous (referred pain) or dermatogenous (radicular pain).

Referred pain occurs when certain structures of mesodermal origin (e.g., muscles, ligaments, periosteum, joint capsule, and annulus) are subjected to abnormal stimuli such as excessive stretching or the injection of hypertonic saline. With these abnormal stimuli, a deep, ill-defined, dull, aching discomfort is noted that may be referred into the lumbosacral or sacroiliac joint as well as the legs and buttocks (Fig. 9–4).[20] The pattern of referral is to the area designated as the sclerotome, which has the same

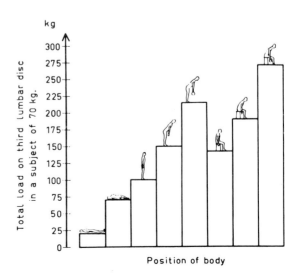

Figure 9–2. This figure illustrates the total load on the third lumbar disc in a subject weighing 70 kg. (From Nachemson A: In vivo discometry in lumbar discs with irregular nucleograms. Acta Orthop Scand 36:426, 1965 ©1965 Munksgaard International Publishers Ltd, Copenhagen, Denmark.)

Experimental flow of fluid in autopsy discs.

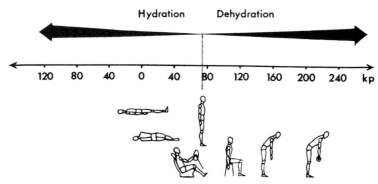

Figure 9–3. Theoretical calculation on the hydration-dehydration points as obtained experimentally by Kramer combined with the findings of intradiscal pressure measurements by Nachemson. (From Nachemson A: Toward a better understanding of low-back pain: A review of the mechanics of the lumbar disc. Rheumatol Rehabil 14(3):129, 1975.)

embryonic origin as the mesodermal tissues stimulated. The referred distribution of pain, however, depends not only on segmental innervation but also on the severity of pain and the extent to which the individual is cognizant of the stimulated components of the axial skeleton.[20] In addition, dull, deep, and boring referred pain can often present concurrently with the sharp, lancinating radicular pain from nerve root tension.

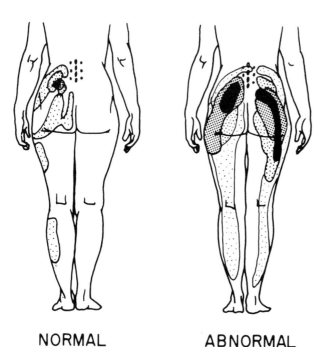

NORMAL   ABNORMAL

Figure 9–4. Pain referral pattern for asymptomatic and symptomatic subjects. This confirms that the pain referral pattern from stimulation of the lumbar facet joint is in the typical locations of lumbago. (From Mooney V, Robertson J: The facet syndrome. Clin Orthop 115:149, 1976.)

Radicular Symptoms

Radicular Pain

In contrast to the ill-defined nature of deep referred pain, superficial or cutaneous pain is clearly localized by the patient. It is sharp and lancinating, and it is restricted to the dermatome of the nerve root involved (Fig. 9–5). Pressure on an inflamed nerve root by a disc fragment, bulging annulus, or compromised lateral recess can produce pain and motor or sensory deficits in the lower extremities. Smyth and Wright demonstrated that an inflamed nerve root is far more sensitive to compression than a normal root and that the longitudinal extension of pain was directly related to the amount of pressure on the root.[37]

The etiologic role of mechanical tension or compression on the nerve root yielding radicular pain is generally accepted; however, whether it causes damage to the intrinsic structure of the neural tissue or its accom-

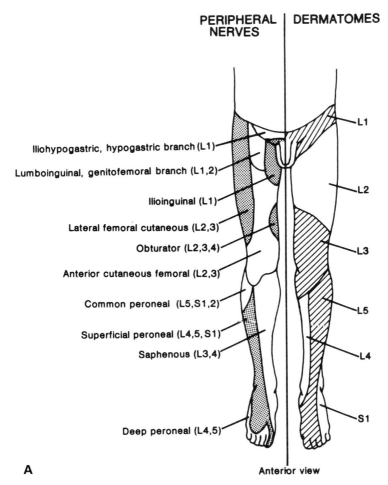

PERIPHERAL NERVES | DERMATOMES

Iliohypogastric, hypogastric branch (L1)
Lumboinguinal, genitofemoral branch (L1,2)
Ilioinguinal (L1)
Lateral femoral cutaneous (L2,3)
Obturator (L2,3,4)
Anterior cutaneous femoral (L2,3)
Common peroneal (L5,S1,2)
Superficial peroneal (L4,5,S1)
Saphenous (L3,4)
Deep peroneal (L4,5)

L1
L2
L3
L5
L4
S1

A   Anterior view

Figure 9–5. *A,* Anterior view of the lower extremities depicting skin areas innervated by nerve roots (*right*) and peripheral nerves (*left*).

Illustration continued on following page

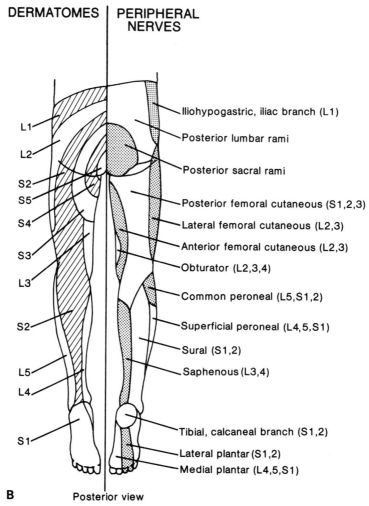

DERMATOMES | PERIPHERAL NERVES

L1
L2
S2
S5
S4
S3
L3
S2
L5
L4
S1

Iliohypogastric, iliac branch (L1)
Posterior lumbar rami
Posterior sacral rami
Posterior femoral cutaneous (S1,2,3)
Lateral femoral cutaneous (L2,3)
Anterior femoral cutaneous (L2,3)
Obturator (L2,3,4)
Common peroneal (L5,S1,2)
Superficial peroneal (L4,5,S1)
Sural (S1,2)
Saphenous (L3,4)
Tibial, calcaneal branch (S1,2)
Lateral plantar (S1,2)
Medial plantar (L4,5,S1)

B   Posterior view

Figure 9–5 *Continued B,* Posterior view of the nerve root (*left*) and peripheral nerve (*right*) areas of the lower extremities. (From Borenstein DG, Wiesel SW: Low Back Pain. Philadelphia, W.B. Saunders, 1989.)

panying vasculature remains unclear.[17,26,29] The inflammatory component of the radicular syndrome described in Chapter 2 is also of significance, but again, the causative agents are still under investigation.

Both the sclerotomes and dermatomes exhibit varying amounts of overlap. However, in the case of dermatomes, the pattern of distribution and spread of pain are usually specific enough to assist in localization of the disc and nerve root involved. The clinical picture may be confusing if the pain distribution is the result of implication of two nerve roots at one level. In this case, bilateral leg symptoms are present. Also, pain may be caused by irritation of two contiguous roots on the same side. This results in the potential for considerable overlap of pain patterns; other physical signs, along with imaging studies, are required to pinpoint the involved levels.

Motor Weakness

On occasion, patients may present with weakness in the lower extremities as their outstanding symptom. The weakness may be present without pain or clinically apparent sphincter disturbances and most commonly involves the L4 or L5 anterior roots. Although these motor deficits may be due to degenerative disc disease, a relatively painless monoradicular or, especially, multiradicular paresis requires a differential diagnosis that includes metabolic or infectious neuropathy or a space-occupying lesion of the spinal cord itself.

Sensory Changes

Sensory alterations in the dermatome of the involved nerve root are frequently observed in lesions of the lumbar discs. However, the patient is often not aware of these abnormalities until the lesion is far advanced. In some cases the patient indicates a feeling of numbness or of "pins and needles" (paresthesias) in an area of dermatome distribution. In addition to impairment of sensation due to irritation or dysfunction of the sensory fibers of a nerve root, patients may report a decrease in position sense in the involved leg. This is indicative of involvement of the proprioceptive nerve fibers in addition to the other fibers of sensation.

HISTORY

Risk Factors

Epidemiologic studies have revealed that only a few factors appear to be important in the pathogenesis of low back pain and sciatica. Recognized risk factors include occupations that require repetitive lifting in the forward bent-and-twisted position, exposure to vibrations from vehicles or industrial machinery, and cigarette smoking.[13] Variations in spinal posture, such as lordosis and scoliosis of less than 60°, do not appear to increase the risk of low back pain or sciatica.[32] The effects of increased body height and weight as well as discrepancies in leg length are controversial.[16] While low back pain is common during pregnancy,[10] the incidence of herniated discs does not appear to be increased.[44]

Injury is a variable feature in the history of lumbar disc problems. The patient frequently will associate the onset of back trouble with a specific injury,—often occurring days or weeks before the onset of severe symptoms. Others may associate the presenting symptoms with a previous trauma that resulted in a minor low back strain that has developed into a serious back disorder. It is likely that trauma can aggravate an already degenerative disc, but it is certainly not a requisite to the onset of low back pain, since a large group of patients deny any history of trauma.

Lumbar Spine Clinical Syndromes

Careful analysis of the history of patients reveals that the manner in which the lumbar disc syndrome first becomes symptomatic varies widely. Nevertheless, several distinct patterns evolve that are characteristic of a lumbar disc lesion in the various stages of the degenerative process.

Back Pain Alone

The most common onset of back pain is characterized by a diffuse continuous pain in the lower lumbar region that begins gradually and is punctuated by periods of more intense pain. These exacerbations are often initiated by some excessive flexion strain of the lumbar spine. The pain is mechanical in nature; it is relieved by rest and aggravated by activity. Discogenic pain usually has the definite mechanical quality of being accentuated with prolonged sitting and standing—a clinical correlation of increased symptoms with positions of increased spinal load. Pain that increases while the patient is in bed at night is more suggestive of a neoplastic or infectious process. The pain of disc disease is characteristically intermittent, and one should be wary when the patient states that from the onset the pain has been unrelenting and progressive. As a rule, most individuals with back pain are able to continue functioning; however, the emotional instability and intolerance to pain of some patients may make them completely incapacitated during exacerbations.

In some patients, sudden severe back pain may be initiated by acute displacement of nuclear disc material. The patient is seized by severe, agonizing pain in the low back that may be completely incapacitating. Generally, the patient maintains an abnormal posture due to severe muscle spasm and moves about cautiously. Fortunately, acute symptoms tend to regress within a few days, but sometimes they can last for several weeks. If a careful inquiry is made, a history of some previous back discomfort can usually be elicited.

Sciatic Pain Without Back Pain

This syndrome varies widely. In some patients, there is a sharp, lancinating pain, starting in the proximal thigh or buttock and radiating the full length of the limb along the dermatome of the involved nerve root. The L5 and S1 spinal nerves are most frequently involved. In a large percentage of patients, the pain comes on slowly, often felt as an ache in one of the buttocks, and gradually spreads distally to involve the calf or the foot. When the progression of symptoms is reversed (i.e., beginning distally and moving proximally), the possibility of thoracic cord involvement must be considered.

It should be pointed out that some patients note focal areas of pain in the lower extremities rather than the typical pattern of dermatome involvement. The primary complaint of these individuals may be pain of the knee, calf, ankle, or heel (Fig. 9–6). In studying pain and spinal root lesions, Friis and colleagues have found that approximately 10 percent of patients with L5 or S1 lesions in particular had asymptomatic areas of dermatome between painful foci.[12]

Although the patient may be free of back pain, there may be marked list, muscle spasm, and limitation of motion of the lumbar spine, especially in extreme lateral lumbar disc herniation. When the sciatic pain is acute, the patient's family may note listing, usually away from the side of the sciatica. Occasionally, if the disc herniation is axillary or central in position, the patient may list toward the side of the sciatica. Both involuntary maneuvers constitute an effort to decrease tension on the nerve root. The limited lumbar mobility, however, may not be purely a defensive maneuver but rather a manifestation of intrinsic neuromuscular pathology.[11]

Sciatic pain is generally not relieved significantly by changes in posture or by rest. The pain is frequently made worse by any action that increases intraspinal pressures, such as the Valsalva maneuver, coughing and sneezing, and bearing down during defecation. Sciatic pain caused by a disc herniation is classically aggravated by maneuvers that flex the lumbar spine and hip, such as sitting. This is in contrast to the sciatic pain re-

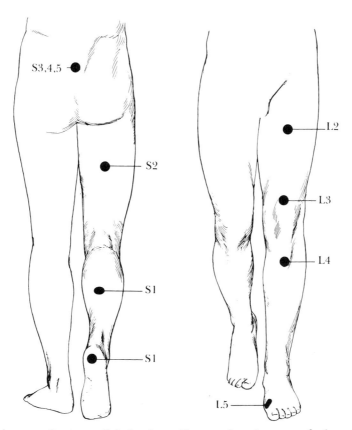

Figure 9–6. Pain may radiate to small, isolated, specific areas along the course of a dermatome. (From Rothman RH, Simeone FA: The Spine. 2nd ed. Philadelphia, W.B. Saunders, 1982.)

sulting from spinal stenosis, which is intensified by extension of the spine. Aggravation of the pain with walking (neurogenic claudication) is more characteristic of spinal stenosis but may occasionally be seen with acute disc herniations. Sciatic pain less commonly may result from degenerative spondylolisthesis in the elderly.

At the onset of sciatica due to disc herniation, back pain may suddenly abate. The mechanical explanation for this is that once the annulus has ruptured, it is no longer placed under tension and is no longer a stimulus for pain. Another interesting phenomenon is occasionally observed in patients with severe sciatica: the pain may suddenly disappear but the motor and sensory deficits remain. This must not be misconstrued as evidence of improvement, however, for it indicates that the physiologic function of the nerve root has been completely interrupted.

Back Pain with Sciatica

In a small group of patients, back pain and sciatica appear simultaneously. The onset may be acute or gradual. The back pain and leg pain may be of equal severity, but generally one overshadows the other. When pain in the back and leg is severe and the onset sudden, a dramatic incapacitation may result.

Recurrent Attacks of Low Back Problems

Wide variations are found in the clinical course of lumbar disc disease. These events vary from patient to patient, as well as in the same patient over time. In general, following an initial episode of low back pain with or without sciatica, the patient will experience repeated attacks that may become more frequent and intense and may lead to more disability. Between acute episodes of back pain, the patient usually experiences stiffness, weakness, or instability that is present at a low but noticeable level. The patient may learn that exacerbations are related to certain types and degrees of activity. When the final stages of disc degeneration have been reached and fibrosis of the disc is complete, symptoms may disappear. However, in some cases, the end stages of degeneration may leave a spinal motion segment unstable, giving rise to further back pain.

Cauda Equina Syndrome

Occasionally, a large midline disc herniation may compress several roots of the cauda equina (Fig. 9–7). This is estimated to occur in only 1 to 2 percent of patients with disc protrusions.[33,39] In young adults, the herniation usually occurs above L4, but in older individuals it may occur at any level. There is a particularly high coincidence of cauda equina syndrome and intradural disc rupture in the high lumbar areas, but these lesions are extremely rare.[31]

If the herniation is large, it may mimic an intraspinal tumor, particularly if it has been slowly progressing. Often back or perianal pain will predominate, and radicular symptoms may be masked. Difficulty with urination, consisting of frequency due to overflow incontinence, may develop relatively early. In males, a history of recent impotence may be elicited. If leg pain develops, it may be followed by numbness of the feet and difficulty in ambulating.

The variety of symptoms occurs because the lesions generally compress several spinal nerve roots. The centrally placed sacral fibers to the lower abdominal viscera produce symptoms that characterize cauda equina compression syndrome. Sensory deficit is typical and is frequently situated higher than the motor level. Perianal numbness and loss of the anal or bulbocavernosus reflex is a sign of advanced cauda equina syndrome.

Cauda equina syndrome is significant in that is must be considered a reason for prompt surgical intervention. Spontaneous neurologic recovery has not been observed. If incontinence is present, only surgery undertaken promptly can offer the chance to decrease the likelihood of permanent urinary drainage problems. Neurologic return, even with surgery, is variable.

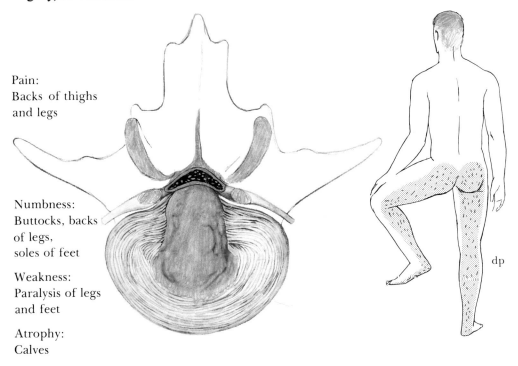

Pain:
Backs of thighs
and legs

Numbness:
Buttocks, backs
of legs,
soles of feet

Weakness:
Paralysis of legs
and feet

Atrophy:
Calves

Paralysis:
Bladder and bowel

Figure 9–7. Massive herniation at the level of the third, fourth, or fifth disc may cause severe compression of the cauda equina. Pain is confined chiefly to the buttocks and the back of the thighs and legs. Numbness is widespread from the buttocks to the soles of the feet. Motor weakness or loss is present in the legs and feet with loss of muscle mass in the calves. The bladder and bowels are paralyzed. dp = distribution of pain and paresthesia. (From DePalma, AF, Rothman, RH: The Intervertebral Disc. Philadelphia, W.B. Saunders, 1970.)

Bladder Symptoms

Intervertebral disc protrusions may occasionally present as an isolated abnormality of bowel and bladder function in patients with minimal or absent back pain and sciatica.[34] Disc disease should be ruled out in patients who develop urinary retention, vesical irritability, or incontinence, especially in the absence of infection or other pelvic abnormalities. This is more common in middle-aged than in older patients.

Four types of bladder abnormalities due to disc degeneration have been described: (1) total urinary retention; (2) chronic partial retention; (3) vesicular irritability; and (4) unawareness of the need to void.[19] The uninhibited type of neuropathic bladder dysfunction without loss of bladder sensation may represent the incipient stage of an evolving bladder disorder due to increasing involvement of the sacral roots.

Bladder dysfunction may also be seen with degenerative spinal stenosis.[35] Although the same abnormalities that can accompany disc herniation may be seen, intermittency of symptoms is common with spinal stenosis. The diagnosis can be confirmed with cystoscopy and cystometrography in conjunction with a lumbar spine imaging study.

Neurogenic Claudication

The clinical presentation of neurogenic claudication is well documented.[41] Vague leg pain, dysesthesias, and paresthesias distributed over the anterior and posterior thighs and calves are classically induced by spinal postures that mechanically compromise the neural canal and foramina. Patients of either sex, usually over 40 years old, will first notice these symptoms on ambulation and will obtain relief on sitting or lying down.[46] The increased lordotic position of the lumbar spine that is assumed with walking, particularly downhill, is most likely causative. Less often, this syndrome is precipitated by increased metabolic and vascular demands of the lower extremities with walking and is caused by compromise of neural blood flow, although a combined mechanism is possible.[8,45]

Although ischemia to the cauda equina is probably the final common pathway in any neurogenic claudication syndrome, it is the postural type of neurogenic claudication that has been best defined. It must be differentiated from vascular claudication resulting from muscle ischemia secondary to aortofemoral disease. The symptomatic relationship to posture has been verified with the bicycle test of van Gelderan, in which claudication symptoms are not produced when the patient is on the bicycle, since there is a reduction of the lumbar lordosis and a subsequent increase in the sagittal central and foraminal dimensions of the canal.[7] In contrast, vascular claudication symptoms will be produced with ambulation on an upgrade and by stress on the bicycle, which increase metabolic demands. Rubor and pallor changes with elevation and the absence of pulses below the hips are classic signs of vascular claudication. In cases in which the diagnosis is unclear, arteriography may be necessary to confirm vascular claudication. Provocation of a neurologic deficit with brisk walking may help indicate neurogenic claudication, and in early stages abnormal neurologic findings may be found only after such a stress test. With progression of the neurogenic claudication syndrome, symptoms may occur at rest, and muscle weakness, atrophy, and asymmetric reflex changes may be present.

The clinical syndrome of intermittent neurogenic claudication is closely associated with lumbar spinal stenosis. The distinction between spinal stenosis and disc protrusion is usually straightforward (Table 9–1). For spinal stenosis, an accepted classification of the syndrome has been developed, and symptoms have been attributed to the anatomic configuration occurring locally, segmentally, or generally in the affected osseous and soft tissues (Fig. 9–8). However, it is important to realize that structural changes in the spinal canal and neural foramina, often exaggerated by posture, are important but not absolute determinants of intermittent claudication.[42] The symptoms manifested may vary significantly in individuals with similar anatomic changes owing to the temporal framework within which the neural compression has occurred, the individual susceptibility of the nerves involved, and the unique functional demands and pain tolerance of the patient.

Salient Historical Points

In summary, several key points must be obtained from the patient's history. Most important is characterization of the pain with respect to quality, location, time of onset, presence of radiation, association with activity, and exacerbating or relieving positions or activities. Also, any history of previous back problems or surgery must be elicited. Presence of motor weakness or sensory abnormalities will help to define the nerve roots involved. Recent changes in bowel or bladder habits may be a harbinger of cauda equina compression. Finally, especially in older patients, a careful history of metabolic, infectious, and malignant disorders is imperative. Knowledge of these key historical points will help direct the physical examination and subsequent diagnostic studies to arrive at a correct diagnosis

Table 9–1. DISC PROTRUSION VS. SPINAL STENOSIS

	Disc Protrusion	Spinal Stenosis
Pain Pattern	Acute	Insidious
	Worse with sitting	Worse with walking
	Worse with flexion	Worse with extension
Response to Conservative Therapy	>90%	50%
Age at Onset	30–50	>60
Radiography	Normal	Narrow canal
Myelography	Asymmetric defect	Symmetric defect
CT, MRI	Herniated disc	Narrow canal/foramina

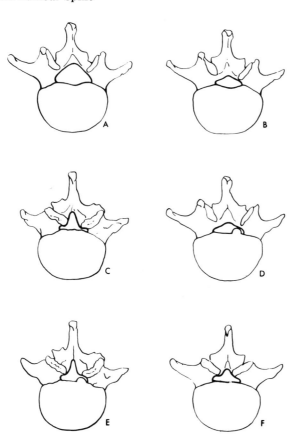

Figure 9–8. Types of lumbar spinal stenosis. *A,* Normal canal. *B,* Congenital/developmental stenosis. *C,* Degenerative stenosis. *D,* Congenital/developmental stenosis with disc herniation. *E,* Degenerative stenosis with disc herniation. *F,* Congenital developmental stenosis with superimposed degenerative stenosis. (From Arnoldi CC, et al: Lumbar spinal stenosis and nerve root entrapment syndromes. Clin Orthop 115:4, 1976.)

PHYSICAL EXAMINATION

Inspection

The gait and stance of patients with acute disc syndromes are striking and characteristic. The patient usually holds the painful leg in a flexed position and is reluctant to place the foot directly on the floor, walking with an antalgic gait. Presumedly, flexion of the leg relaxes the sciatic nerve roots and is an involuntary effort at root decompression. The lumbar spine is flattened due to a reduction or reversal of the normal lumbar lordosis.

When the involved nerve root is under severe tension, the patient usually lists away from the side of the sciatica, producing a "sciatic scoliosis" (Fig. 9–9). When the disc herniation is lateral to the nerve root, the patient will incline away from the side of the irritated nerve in an attempt to draw the nerve root away from the disc fragment. This is most dramatic in patients with extreme lateral disc herniations, such that lateral bending toward the side of the lesion will markedly exaggerate the patient's pain and paresthesias.[1,22] In contrast, when the herniation is in an axillary position medial to the nerve root, the patient will list toward the

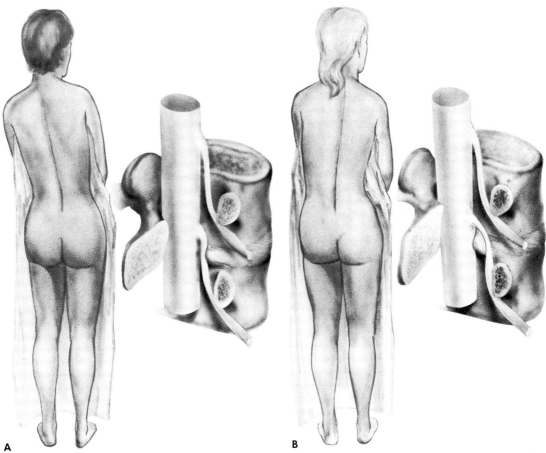

Figure 9–9. *A,* Herniation of the disc lateral to the nerve root. This will usually produce a sciatic list away from the side of the irritated nerve root. *B,* Herniation of the disc medial to the nerve root and in an axillary position. This will usually produce a sciatic list toward the side of the irritated nerve root. (From Rothman RH, Simeone FA: The Spine. 2nd ed. Philadelphia, W.B. Saunders, 1982.)

side of the lesion. In many cases, the deviation of the trunk to one side is so insignificant that it may be unnoticed by the patient. However, the list may become more apparent when the patient bends forward.

Limitation of motion is usually noted during the symptomatic phase of lumbar disc disease. Flexion of the lumbar spine is more seriously impaired than extension. Some restriction of lateral flexion (often asymmetric) is detectable, but severe impairment rarely occurs. Rotation of the spine is less affected than lateral bending. Motion in all directions should be evaluated according to the patient's tolerance.

Palpation and Percussion

Palpation of the lumbar spine in the midline usually elicits pain at the level of the symptomatic degenerative disc. It is not unusual to also find tenderness laterally along the iliac crest and the iliolumbar ligament as well as over the sacroiliac joint. In many instances, the tenderness does not reflect disease in these lateral areas, but rather hyperesthesia secondary to nerve root irritation. Occasionally, no tenderness is elicited with palpation of the lumbar spine in the erect position, and it is necessary to have the patient flex the spine, to apply pressure in the midline, and then to direct the patient to extend the spine. This maneuver may produce marked pain in some instances.

When muscle spasm is present, palpation will reveal significant hardness in the contracted muscle mass. The area will frequently be exquisitely tender on firm palpation. In less marked cases of paravertebral muscle spasm, palpation should not be directed over the muscle belly but should start in the midline with pressure exerted laterally to appreciate subtle differences in muscle tone.

Palpation over the facet joints 1 to 3 cm from the midline will frequently elicit tenderness, particularly in patients who have symptomatic degenerative joint disease with or without symptoms of spinal stenosis. This tenderness is exaggerated on palpation with extension of the spine, which increases the lumbar lordosis.

Palpation should also be performed in the sciatic notch and along the course of the sciatic nerve itself. Hyperesthesia along the nerve is common. When pain is localized to a specific area along the course of the sciatic nerve, careful regional examination is warranted to rule out local lesions irritating the sciatic nerve such as abscess, neurofibroma, glomus tumor, lipoma, or sterile abscess following local drug injections.

Percussion of the lumbar spine may elicit local pain. More significantly, it may reproduce sciatica when nerve root compression is present. As with many of the physical findings, it is suggestive, but not pathognomonic, of a herniated disc.

The presence of tender motor points in the lower extremities may be of both diagnostic and prognostic importance. These points represent the main neuromuscular junctions in the involved muscle groups corresponding to the segmental level of nerve root involvement.[14] In the absence or presence of true radicular signs, back pain patients with tender motor points may have a longer disability period. It is important that this tenderness not be mistaken for thrombophlebitis, especially when it is in the calf.

Neurologic Examination

A meticulous neurologic examination will yield objective evidence of nerve root compression if present. It will also suggest the level of involvement, but it is not conclusive in this regard. The most frequent levels of disc herniation are L4-5 and L5-S1, followed by L3-4. Disc herniations at L5-S1 will usually compromise the first sacral nerve root. Similarly, a disc herniation at L4-5 will most often compress the fifth lumbar root, whereas herniation at L3-4 will most frequently involve the fourth lumbar root (Table 9–2).

Table 9–2. CLINICAL FEATURES OF HERNIATED LUMBAR DISCS

L3-4 Disc; L4 Nerve Root

Pain	Lower back, hip, posterolateral thigh, across patella, anteromedial aspect of leg
Numbness	Anteromedial thigh and knee
Weakness	Knee extension
Atrophy	Quadriceps
Reflexes	Knee jerk diminished

L4-5 Disc; L5 Nerve Root

Pain	Sacroiliac region, hip, posterolateral thigh, anterolateral leg
Numbness	Lateral leg, first webspace
Weakness	Dorsiflexion of great toe and foot
Atrophy	Minimal anterior calf
Reflexes	None, or absent posterior tibial tendon reflex

L5-S1 Disc; S1 Nerve Root

Pain	Sacroiliac region, hip, posterolateral thigh/leg
Numbness	Back of calf; lateral heel, foot, and toe
Weakness	Plantarflexion of foot and great toe
Atrophy	Gastrocnemius and soleus
Reflexes	Ankle jerk diminished or absent

Due to variation in root configuration and the position of the herniated material, L4-5 herniations can affect not only the fifth lumbar nerve but also the first sacral nerve. In extreme lateral herniations, the nerve exiting at the same level as the disc will be compressed on its course out of the neural foramen at that level. The pattern of neurologic involvement may be more confusing when, in addition to a disc herniation, there is superimposed facet arthritis with lateral encroachment of the foramina. For example, with the most typical pattern of spinal stenosis at the L4-5 level, there may be compression of the L4 nerve root far laterally in the foramen between the arthritic facet joint, the bulging annulus, and the minor subluxation of the bodies of L4 and L5 that are frequently seen. Somewhat more medially, the L5 nerve root may also be compromised at this level by the arthritic and subluxed facet joints in the area of the lateral recess. Accordingly, physical findings always require confirmation with imaging studies prior to surgical intervention.

Motor Findings

Clinical assessment of the motor strength in any group of muscles is best accomplished by testing the muscle group against resistance. The hips must be tested for flexion, extension, abduction, and adduction; the knee for flexion and extension; the ankle for dorsiflexion and plantarflexion, inversion, eversion; and the toes for dorsiflexion and plantarflexion.

Compression of the motor fibers of the nerve roots results in weakness or paralysis of the muscle group associated with loss of tone and mass. Usually, a group rather than a single muscle is involved. The patient may not be aware of any weakness until the loss is rather profound. With compression of the first sacral nerve root, little motor involvement is noted other than an occasional weakness in flexion of the foot and great toe. With compromise of the fifth lumbar nerve root weakness, primarily of the great toe and other toe extensors and less often of the evertors and dorsiflexors of the foot, is noted. Atrophy of the anterior and lateral compartments of the leg may also be seen. With compression of the fourth lumbar nerve root, the quadriceps muscles are frequently affected, and the patient may notice weakness of extension and, more often, instability of the knee. If such symptoms are present, atrophy is usually prominent. Involvement of the third lumbar root is less common; it affects the abductors, internal rotators, and flexors of the hip joint as well as the extensors of the knee joint.

Sudden, partial, or complete paresis of all the roots of the cauda equina, associated with loss of function of the sphincter muscles, is indicative of severe compression of the cauda equina and may be produced by a massive extrusion of disc material from any of the lumbar discs. The clinical picture produced by a massive extrusion is similar to that caused by an intraspinal tumor located at the same interspace. Bilateral motor and sensory deficits are more commonly the result of intraspinal tumors, and such deficits have an insidious onset in contrast to the sudden onset so characteristic of massive nuclear extrusions.

One must also consider that motor weakness may be a manifestation of a metabolic peripheral neuropathy such as with diabetes. The differentiation can be made clinically, since the paresis associated with compromise of the fifth spinal nerve will frequently spare the tibialis anterior muscle, while it will usually be involved in diabetic peripheral neuropathy of the peroneal nerve. Furthermore, the Trendelenburg sign due to gluteus medius denervation resulting from fifth lumbar radiculopathy is not present in diabetic peroneal neuropathy. Electromyography (EMG) is also helpful in differentiating a diabetic peripheral neuropathy from the L5 nerve root syndrome. Usually, a more diffuse pattern of involvement may be evident on EMG than can be detected clinically, suggesting a metabolic etiology.

Sensory Changes

Abnormal objective sensory manifestations may or may not be associated with involvement of a nerve root in lumbar disc lesions. However, when present, because of overlap in the dermatomes of spinal nerves, it may be difficult to identify the specific root involved. The sensory pattern in the foot and leg is more specific than in the thigh and buttock.

Testing is most easily performed by having the patient compare sensation of the sharp and blunt ends of a pin in adjacent cutaneous areas. With compression of the fourth lumbar nerve root, sensory abnormalities may be noted in the anteromedial aspect of the leg. With compromise of the L5 root, sensory changes may be experienced in the anterolateral portion of the leg and along the medial aspect of the foot to the great toe.

Radiculopathy of the S1 nerve root usually involves sensory abnormalities in the posterior aspect of the calf and lateral aspect of the foot. In general, sensory changes are only of clinical significance if they correlate with the patient's pattern of referred pain and motor deficits.

Reflex Changes

The deep tendon reflexes are frequently altered in nerve root compression syndromes. The Achilles reflex is diminished or absent with compression of the first sacral nerve root, although disc herniation is more frequent among those with an absent Achilles reflex than in those in whom this reflex is simply diminished.[15] Compression of the fifth lumbar nerve root most commonly causes no reflex changes, but on occasion, an asymmetric diminished posterior tibial reflex can be observed. Involvement of the fourth lumbar nerve root from an L3–4 disc herniation classically results in a decreased or absent patellar tendon reflex; however, it is possible for an L4-5 disc herniation to result in this reflex abnormality. It is important to note that the absence of any reflex must be asymmetric to have any clinical significance.

When eliciting a reflex, it is suggested that several tendon taps be performed in order to assess the amplitude of the response. Frequently, a reflex response may fatigue when the involved reflex arc is compromised from disc herniation. Finally, many abnormalities other than disc herniation can produce deep tendon reflex changes. Accordingly, the absence of the Achilles reflex is more often a concomitant of advanced age than of radiculopathy.

Nerve Root Irritation Signs

There are several maneuvers that tighten the sciatic nerve, and in doing so, further compress an inflamed lumbar nerve root against a herniated disc or bony spur.[35] With the straight leg raising maneuver, the L5 and S1 nerve roots move 2 to 6 mm at the level of the foramina. When the straight leg raising test is performed in a patient with ventral compromise of the canal or a foramen, the involved nerve root is subject to both tensile and secondary compressive forces to which it cannot accommodate without producing radicular symptoms.[2] The L4 nerve root moves a shorter distance, and the more proximal lumbar roots show little motion with straight leg raising. Thus the straight leg raising test is of most value in lesions involving the fifth lumbar and first sacral nerve roots.

The conventional straight leg raising test is performed with the patient supine and the head flat or on a thin pillow. The examiner's hand is placed on the ilium to stabilize the pelvis, and the other hand slowly elevates the leg by the heel with the knee kept straight. The patient should be questioned as to whether this produces leg pain, particularly pain below the knee. This test is considered positive only when leg pain or radicular symptoms are produced; back pain alone does not constitute a positive finding. The majority of tension in the lower lumbar roots is generated with the leg at 35 to 70° of elevation, and any radicular pain produced at or above 70° is due to sciatic nerve deformation distal to the roots and should not be attributed to nerve root irritation (Fig. 9–10).[9]

The reliability of the straight leg raising sign is somewhat dependent on patient age. In a review of 2000 patients with surgically confirmed disc herniations, younger patients showed a marked propensity for a positive straight leg raising test.[38] Although a positive test alone is not pathognomonic, a negative test in a younger patient most probably excludes the possibility of a herniated disc. After the age of 30, however, the negative straight leg raising sign no longer reliably excludes this diagnosis (Fig. 9–11).

Several variations of the straight leg raising test have been described. The knee may first be flexed to 90° and the hip then flexed to 90°. Next, the knee is gradually extended. If this maneuver produces leg pain, the test is considered positive. Lasegue is credited with this test, which bears his name, and the straight leg raising test. There is another variation in which the foot is dorsiflexed. This not only may produce exacerbation of the pain generated in the straight leg raising test, but it also may reproduce radicular pain when the conventional straight leg raising test is negative.

MacNab feels the most reliable test of nerve root tension is the bowstring sign.[24] The straight leg raising test is performed until pain is elicited; then the knee is flexed, which will usually reduce symptoms.

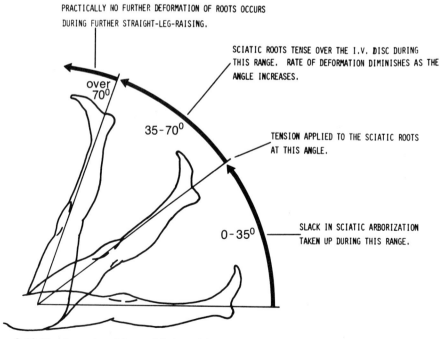

PRACTICALLY NO FURTHER DEFORMATION OF ROOTS OCCURS DURING FURTHER STRAIGHT-LEG-RAISING.

SCIATIC ROOTS TENSE OVER THE I.V. DISC DURING THIS RANGE. RATE OF DEFORMATION DIMINISHES AS THE ANGLE INCREASES.

over 70°

35-70°

TENSION APPLIED TO THE SCIATIC ROOTS AT THIS ANGLE.

0-35°

SLACK IN SCIATIC ARBORIZATION TAKEN UP DURING THIS RANGE.

Figure 9–10. The dynamics of the straight leg raising test. (Modified from Fahrni WH: Observations on straight leg raising, with special reference to nerve root adhesions. Originally published in *Canadian Journal of Surgery,* Vol. 9, January 1966.)

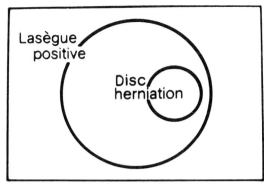

Age: under 30 years

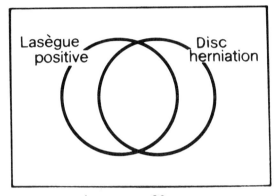

Age: over 30 years

Figure 9–11. These Venn diagrams illustrate the marked propensity for a positive Lasègue test with disc herniation in the young. Over the age of 30, the propensity decreases, although the specificity increases for this test in disc herniation. (From Spangfort E: Lasègue's sign in patients with lumbar disc herniation. Acta Orthop Scand 42:A59, 1971. ©1971 Munksgaard International Publishers Ltd, Copenhagen, Denmark.)

When finger pressure is applied to the popliteal space over the terminal aspect of the sciatic nerve the painful radicular symptoms reappear.

The sitting root test is yet another variation on this theme. With the patient sitting and the cervical spine flexed, the knee is extended while the hip remains flexed to 90°. The patient may complain of leg pain or may attempt to extend the hip, again indicating nerve root tension. This test is often useful to distinguish malingerers who may have been through enough examinations to fake a positive conventional straight leg raising sign.

The contralateral straight leg raising test is performed in the same manner as the conventional straight leg raising test, except that the nonpainful leg is raised. If this produces sciatica in the opposite extremity, the test is considered positive. This sign is very suggestive of a herniated disc and also is an indication of the location of the extrusion.[18] The prolapse is often large and is usually medial to the nerve root in the axilla (Fig. 9–12).

The reverse straight leg raising test (femoral nerve stretch test) is performed when the roots of the femoral nerve are involved. These higher lumbar nerve roots are tensed by the opposite of the conventional straight leg raising maneuver, that is, by hip extension and knee flexion.[6] This is

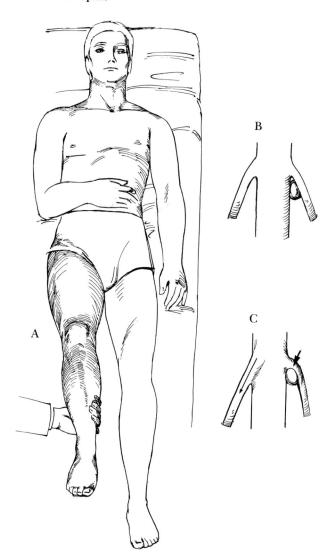

Figure 9–12. Movement of nerve roots when the leg on the opposite side is raised. *A,* When the leg is raised on the unaffected side the roots on the opposite side slide slightly downward and toward the midline. *B* and *C,* In the presence of a disc lesion, this movement increases the root tension. (From DePalma AF, Rothman RH: The Intervertebral Disc. Philadelphia, W.B. Saunders, 1970.)

usually performed while the patient is prone or positioned laterally with the unaffected side down. As with the straight leg raising test, there is a contralateral femoral traction sign.

Peripheral Vascular Examination

No examination of a patient with back or leg pain can be considered complete without evaluation of the peripheral circulation. There should be an assessment of pulses in the dorsalis pedis and posterior tibial arteries, as well as a determination of skin temperature and an inspection for the presence of atrophic changes seen with vascular insufficiency.

It is essential to differentiate vascular claudication from intermittent neurogenic claudication, both of which occur in the aging population. In the unusual case in which the patient's history and physical findings are consistent with both types of claudication, quantitative studies of the aortofemoral arterial system may be indicated. Both processes can be present simultaneously.[5]

Hip Joint Evaluation

It is also important to differentiate intra-articular hip disease from symptomatic spinal degenerative disease. Limitation of motion of the hip, along with groin discomfort, is most indicative of hip disease. The hips are best examined with the patient supine by flexing the hip and knee to 90° and checking the range of internal and external rotation of the hip. This maneuver should not elicit any signs indicative of nerve root tension. Reproduction of the patient's symptom complex in the thigh and leg with rotation of the hip suggests hip pathology rather than nerve root compression as the causative factor. On occasion, degenerative hip disease can be found concurrently in patients with low back pain.[25]

The piriformis muscle, an external rotator of the hip, has been implicated as a cause of sciatic-like symptoms.[21,30] This muscle runs in proximity to the sciatic nerve, and any injury to the muscle could precipitate local pain over the sciatic notch as well as irritation along the course of the nerve. Tenderness over the piriformis muscle on rectal or vaginal examination, along with local and referred pain with weakness when the hip is abducted and externally rotated against resistance is most suggestive of this syndrome.

Abdominal and Rectal Examination

Many intra-abdominal and retroperitoneal abnormalities can result in low back and leg pain. Careful palpation of the abdomen together with rectal and pelvic examinations will disclose many of these lesions. In older men, prostate tumor should also be ruled out. Also, costovertebral angle tenderness should be assessed to help exclude pyelonephritis. In general, most of these other entities will lack the typical mechanical features of low back pain caused by degenerative spinal disease.

Salient Objective Findings

The physical examination of the low back pain patient must first establish that the problem emanates from the low back and not from intra-abdominal, pelvic, or hip structures. Next, the presence or absence of objective findings such as sensory, motor, or reflex changes as well as nerve root tension signs is assessed. Then after a careful history and physical examination, the physician should be relatively certain of the etiology of the patient's complaints. The next step is to confirm the working diagnosis by using the appropriate combination of confirmatory diagnostic studies.

References

1. Abdullah AF, Ditto EW, Byrd EB, et al: Extreme lateral disc herniations. J Neurosurg 41:229–234, 1974.
2. Breig A, Marions O: Biomechanics of the lumbosacral nerve roots. Acta Radiol 1:1141–1160, 1963.
3. Brown MD, Tsaltas TT: Studies on the permeability of the intervertebral disc during skeletal maturation. Spine 4:240–244, 1976.
4. Deyo RA, Tsui-Wu YJ: Descriptive epidemiology of low-back pain and its related medical care in the United States. Spine 12:264–268, 1987.
5. Dodge LD, Bohlman HH, Rhodes RS: Concurrent lumbar spinal stenosis and peripheral vascular disease. Clin Orthop 230:141–148, 1988.
6. Dyck P: The femoral nerve traction test with lumbar disc protrusions. Surg Neurol 6:163–166, 1976.
7. Dyck P, Doyle JB: "Bicycle test" of van Gelderan in diagnosis of intermittent cauda equina compression syndrome. J Neurosurg 46:667–670, 1977.
8. Evans JG: Neurogenic intermittent claudication. Br Med J 5415:985–987, 1964.
9. Fahrni WH: Observations on straight leg raising with special reference to nerve root adhesions. Can J Surg 9:44–48, 1970.
10. Fast A, Shapiro D, Ducommun EJ, et al: Low-back pain in pregnancy. Spine 12:368–371, 1987.
11. Fidler MW, Jowett RL, Trouup JDG: Myosin ATPase activity in multifidus muscle from cases of lumbar spinal derangement. J Bone Joint Surg 57B:220–227, 1975.
12. Friis ML, Gulliksen GC, Rasmussen P, et al: Pain and spinal root compression. Acta Neurochir 39:241–249, 1977.
13. Frymoyer JW: Back pain and sciatica. N Engl J Med 318:291–300, 1988.
14. Gunn CC, Chir B, Milbrand WE: Tenderness at motor points: A diagnostic and prognostic aid to low back injury. J Bone Joint Surg 58A:815–825, 1976.
15. Hakelius A, Hindmarsh J: The significance of neurological signs and myelography findings in the diagnosis of lumbar root compression. Acta Orthop Scand 43:234–238, 1972.
16. Heiovaara M: Body height, obesity, and risk of herniated lumbar intervertebral disc. Spine 12:469–472, 1987.
17. Hoyland JA, Freemont AJ, Hayson MIV: Intervertebral foramen venous obstruction. A cause of periradicular fibrosis? Spine 14:558–568, 1989.
18. Hudgins WR: The crossed straight leg raising test. N Engl J Med 297:1127, 1977.
19. Jones DL, Moore T: The types of neuropathic bladder dysfunction associated with prolapsed lumbar intervertebral discs. Br J Urol 45:39–43, 1973.
20. Kellgren JH: The anatomical source of back pain. Rheumatol Rehabil 16:3–12, 1977.
21. Kirkaldy-Willis WH, Hill RJ: A more precise diagnosis for low back pain. Spine 4:102–104, 1979.
22. Kornberg M: Extreme lateral lumbar disc herniations. Clinical syndrome and computed tomography recognition. Spine 586–589, 1987.
23. Kulak RF, Schultz AB, Belytschko TB: Biomechanical characteristics of vertebral motion segments and intervertebral discs. Orthop Clin North Am 6:121–133, 1975.
24. MacNab I: Backache. Baltimore, Williams & Wilkins, 1983.
25. Magora A: Investigation of the relation between low back pain and occupation. VII. Neurologic and orthopaedic conditions. Scand J Rehab Med 7:146–151, 1975.
26. Murphy RW: Nerve roots and spinal nerves in degenerative disk disease. Clin Orthop 129:46–60, 1977.
27. Nachemson A: In vivo discometry in lumbar disc with irregular nucleograms. Acta Orthop Scand 36:418–434, 1965.
28. Nachemson A: Towards a better understanding of low-back pain: A review of the mechanics of the lumbar disc. Rheumatol Rehabil 14:129–143, 1975.
29. Olmarker K, Rydevik B, Holm S: Edema formation in spinal nerve roots induced by experimental, graded compression. Spine 14:569–573, 1989.
30. Pace JB, Neagle D: Piriformis syndrome. West J Med 124:435–439, 1976.
31. Peyser E, Harari A: Intradural rupture of lumbar intervertebral disk: report of two cases with review of the literature. Surg Neurol 8:95–98, 1977.
32. Pope MH, Bevins T, Wilder DG, et al: The relationship between anthropometric, postural, muscular, and mobility characteristics of males age 18–55. Spine 10:644–648, 1985.
33. Raaf J: Some observations regarding 905 patients operated upon for protruded lumbar intervertebral disc. Am J Surg 97:388–399, 1959.
34. Ross JC, Jameson RM: Vesical dysfunction due to prolapsed disc. Br Med J 3:752–754, 1971.
35. Scham S, Taylor T: Tension signs in lumbar disc prolapse. Clin Orthop 44:163–170, 1966.
36. Sharr MM, Garfield JS, Jenkins JD: The association of bladder dysfunction with degenerative lumbar spondylosis. Br J Urol 45:616–620, 1973.
37. Smyth MJ, Wright VJ: Sciatica and the intervertebral disc. An experimental study. J Bone Joint Surg 40A:1401–1418, 1958.
38. Spangfort E: Lasègue's sign in patients with lumbar disc herniation. Acta Orthop Scand 42:459–460, 1971.

39. Spangfort EV: The lumbar disc herniation. A computer-aided analysis of 2504 operations. Acta Orthop Scand (Suppl) 142:1–95, 1972.
40. Svensson HO, Andersson GB, Johansson S, et al: A retrospective study of low-back pain in 38- to 64-year-old women. Spine 13:548–552, 1988.
41. Verbiest H: Radicular syndrome from developmental narrowing of the lumbar vertebral canal. J Bone Joint Surg 36B:230–237, 1954.
42. Verbiest H: Pathomorphologic aspects of developmental lumbar stenosis. Orthop Clin North Am 6:177–196, 1975.
43. Weber H: Lumbar disc herniations. A prospective study of prognostic factors including a controlled trial. J Oslo City Hosp 28:36–61, 89–103, 1978.
44. Weinreb JC, Wolbarsht LB, Cohen JM, et al: Prevalence of lumbosacral intervertebral disc abnormalities on MR images in pregnant and asymptomatic nonpregnant women. Radiology 170:125–128, 1989.
45. Wilson CB, Ehni G, Grollimus J: Neurogenic intermittent claudication. Clin Neurosurg 18:62–85, 1971.
46. Wiltse LL, Kirkaldy-Willis WH, McIvor GW: The treatment of spinal stenosis. Clin Orthop 115:83–91, 1976.

CHAPTER 10

Confirmatory Diagnostic Studies in the Lumbar Spine

Diagnostic tests should be used to confirm the core of information gathered from a thorough history and physical examination. Several lumbosacral imaging modalities are currently available, including plain film radiography, venography, discography, myelography, computerized tomography (CT), and magnetic resonance imaging (MRI). While each of these tests has a place in the temporal sequence of the evaluation of back problems, none should be used for general screening, since most are overly sensitive and relatively unselective. Many of the iatrogenic catastrophes in the management of acute low back pain can be attributed directly to excessive reliance on diagnostic studies without positive clinical correlation.

To evaluate the true clinical value of any diagnostic study, one must know its sensitivity (false negatives) and specificity (false positives). The specificity, or false-positive rate, is usually measured in a population of symptomatic patients who have undergone surgery; however, often there is a much higher rate of false positives when an asymptomatic group is studied. The accuracy of any single test increases when it is combined with a second or third diagnostic study.[43] The physician's challenge is to select diagnostic tests on the basis of their performance characteristics so that the correct diagnosis is obtained with the least cost and morbidity. The studies most frequently utilized in the diagnostic assessment of low back pain will be described and critically analyzed with this in mind. Diagnostic modalities coming into vogue as well as those falling out of favor will also be briefly discussed.

PLAIN RADIOGRAPHS

The diagnosis of disc herniation can usually be made on the basis of history and physical examination. Plain radiographs of the lumbosacral spine will rarely add any information, but must be obtained in the appropriate setting to rule out other pathologic conditions such as infection or tumor. Plain radiographs are valuable for making the diagnosis of spinal stenosis, spondylolisthesis, gross segmental instability, or fracture.

The radiograph must be of excellent quality and taken with attention to detail. In general, three views are all that are required to assess the lumbosacral spine: an anteroposterior (AP) view, a lateral view, and a coned-down lateral view of the lower two interspaces. On occasion, two oblique views are also taken to identify subtle spondylolysis or pars interarticularis defects. However, oblique views provide limited information and should not be routinely included.

The AP view allows visualization of the vertebral bodies, spinous and transverse processes, pedicles, facet joints, and laminae (Fig. 10–1A). Malalignment of the spinous processes is a reflection of rotation or lateral movement of the spine. The pedicles are seen end-on in the AP projection, and the loss of the pedicle margin (winking-owl sign) may be seen in patients with metastatic disease. The primary soft tissue structure seen in the AP view is the psoas muscle. Asymmetric visualization or absence of the psoas shadow may indicate retroperitoneal pathology.

The lateral radiograph displays the lumbar lordosis (Fig. 10–1B). In this projection, the spinous processes and posterior margins of the vertebral bodies should form a smooth curve. Displacement of one vertebral body anterior or posterior to the rest may be an indication of spinal instability. Normally, the disc space height increases gradually from L1 to L5. In contrast, the L5-S1 disc space and intervertebral foramen are narrower than the other lumbar vertebrae.

The oblique views of the lumbar spine are obtained to demonstrate the facet joints and pars interarticularis (Fig. 10–1C). These views may demonstrate facet arthritis or spondylolysis and are not required as part of the routine radiographic series.

Although plain films are useful for surveying the bony elements of the spine and paraspinal soft tissues, the contents of the spinal canal, including cord, dura, ligaments, and encroaching disc, are not visualized. In addition, bony lesions may not be apparent until 50 percent of the cancellous bone has been destroyed.[2]

Degenerative changes, such as disc space narrowing, traction osteophytes, vacuum disc phenomenon,[17] and end-plate sclerosis, are quite prevalent in older individuals (Fig. 10–2). Unfortunately, these radiographic findings show a poor correlation with clinical symptoms. Bone spurs are not pathognomonic for disc degeneration and must be differentiated from other conditions such as Reiter's syndrome, ankylosing spon-

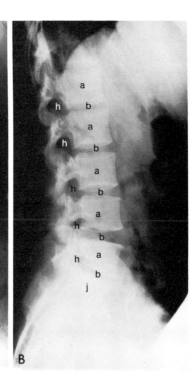

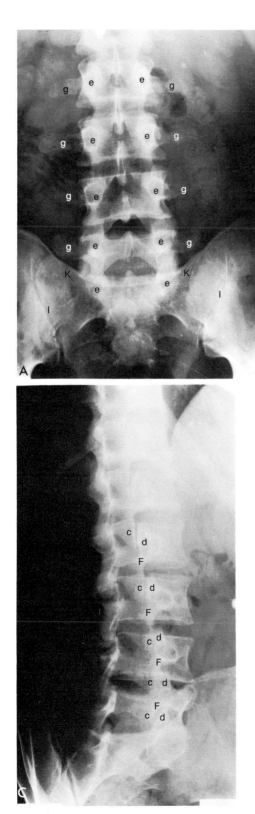

Figure 10–1. *A,* AP, *B,* lateral, and *C,* oblique views of a normal lumbar spine with anatomy labeled: (a) lumbar vertebra; (b) intervertebral disc; (c) inferior facet; (d) superior facet; (e) pedicle; (F) pars interarticularis; (g) transverse process; (h) neural foramina; (i) sacroiliac joint; (j) sacrum; and (K) sacral ala. (From Wiesel SW, Bernini PA, Rothman RH: The Aging Lumbar Spine. Philadelphia, W.B. Saunders, 1982.)

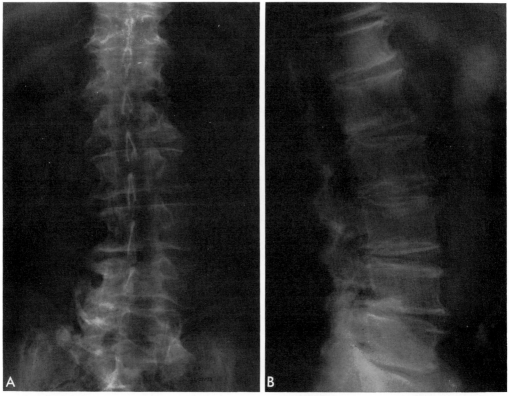

Figure 10–2. Radiographs of the lumbar spine illustrate advanced multilevel disc degeneration with loss of height of the disc space, marked osteophyte formation, and sclerosis of the end plates. Foraminal encroachment is present. (From Rothman RH, Simeone FA: The Spine, 2nd ed. Philadelphia, W.B. Saunders, 1982.)

dylitis, and diffuse idiopathic skeletal hyperostosis. Osteophytes are usually more prominent anterolaterally than posterolaterally, and their presentation is most likely a result of annular and ligamentous attachments to the vertebral bodies above and below a degenerative disc.[49] A traction spur, or horizontal osteophyte, is found 2 to 3 mm from the disc space and is thought to arise from stress at the sites of ligament insertion during the hypermobile phase of disc degeneration (Fig. 10–3).

In addition to posteriorly directed disc herniations, protrusion directly into the verterbral body (Schmorl's node) can also occur.[41] This type of herniation is most commonly seen in the central and posterocentral portion of the body and is surrounded by a rim of sclerotic bone. It is possible that herniation follows the residual embryonic channels through the cartilaginous vertebral end plate. A relative weakness at the interface between the cartilaginous end plate and the vertebral body may be a predisposing factor to this type of herniation. Other pathologic states such as trauma, infection, congenital defects, or metabolic disease that may weaken the vertebral end plate must also be considered as a cause of intervertebral herniation.

During the course of spinal degeneration and aging, derangement in the alignment of vertebrae as well as alterations in their normal motion may occur. Ultimately, degenerative spondylolisthesis may de-

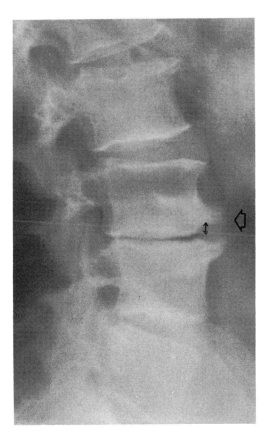

Figure 10–3. Radiograph illustrates traction osteophyte at the L3-4 level. Note that the osteophyte is horizontally oriented and 2 mm away from the disc space. Note also the marked narrowing of the disc space and the vacuum phenomena at L3-4. (From Rothman RH, Simeone FA: The Spine, 2nd ed. Philadelphia, W.B. Saunders, 1982.)

velop with anterior slippage of one vertebral body on another.[16,48] In determining radiographic instability, a host of techniques ranging from simple one-plane measurements to three-dimensional computerized stereoradiography have been attempted. Quantitation of instability is hampered by variations in measurement techniques, poor definition of the "normal" range of motion, and variable reproducibility of measurements.[36,40,47]

Instability at a spinal segment may be visualized on weight-bearing flexion-extension bending films (Fig. 10–4). Guidelines have been established from cadaveric experiments to quantify lumbar instability, but these remain to be correlated in vivo with clinical symptoms (Table 10–1).[39] The instability checklist uses, in part, measurements of the relative AP translation between two vertebrae measured on either a flexion or an extension radiograph. Alternatively, calculation of dynamic AP translation, defined as the change in relative vertebral positions from flexion to extension, may provide a more accurate assessment of vertebral motion than measurement of static displacement on the flexion or extension view alone (Figs. 10–5, 10–6). A recent study has shown that although 42 percent of normal subjects had at least one level with a static listhesis greater than 3 mm in either flexion or extension, only 5 percent of normals had a dynamic AP translation greater than 3 mm.[6] Further studies with this and other methods are required to assess correlation of radiographic instability with clinical symptoms.

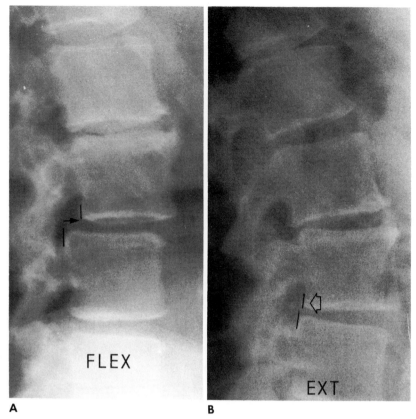

Figure 10–4. Radiographs illustrate segmental instability due to disc degeneration on flexion and extension views. *A,* Note that in flexion there is a 3.5 mm anterior migration of the cranial vertebra. *B,* In extension there is almost complete alignment of the vertebral body. This was productive of both back pain and sciatica. (From Rothman RH, Simeone FA: The Spine, 2nd ed. Philadelphia, W.B. Saunders, 1982.)

Table 10–1. CHECKLISTS FOR DIAGNOSIS OF CLINICAL INSTABILITY IN THE LUMBAR SPINE AND AT THE LUMBOSACRAL JUNCTION*

Lumbar Spine (L1–L5)		Lumbosacral Spine (L5–S1)	
Condition	*Points*	*Condition*	*Points†*
Damage to cauda equina	3	Damage to cauda equina	3
Relative flexion sagittal plane translation 8%, or extension sagittal plane translation 9%	2	Relative flexion sagittal plane translation 6%, or extension sagittal plane translation 9%	2
Relative sagittal plane rotation 9%	2	Relative sagittal plane rotation 1%	2
Destruction of anterior elements	2	Destruction of anterior elements	2
Destruction of posterior elements	2	Destruction of posterior elements	2
Dangerous loading expected	1	Dangerous loading expected	1

*(From Posner I, White AA, Edwards WT, et al: A biomechanical analysis of the clinical stability of the lumbar and lumbosacral spine. Spine 7:374–389, 1982.)
†Damage to the cauda equina equals 3 points, of which 2 points denote destruction of all anterior or posterior elements, and 1 point for anticipation of dangerous loads. A total of 5 or more points indicates clinical instability.

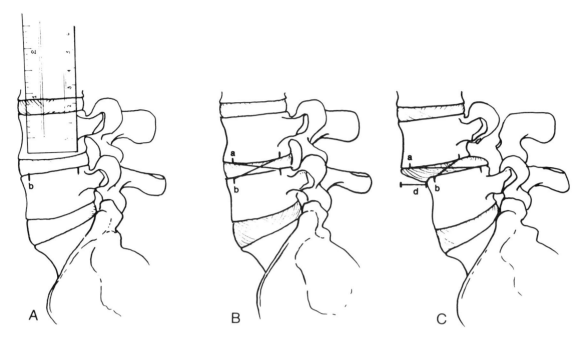

Figure 10–5. Calculation of relative slip (d) of superior on inferior vertebral body. *A,* A ruler slightly narrower than the vertebral body is vertically positioned parallel to and centered between the anterior and posterior vertebral cortices. The intersection of the sides of the ruler with the end plate is marked. *B,* Diagonal lines a and b are drawn to connect the end-plate marks and their dimensions are measured. *C,* Static slip (d) is calculated as $1/2(a - b)$. Dynamic translation is the relative difference between the static slip calculated in flexion and in extension. (From Boden SD, Wiesel SW: Lumbosacral segmental motion in normal individuals. Spine 15:571–576, 1990.)

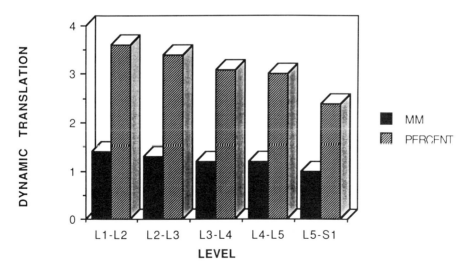

Figure 10–6. Dynamic A-P translation expressed as absolute millimeters (MM) and as a percentage of the width of the superior vertebral body (PERCENT). Dynamic translation is defined as the difference between the relative slip in flexion and the slip in extension between two vertebrae. (From Boden SD, Wiesel SW: Lumbosacral segmental motion in normal individuals. Spine 15:571–576, 1990.)

EPIDURAL VENOGRAPHY

Lumbar epidural venography initially was popular because of its high sensitivity at the L5-S1 interspace, its ease of performance, and its low complication rate, compared to the oil-based myelography done at that time. The abnormal filling of epidural veins in close proximity to the neural elements is presumed to reflect encroachment of a nerve. In a study of 30 surgically confirmed cases, the sensitivity and specificity of epidural venography were found to be 83 percent and 88 percent, respectively.[22] The accuracy of metrizamide myelography has since been shown to exceed that of epidural venography in the diagnosis of lumbar disc herniation and spinal stenosis. Epidural venography, like myelography, can identify a mechanical obstruction but often offers few clues to the etiology of the abnormality. Venography may still be useful as a secondary contrast technique in patients with a congenitally short or tapered dural sac, a situation in which the L5-S1 interspace is difficult to evaluate with myelography. However, with the current availability of noninvasive tests with greater sensitivity, this procedure has become all but obsolete.

DISCOGRAPHY

Since lumbar discography was introduced in 1948, its predictive value in the diagnosis of low back pain and sciatica has been disputed. The test is performed by a percutaneous posterolateral injection of dye into the disc space and is believed not to injure normal discs.[25] It was originally hoped that the demonstration of posterior extravasation of dye from the disc would indicate disc rupture (Fig. 10–7). However, it is now known that small asymptomatic tears in the annulus fibrosus are often associated with disc aging and may permit dye extravasation in the absence of disc rupture.[50,56]

In 1968, Holt concluded that discography was a nonspecific and unreliable test when he found that 37 percent of asymptomatic young men had positive discograms.[21] This conclusion continues to be challenged.[45] Since that study, correlation of radiographic dye extravasation with reproduction of the patient's pain during disc injection has added an important diagnostic dimension to the discogram. In a prospective investigation, it has been shown that addition of the pain reproduction criteria decreases the false-positive rate to nearly zero.[52] Another recent study examined CT scanning after lumbar discography in patients with negative EMG, plain CT, and/or myelography. Positive correlation between the CT discogram image and symptoms produced during the discogram injection occurred in 90 percent.[21] Currently, discography is best reserved as a secondary diagnostic adjunct to be used when less invasive tests are negative or equivocal in the presence of persistent pain.

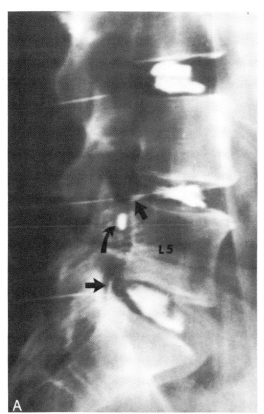

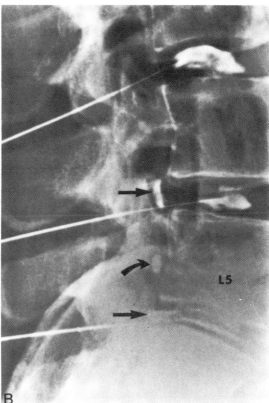

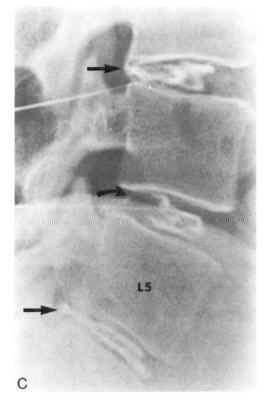

Figure 10–7. Abnormal discograms. *A,* Posterior extravasation at L4-5 and L5-S1 (*straight arrows*). Normal discogram at L3-4. Small amount of residual iophendylate (Pantopaque) is present behind the body of L5 (*curved arrow*). The extravasated contrast agent at L4-5 is less dense than this residual oil drop. *B,* Posterior extravasation at L4-5 and L5-S1 (*straight arrows*). Normal discogram at L3-4. Minimal residual Pantopaque (*curved arrow*). *C,* Posterior extravasation at L5-S1 and minimal posterior extravasation at L3-4 (*straight arrows*). Moderate degenerative changes at L4-5 without extravasation (*curved arrow*). (From Kricun ME: Imaging Modalities in Spinal Disorders. Philadelphia, W.B. Saunders, 1988.)

MYELOGRAPHY

Myelography has long been the "gold standard" for evaluating neural compression. Dye is injected into the dural sac and mixes with the spinal fluid. The outline of the contents of the spinal canal can be visualized on x-ray films; any extradural mass such as a herniated disc will show up as a filling defect in the dye column, while an intrathecal mass will appear as an outward protrusion. Myelography is unable to differentiate disc protrusion from bony, malignant, infectious, or other extradural encroachment on the spinal canal. The diagnostic accuracy of myelography is also questionable in cases of far lateral disease and at the L5-S1 level where the epidural space may be large.

As an invasive procedure that usually requires overnight hospitalization, myelography should not be taken lightly. Complications include severe headache, nausea, vomiting, and, rarely, seizures.[3] Prior to the utilization of the water-soluble dye metrizamide, the oil-based agent Pantopaque had a much higher incidence of complications and was known to cause a crippling arachnoiditis. Newer contrast agents are now available that are reported to have fewer side effects.[26,29,46]

Various patterns of myelographic abnormalities may be observed. The defects that are most often noted with posterolateral disc herniations are incomplete filling or elevation of the spinal nerve root sleeve, lateral indentation of the dural sac, and a double density of the sac noted on the lateral projection (Fig. 10–8). A large lateral herniation can also produce a complete myelographic block at the level of the disc space. Elevation of the nerve sleeve may be the only abnormality noted, but it is the least reliable of the findings. With water-soluble dye, subtle changes in the contour or location of nerve roots are more meaningful, particularly if there is asymmetric proximal swelling of the nerve within the central dye column. Indentation of the dural sac seen in the AP or oblique projections and the double density seen on the lateral view (Fig. 10–9) are more convincing findings.

Large central disc herniations may produce a complete myelographic block (Fig. 10–9) at the level of the involved disc space. In the AP projection, the block will show an irregular saw-tooth or paintbrush appearance. The lateral view will reveal compression and elevation of the anterior portion of the dural sac due to ventral pressure from the herniated disc. A stenotic effect may be observed with smaller central discs, which force the nerve sleeve origins laterally, preventing dye from filling the central area. More commonly, such defects are associated with spinal stenosis, with or without disc herniations.

Free or sequestered disc fragments may migrate in a caudal or cranial direction and may result in symptomatic involvement of an additional nerve root. Free fragments are seen as well-circumscribed filling defects of varying diameters above or below the disc space (Fig. 10–10).

Chronic disc degeneration will frequently be associated with spinal stenosis and will produce myelographic defects caused by diffuse

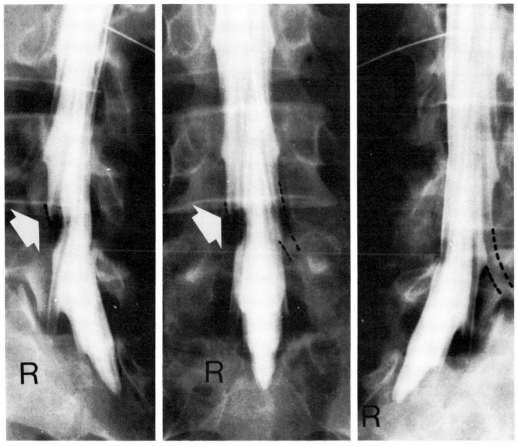

Figure 10–8. Metrizamide myelogram illustrating a herniated disc at L4-5 on the right (*arrows*). Note amputation of the nerve root sleeve and indentation of the dural sac. (From Rothman RH, Simeone FA: The Spine, 2nd ed. Philadelphia, W.B. Saunders, 1982.)

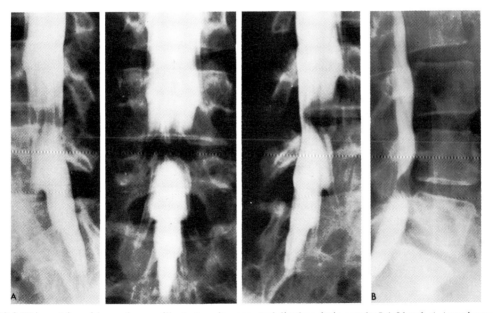

Figure 10-9. This metrizamide myelogram illustrates a large central disc herniation at the L4-5 level. *A*, Anterior-posterior and oblique views reveal this prominent defect more marked on the right. *B*, This lateral view illustrates a "double-density" prominent ventral indentation of the dye column. (From Rothman RH, Simeone FA: The Spine, 2nd ed. Philadelphia, W.B. Saunders, 1982.)

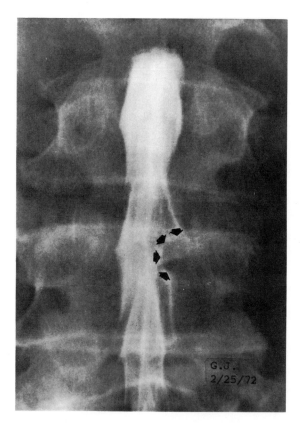

Figure 10–10. Free fragments of disc material produce a myelographic defect characterized by smooth, well-circumscribed indentations in the dye column (*arrows*). They may be at the level of the disc space or migrate at a distance, and may be difficult to differentiate from neurofibromata. Oil was the contrast medium in this illustration. (From Rothman RH, Simeone FA: The Spine, 2nd ed. Philadelphia, W.B. Saunders, 1982.)

posterior bulging of the annulus, hypertrophy and redundancy of capsular and ligamentous tissue, and hypertrophic osteophyte formation. In the AP projection, a symmetric "hourglass" waisting of the dye column will be noted, resulting from obliteration of the lateral recess (Fig. 10–11). In the lateral projection, indentation of the dye column will be seen at the level of the disc space. If no osteophytes are present, the indentation will be 2 to 3 mm in depth; if osteophytes have formed, they are easily seen and coincide with the dye column defects.

In patients whose symptoms are dynamically exaggerated in flexion or extension, myelography in both positions may reveal pathology that is worsened by postural changes. This is most common in degenerative spondylolisthesis and spinal stenosis (Fig. 10–12).

Several artifacts may create myelographic defects and mimic disc herniations. The spinal needle used to introduce the dye can produce a defect that varies greatly in size. Similarly, an epidural hematoma from a spinal needle advanced too far anteriorly can mimic an epidural mass. For this reason, the lumbar puncture is generally performed at the L2-3 interspace. Artifacts may also be seen in individuals who have had previous oil contrast media myelography, particularly in the presence of previous surgery. A variety of epidural and arachnoid scarring patterns may be seen in these instances (Fig. 10–13).[38]

Hitselberger found that despite its historical role as the standard, myelography was abnormal in 24 percent of asymptomatic people.[23]

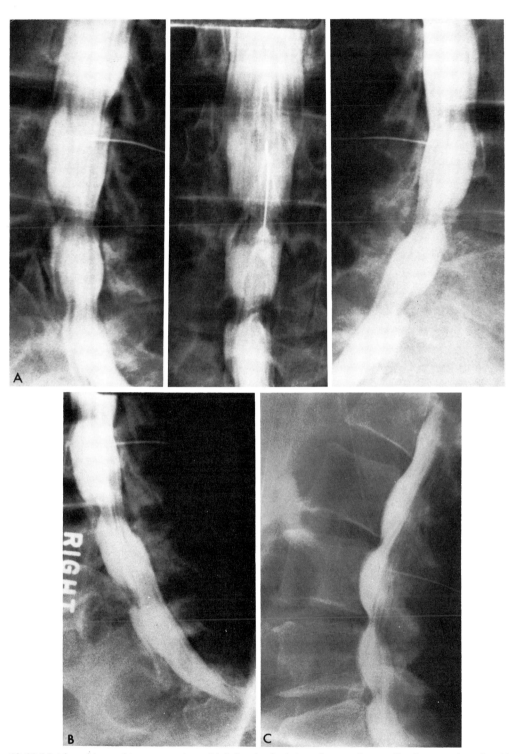

Figure 10–11. Metrizamide myelogram reveals multiple-level spinal stenosis secondary to disc degeneration. *A* and *B,* The AP and oblique views reveal the multiple wasting defects typical of spinal stenosis. *C,* Lateral view illustrates multiple ventral defects due to diffuse bulging at the annulus. (From Rothman RH, Simeone FA: The Spine, 2nd ed. Philadelphia, W.B. Saunders, 1982.)

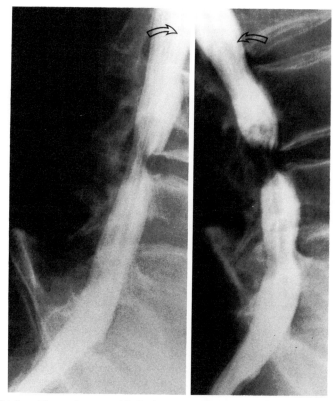

Figure 10–12. Metrizamide myelogram with flexion-extension lateral views reveals a partial block in flexion and a complete block in extension (*arrows*). Patient became markedly paretic in extension. This illustrates classic spinal stenosis secondary to disc degeneration. (From Rothman RH, Simeone FA: The Spine, 2nd ed. Philadelphia, W.B. Saunders, 1982.)

For this reason, if the myelogram is used as a "screening test" in the absence of objective clinical findings, exploratory surgery and disaster can result. When indicated, one particular advantage of the myelogram over conventional CT is that it can evaluate the lower thoracic spine without additional radiation. Acute radiculopathies can be caused by intradural extramedullary tumors in the lower thoracic area. However, now multiplanar CT and MR can also image this area and can generate three-dimensional images quite similar in appearance to a myelogram.

The trained spine surgeon has until recently reserved the myelogram for preoperative assurance—to confirm the location of the damaged disc or to check for a congenitally anomalous nerve root, tumor, or double disc. Although most studies report the accuracy of CT and myelography to be comparable, a carefully controlled and blinded investigation determined that myelography was more accurate than CT (83% vs. 72%) in the diagnosis of herniated lumbar discs.[5] Furthermore, Zsernaviczky and Juppe found myelography to have a lower false-positive rate and a higher false-negative rate than CT.[57] However, its expense (with hospitalization), inability to diagnose foraminal pathology, and complication rate have rendered myelography a distant second choice in centers where CT and MR are readily available. Myelography can still play a role

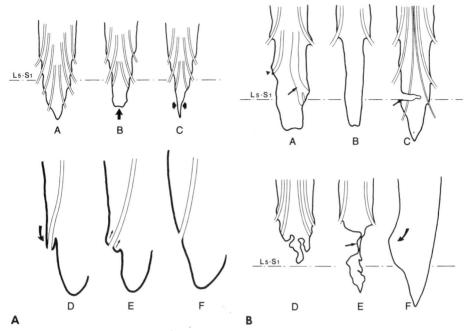

Figure 10–13. *A,* Arachnoid scarring. Stage 1. (A) Diagram of normal appearances. (B) Short and blunted theca. (C) Narrowed, filiform cul-de-sac—lesions of the nerve roots. (D) Vertical position of the nerve roots and approximation to the theca. (E) Retraction of the subarachnoid extensions above and below the nerve root, giving a "stump" appearance. (F) Total effacement of the root sheath. *B,* Arachnoid scarring. Stage 2. (A) Shortening of the thecal lesions above L5–S1. "Enlarged roots" (*arrow*). Stumplike root sheath (*arrowhead*). (B) Tubular appearance. The root sheaths are completely obliterated. Epidural lesions. (C) Characteristic "pinched" appearance. Mixed arachnoid and epidural lesions. (D) Ragged lower end to an amputated theca. (E) Persistent stenosis—postoperative meningocele. (From Picard L, Roland J, Blanchot P, et al: Scarring of the theca and the nerve roots as seen in radiculography. J Neuroradiol 4:29, 1977.)

in confirming the diagnosis of arachnoiditis when the diagnosis is otherwise uncertain and in imaging the postoperative spine when metal hardware would distort or prevent imaging by CT or MR.

COMPUTED TOMOGRAPHY

Computed tomography (CT) is currently the most versatile and widely available noninvasive modality for evaluating abnormalities of the lumbosacral spine. Multiple cross-sectional (axial) images of the spine are made at various levels and with reformatting, coronal, sagittal, and three-dimensional images may be created. The CT scan demonstrates not only the bony spinal configuration but also the soft tissue in graded shading, so that ligaments, nerve roots, free fat, and intervertebral disc protrusions can be evaluated as they relate to their bony environment.

A CT section of the lumbar spine will contain different anatomic structures depending on the precise level of the cross section (Fig. 10–14). The lumbar nerve roots are best visualized on an axial section through the inferior third of the vertebral body (Fig. 10–15). The strength

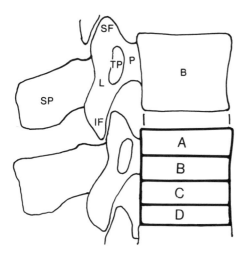

Figure 10–14. The four basic CT sections of the lumbar spine. The structures imaged by the scan include the spinous process (SP), inferior articular facet (IF), laminae (L), transverse process (TP), superior articular facet (SF), pedicle (P), and body (B). (From Borenstein DG, Wiesel SW: Low Back Pain: Medical Diagnosis and Comprehensive Management. Philadelphia, W.B. Saunders, 1989.)

of CT as a lumbosacral imaging technique is not its resolution of structures, but rather its demonstration of spatial relationships of anatomic structures on axial images.

The full spectrum of the age-related changes in the lumbar spine can be readily visualized with the CT scan. In younger patients, simple posterolateral (Fig. 10–16) or central (Fig. 10–17) herniated discs are seen as a focal soft-tissue density protruding from the disc space posteriorly. In the older population, spinal stenosis may be seen (Fig. 10–18) with associated hypertrophy of the facet joints, resulting in lateral recess stenosis (Fig. 10–19) or neural foraminal stenosis (Fig. 10–20). In addition, redundant or hypertrophic ligamentum flavum and annular bulging may be seen. CT is also useful for localizing and defining the extent of neoplastic or infectious processes in the spine.

Several prospective comparisons of CT with myelography have demonstrated that CT is at least as sensitive (97% vs. 93%) and specific (80% vs. 76%) in the diagnosis of herniated lumbar discs.[21] The sensitivity of CT appears to be enhanced by the addition of intradural metrizamide contrast, which has been shown to demonstrate additional pathology in up to 30 percent of cases.[1,10,14,51] The routine axial CT scan is often unable to demonstrate foraminal disc herniation, facet hypertrophy, or end-plate osteophytes. Camp reports these abnormalities in 15 percent of operative patients, and if unrecognized, they may be responsible for failed back surgery.[11] The use of multiplanar reformatting, and in some complex cases three-dimensional reconstruction, can minimize the frequency of such diagnostic errors. The primary weakness of CT scanning remains its inability to reliably demonstrate intrathecal pathology (e.g., tumors).

The CT scan is an extremely valuable diagnostic tool when it is used appropriately to confirm the patient's clinical findings. However, recent studies reveal the pitfalls of making clinical decisions on the basis of isolated CT scan findings. Despite many reports in the literature indicating that CT scanning has a mean accuracy of 90 percent in symptomatic patients,[15,51] 34 percent of asymptomatic people had abnormal CT scans

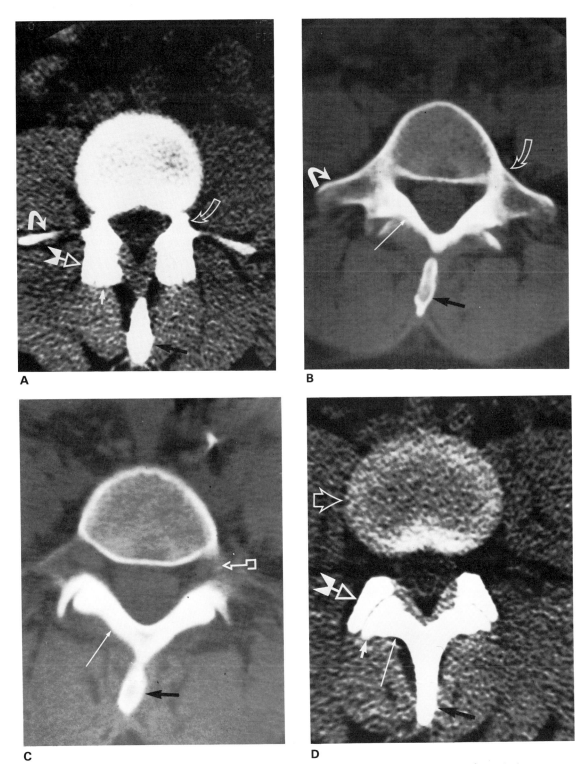

Figure 10–15. *A,* CT scan showing the superior third of the vertebral body, the pedicles (*open curved arrow*), the transverse processes (*curved arrow*), the superior facets (*arrow with tail*), the spinous process (*black arrow*), and the inferior facet of the next higher vertebra (*short arrow*). *B,* The middle third of the vertebral body, the pedicles (*open curved arrow*), the laminae (*long arrow*), and the spinous process (*black arrow*) are shown. *C,* The lower third of the vertebral body, the neural foramina and nerve roots (*arrow with square*), the laminae (*long arrow*), and the spinous process (*black arrow*) are shown. *D,* This section of the scan contains the intervertebral disc (*open arrow*) and the facet joints. The imaged osseous structures include the superior facet of the vertebra below the disc (*arrow with tail*) and the inferior facet (*short arrow*), the laminae (*long arrow*), and the spinous process (*black arrow*) of the vertebra above the disc. (From Borenstein DG, Wiesel SW: Low Back Pain: Medical Diagnosis and Comprehensive Management. Philadelphia, W.B. Saunders, 1989.)

143

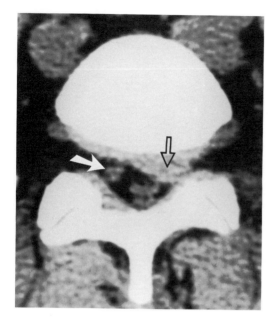

Figure 10–16. Posterolateral disc herniation. A posterolateral disc herniation at L5-S1 on the left (*open arrow*) is encroaching on epidural fat and compressing the S1 nerve root. Notice the uninvolved S1 nerve root on the right (*white arrow*), which is surrounded by epidural fat. (From Kricun ME: Imaging Modalities in Spinal Disorders. Philadelphia, W. B. Saunders, 1988.)

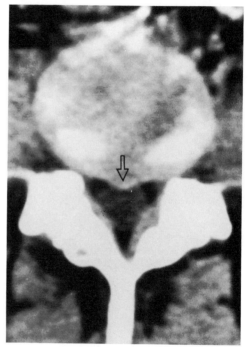

Figure 10–17. Central disc herniation. On this axial CT scan at L4-5, there is a small, central, focal protrusion of the disc (*arrow*). (From Kricun ME: Imaging Modalities in Spinal Disorders. Philadelphia, W. B. Saunders, 1988.)

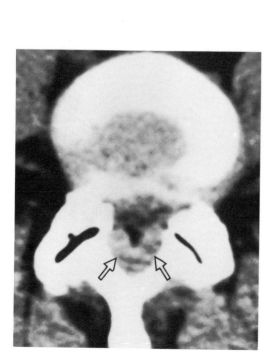

Figure 10–18. Spinal stenosis. The size of the thecal sac is diminished owing to thickening of the ligamenta flava (*arrows*). Gas within the facet joints (vacuum facet) is evident. (From Kricun ME: Imaging Modalities in Spinal Disorders. Philadelphia, W. B. Saunders, 1988.)

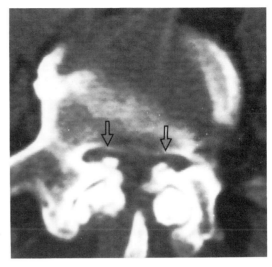

Figure 10-19. Lateral recess stenosis. Axial CT scan demonstrates narrowing of the lateral recesses (*arrows*) that is caused by osteophytes of the articular processes. In addition, there is central spinal stenosis. (From Kricun ME: Imaging Modalities in Spinal Disorders. Philadelphia, W. B. Saunders, 1988.)

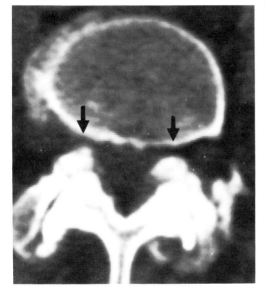

Figure 10-20. Neural foraminal stenosis. Axial CT scan at L4 demonstrates narrowing of the neural foramina (*arrows*) that is caused by osteophyte formation of the superior articular processes at this level. Mild central stenosis can also be observed. (From Kricun ME: Imaging Modalities in Spinal Disorders. Philadelphia, W. B. Saunders, 1988.)

when reviewed by three independent expert interpreters.[55] The implication is that a patient with a negative history and physical examination for a spinal lesion has a 1-in-3 chance of having an abnormal CT scan. If the decision for surgery is based only on scan results, there is a 30 percent chance that the patient will undergo an unnecessary and unsuccessful operation. However, if the patient's clinical picture correlates with the CT scan abnormalities, CT can be a useful confirmatory diagnostic tool.

MAGNETIC RESONANCE IMAGING

Magnetic resonance imaging (MRI) is the newest diagnostic imaging modality for the spine. The image of different tissues is obtained by the detection of extremely small differences in proton density in a magnetic field bombarded with short pulses of radio waves causing atoms to vibrate at an angle out of the field. Variations in proton density, radio frequency, and relaxation time to the nonexcited state will modify the MR image to highlight different tissues. Unlike CT and myelography, this approach does not require ionizing radiation or contrast agents. Multiplanar images are directly available.

The normal MR image of the lumbosacral spine shows the vertebral column, intervertebral discs, and spinal canal with the spinal cord in the sagittal view (Fig. 10–21). On T2-weighted images (long relaxation and echo times), the intervertebral disc normally has high signal (white) but loses it with dehydration and early disc degeneration. The axial view shows the paravertebral soft tissue, the disc or vertebral body, the spinal cord, and the nerve roots at the appropriate level (Fig. 10–21B).

The excellent resolution of MRI facilitates description of disc pathology as (1) herniation, (2) contained by the posterior longitudinal ligament, (3) noncontained, or (4) a diffuse bulge. Correlation of neural element encroachment evaluated on the axial views is essential to assess the position and severity of protrusions commonly seen on the sagittal views (Fig. 10–22). MRI is useful for assessing canal encroachment in spinal stenosis and is the imaging modality of choice for evaluating intraspinal tumors.

Numerous investigations are underway to determine the sensitivity and specificity of MRI in the diagnosis of lumbar spine disorders. Early studies that used scanners with poor resolution due to smaller magnets and body coils that did not allow thin imaging slices often concluded

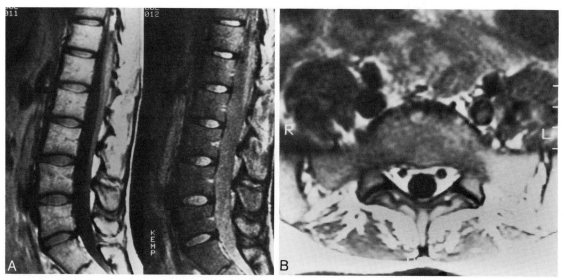

Figure 10–21. *A,* Normal MRI scan of the lumbar spine, sagittal view. The T1-weighted image (*left*) demonstrates bone marrow and fat as whiter structures with vertebral end plates (cortical bone) and ligaments as blacker images. The intervertebral discs are of intermediate density. The T2-weighted image (*right*) demonstrates CSF and nucleus pulposus as whiter structures, with the annulus fibrosus and posterior longitudinal ligament seen as blacker images. *B,* Normal MRI scan of the lumbosacral junction, axial view. T1-weighted image demonstrates surrounding soft tissue structures, with the cauda equina and S1 nerve roots surrounded by epidural fat (*white*).

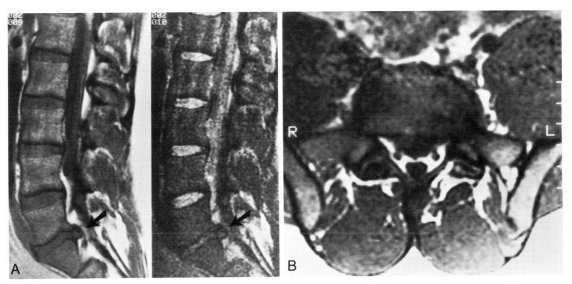

Figure 10–22. *A,* MRI scan of a herniated disc, sagittal view. T1-weighted image (*left*) demonstrates a herniated disc (*arrow*) at the L5-S1 level. The T2-weighted image (*right*) shows loss of the normal white signal within the nucleus pulposus (*arrow*), a sign of degenerative disc disease. (From Boden SD, Davis DO, Dina TS, et al: Abnormal lumbar spine MRI scans in asymptomatic subjects: A prospective investigation. J Bone Joint Surg 72A: 403–408, 1990.) *B,* MRI scan of a herniated disc, axial view. T1-weighted image at the L5-S1 disc space demonstrates a large central herniated disc with lateral displacement of both S1 nerve roots and posterior displacement of the cauda equina.

that CT was the superior technique.[30] With the advent of surface coils, stronger magnets, and newer pulse sequences, MR scans now have much improved resolution. The most recent data suggest that MRI is more accurate in the detection of degenerative disc disease than discography or myelography.[18,53] Compared to CT, MRI is at least as accurate for diagnosing spinal stenosis, sequestered lumbar intervertebral discs, and far lateral disc herniation.[33,35,42] MRI, especially with gadolinium-DTPA contrast enhancement, has clear advantages for demonstrating intraspinal tumors and for distinguishing recurrent disc herniation from postoperative scar.[8,34] In a prospective investigation of operative low back pain patients, the greatest correlation of imaging studies (myelography, CT, MRI) with surgical findings was 93 percent, achieved by the combination of CT and MRI.[33]

As with the other diagnostic imaging modalities discussed, MRI also has been shown to have a significant clinical false-positive rate in asymptomatic individuals. In one prospective and blinded study, 22 percent of the asymptomatic subjects under age 60 and 57 percent of those over age 60 had significantly abnormal scans.[5] In addition, the prevalence of disc degeneration on the T2-weighted MR images was found to approach 98 percent in subjects over age 60 (Fig. 10–23).

Additional carefully controlled, blinded studies with surgical confirmation will yield much needed information.[13] There is no doubt that the role of MRI in the lumbar spine diagnostic arsenal will continue to evolve as the technology improves and the cost decreases.

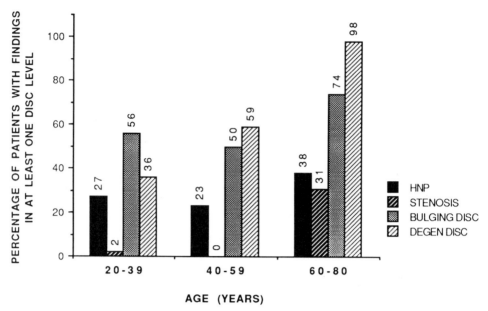

Figure 10–23. MRI scan findings in asymptomatic subjects. Graph demonstrates the prevalence of at least one lumbar level with the indicated abnormality assessed from a population of subjects with no history of back pain, sciatica, or neurogenic claudication. (From Boden SD, Davis DO, Dina TS, et al: Abnormal lumbar spine MRI scans in asymptomatic subjects: A prospective investigation. J Bone Joint Surg 72A:403–408, 1990.)

ELECTRODIAGNOSTIC TESTING

The electromyogram (EMG) is performed by placing needles into muscles to determine if there is an intact nerve supply to that muscle. An abnormal EMG can demonstrate impaired nerve transmission to a specific muscle and isolate the nerve root involved. Initially, the EMG will be negative in spite of nerve entrapment and will only show muscle irritability. After 3 weeks of significant pressure on a nerve root, signs of denervation with fibrillation can be observed.

The EMG, like all of the other confirmatory tests already discussed, is not a screening tool. In fact, when dealing with the average low back problem, the EMG rarely provides any information that cannot be derived from a careful physical examination. It may even confuse the picture, since an EMG may be abnormal from diabetic neuropathy, previous peripheral nerve involvement, or trauma. In cases in which the correlation of clinical signs and imaging is equivocal—especially with chronic unexplained sciatica—nerve conduction studies and electromyography may be helpful.[20] EMG can also detect the involvement of a secondary nerve root in cases of complex back injury preoperatively, sometimes prompting a more extensive operation.

A new noninvasive approach to the diagnosis of herniated lumbar discs, dermatomal somatosensory evoked potentials (DSSEPs), is currently under investigation. This technique stimulates the L5 or S1 dermatome in both legs and simultaneously compares the DSSEPs from both hemispheres of the brain (using scalp electrodes) to detect even slight asymmetry. In assessing 40 patients with lumbosacral disc disease, DSSEPs had 97 percent sensitivity and 100 percent specificity.[27] This technique is experimental and awaits further clinical testing with expansion of the normal data base to include measurement of additional lumbar levels.

THERMOGRAPHY

Thermography records changes in skin temperature. Areas that are "hotter" than normal are believed to represent increased skin blood flow due to irritation of the autonomic component of spinal nerves.[37] Although thermography is estimated to have a sensitivity of 100 percent, the prospective studies performed to date have demonstrated a specificity as low as 60 percent.[12,24] Due to the high rate of false-positive results, the diagnostic value of a positive thermogram in evaluation of back and leg pain is controversial.[9,19,28,32] Thermography may provide a cost-effective method of ruling out anatomic pathology in the compensation patient with no objective findings,[54] and it may also be valuable for diagnosis of entities such as reflex sympathetic dystrophy and facet syndrome.[44] Prospective investigations of thermography are underway to further evaluate its sensitivity, specificity, and correlation with recognized techniques. Unfortunately, this less-than-perfect test—with its colorful and vivid displays—may find its way into the medicolegal armamentarium. However, until the value and role of thermography are clarified, its usefulness remains in question.

References

1. Anand AK, Lee BC: Plain and metrizamide CT of lumbar disk disease: Comparison with myelography. Am J Neuroradiol 3:567–571, 1982.
2. Ardan GM: Bone destruction not demonstrable by radiography. Br J Radiol 24:107–109, 1951.
3. Baker RA, Hillman BJ, McLennan JE, et al: Sequelae of metrizamide myelography in 200 examinations. Am J Roentgenol 130:499–502, 1978.
4. Bell GR, Rothman RH, Booth RE, et al: A study of computer-assisted tomography. II. Comparison of metrizamide myelography and computed tomography in the diagnosis of herniated lumbar disc and spinal stenosis. Spine 9:552–556, 1984.
5. Boden SD, Davis DO, Dina TS, et al: Abnormal lumbar spine MRI scans in asymptomatic subjects: A prospective investigation. J Bone Joint Surg 72A: 403–408, 1990.
6. Boden SD, Wiesel SW: Lumbosacral segmental motion in normals. Spine 15:571–576, 1990.
7. Bogduk N, Cherry D: Epidural corticosteroid agents for sciatica. Med J Aust 143:402–406, 1985.
8. Breger RK, Williams AL, Daniels DL, et al: Contrast enhancement in spinal MR imaging. Am J Neuroradiol 10:633–637, 1989.
9. Brown RK, Bassett LW, Wexler CE, et al: Thermography as a screening modality for nerve fiber irritation in patients with low back pain. Proceedings of the Second Annual Meeting of the Academy of Neuromuscular Thermography, May 1986. Mod Med (Suppl), September 1987, pp. 86–88.
10. Byrd SE, Cohn ML, Biggers SL, et al: The radiographic evaluation of the symptomatic postoperative lumbar spine patient. Spine 10:652–661, 1985.

11. Camp PE: Invasive procedures for treating herniated discs: Clinical and cost considerations. Occup Med: State Art Rev 3(1):75–90, 1988.
12. Chafetz N, Wexler CE, Kaiser JA: Neuro-muscular thermography of the lumbar spine with CT correlation. Spine 13:922–925, 1988.
13. Cooper LS, Chalmers TC, McCally M, et al: The poor quality of early evaluations of magnetic resonance imaging. JAMA 259:3277–3280, 1988.
14. Dublin AB, McGahan JP, Reid MH: The value of computed tomographic metrizamide myelography in the neuroradiological evaluation of the spine. Radiology 146:79–86, 1983.
15. Firooznia H, Benjamin V, Kricheff II, et al: CT of lumbar spine disk herniation: Correlation with surgical findings. Am J Neuroradiol 5:91–96, 1984.
16. Fitzgerald JAW, Newman PH: Degenerative spondylolisthesis. J Bone Joint Surg 58B:184–192, 1976.
17. Ford LT, Gilula LA, Murphy WA, et al: Analysis of gas in vacuum lumbar disc. Am J Roentgenol 128:1056–1057, 1977.
18. Gibson MJ, Buckley J, Mawhinney R, et al: Magnetic resonance imaging and discography in the diagnosis of disc degeneration. J Bone Joint Surg 68B:369–373, 1986.
19. Green J, Coyle M, Becker C, et al: Abnormal thermographic findings in asymptomatic volunteers. Thermology 2:13–15, 1986.
20. Haldeman S, Shouka M, Robboy S: Computed tomography, electrodiagnostic and clinical findings in chronic workers' compensation patients with back and leg pain. Spine 13:345–350, 1988.
21. Haughton VM, Eldevik OP, Magnaes B, et al: A prospective comparison of computed tomography and myelography in the diagnosis of herniated lumbar disks. Radiology 142:103–110, 1982.
22. Herkowitz HN, Wiesel SW, Booth RE, et al: Metrizamide myelography and epidural venography: Their role in the diagnosis of lumbar disc herniation and spinal stenosis. Spine 7:55–63, 1982.
23. Hitselberger WE, Witten RM: Abnormal myelograms in asymptomatic patients. J Neurosurg 28:204–206, 1968.
24. Hubbard J, Maultsby J, Wexler CE: Lumbar and cervical thermography for nerve fiber impingement: A critical review. Clin J Pain 2:131–137, 1986.
25. Johnson RG: Does discography injure normal discs? An analysis of repeat discograms. Spine 14:424–426, 1989.
26. Laasonen EM: Iohexol and metrizamide in lumbar myelography. Comparison of side effects. Acta Radiol 26:761–765, 1985.
27. Machida M, Asai T, Sato K, et al: New approach for diagnosis in herniated lumbosacral disc: Dermatomal somatosensory evoked potentials (DSSEPs). Spine 11:180–184, 1986.
28. Mahoney L, McCulloch JA, Csima A: Thermography in back pain. I. Thermography as a diagnostic aid in sciatica. Thermology 1:43–50, 1985.
29. Maly P, Bach-Gansmo T, Elmqvist D: Risk of seizures after myelography: Comparison of iohexol and metrizamide. Am J Neuroradiol 9:879–883, 1988.
30. Maravilla KR, Lesh P, Weinreb JC, et al: Magnetic resonance imaging of the lumbar spine with CT correlation. Am J Neuroradiol 6:237–245, 1985.
31. McCutcheon ME, Thompson WC: CT scanning of lumbar discography: A useful diagnostic adjunct. Spine 11:257–259, 1986.
32. Mills GH, Davies GK, Getty CJ, et al: The evaluation of liquid crystal thermography in the investigation of nerve root compression due to lumbosacral lateral spinal stenosis. Spine 11:427–432, 1986.
33. Modic MT, Masaryk T, Boumphrey F, et al: Lumbar herniated disk disease and canal stenosis: Prospective evaluation by surface coil MR, CT, and myelography. Am J Neuroradiol 7:709–717, 1986.
34. Nguyen CM, Ho KC, Yu S, et al: An experimental model to study contrast enhancement in MR imaging of the intervertebral disc. Am J Neuroradiol 10:811–814, 1989.
35. Osborn AG, Hood RS, Sherry RG, et al: CT/MR spectrum of far lateral and anterior lumbosacral disk herniations. Am J Neuroradiol 9:775–778, 1988.
36. Penning L, Wilmink JT, van Woerden HH: Inability to prove instability: A critical appraisal of clinical-radiological flexion-extension studies in lumbar disc degeneration. Diagn Imag Clin Med 53:186–192, 1984.
37. Perelman RB, Adler D, Humphrey M: A comparison of lumbosacral thermograms with CT scans. Presented at the 13th Annual Meeting of the American Academy of Thermology, June 1984.
38. Picard L, Roland J, Blanchot P, et al: Scarring of the theca and the nerve roots as seen at radiculography. J Neuroradiol 4:29–48, 1977.
39. Adapted from Posner I, et al: Spinal Stability Criteria, Lumbar Spine. Presented before the Eastern Orthopaedic Association, 1980.
40. Quinnell RC, Stockdale HR: Flexion and extension radiography of the lumbar spine: A comparison with lumbar discography. Clin Radiol 34:405–411, 1983.
41. Resnick D, Niwayama G: Intervertebral disk herniations: cartilaginous (Schmorl's) nodes. Radiology 126:57–65, 1978.
42. Schnebel B, Kingston S, Watkins R, et al: Comparison of MRI to contrast CT in the diagnosis of spinal stenosis. Spine 14:332–337, 1989.

43. Schoedinger GR: Correlation of standard diagnostic studies with surgically proven lumbar disk rupture. South Med J 80:44–46, 1987.
44. Sherman RA, Barja RH, Bruno GM: Thermographic correlates of chronic pain: Analysis of 125 patients incorporating evaluations by a blind panel. Arch Phys Med Rehabil 68:273–279, 1987.
45. Simmons JW, Aprill CN, Dwyer AP, et al: A reassessment of Holt's data on "The question of lumbar discography." Clin Orthop 237:120–124, 1988.
46. Skalpe IO, Nakstad P: Myelography with iohexol (Omnipaque): A clinical report with special reference to the adverse effects. Neuroradiology 30:169–174, 1988.
47. Stokes IAF, Frymoyer JW: Segmental motion and instability. Spine 12:688–691, 1987.
48. Taillard W: Etiology of spondylolisthesis. Clin Orthop 117:30–39, 1976.
49. Torgenson WR, Dotter WE: Comparative roentgenographic study of the asymptomatic and symptomatic lumbar spine. J Bone Joint Surg 58A:850–853, 1976.
50. Vanharanta H, Sachs BL, Ohnmeiss DD, et al: Pain provocation and disc deterioration by age. A CT/discography study in a low-back pain population. Spine 14:420–423, 1989.
51. Voelker JL, Mealey J, Eskridge JM, et al: Metrizamide-enhanced computed tomography as an adjunct to metrizamide myelography in the evaluation of lumbar disc herniation and spondylosis. Neurosurgery 20:379–384, 1987.
52. Walsh TR, Weinstein JN, Spratt KF, et al: Lumbar discography: A controlled, prospective study of normal volunteers to determine the false-positive rate. Presented at the annual meeting of the International Society for Study of the Lumbar Spine, May 19, 1989, Kyoto, Japan.
53. Weisz GM, Lamond TS, Kitchener PN: Spinal imaging: Will MRI replace myelography? Spine 13:65–68, 1988.
54. Wexler CE, Chafetz N: Cervical, thoracic, and lumbar thermography in the evaluation of symptomatic workers' compensation patients. Proceedings of the Second Annual Meeting of the Academy of Neuro-Muscular Thermography, May 1986; Mod Med (Suppl), September 1987, pp. 53–57.
55. Wiesel SW, Bell GR, Feffer HL, et al: A study of computer-assisted tomography: I. The incidence of positive CAT scans in an asymptomatic group of patients. Spine 9:549–551, 1984.
56. Yu S, Sether LA, Ho PS, et al: Tears of the annulus fibrosus: Correlation between MR and pathologic findings in cadavers. Am J Neuroradiol 9:367–370, 1988.
57. Zsernaviczky J, Juppe M: A comparison of myelography and computer tomography in lumbar disc herniation. Int Orthop 13:51–55, 1989.

CHAPTER 11

Standardized Approach to the Diagnosis and Treatment of Low Back and Leg Pain

Low back pain patients present with a set of symptoms; they do not come labeled with a specific diagnosis. The task confronting the examining physician is to integrate the patient's symptoms, physical signs, and diagnostic test results into a logical diagnosis and then to develop an efficient treatment plan. Often this can be quite confusing because the symptom complex and diagnostic information are not straightforward. In addition, findings that are part of normal age-related spinal degeneration must be distinguished from more significant pathology. Therefore, the purpose of this chapter is to present a standardized approach to the diagnosis and treatment of problems that may occur in the aging lumbar spine. This discussion will provide insight into the thought processes helpful in assessing low back problems.

Each low back pain patient will have an associated set of circumstances unique to his or her case. There are, however, a number of common objectives a physician should keep in mind when managing this population. These goals will be reviewed first, and then the diagnostic and treatment protocol will be discussed.

TREATMENT GOALS

The first and most important objective is the prompt return of normal function. Unfortunately, total relief of pain is not always achieved, especially in older patients. Those patients with residual pain must be encouraged to resume as much activity as possible. Patient education is germane to this goal. Many people refrain from work, recreation, or household chores simply because increased activity produces mild discomfort. In their minds, any pain is a signal that they are causing damage to their backs. These patients need to be reassured that the diagnosis of lumbar disc disease does not herald the onset of a progressive crippling disorder and that disc degeneration is a normal consequence of aging. In many cases this information will keep patients functioning and prevent psychological impairment as well.

The second goal is the efficient and precise use of diagnostic studies. With the availability of computed tomography, magnetic resonance imaging, psychological profiles, and specialty consultants—each with his own battery of tests—the physician must resist the impulse to utilize every test available and to meet the often insistent demands of the patient for "the latest study." There is a proper time and indication for each of these diagnostic measures. Decision-making actually can be more difficult and less beneficial when too much information is made available too early in the treatment process.

The third goal is to avoid unnecessary surgery. Surgical intervention that is premature and thus, by definition, not appropriate for attaining the desired goal, has been a terrible burden to the spine surgeon, the luckless patient, and society. The sorrowful saga of the thousands of patients who have undergone multiple spine operations with poor results bears witness to the disastrous overuse of spine surgery in the past. As evidence, one need only look at the review published by Aitken and Bradford in 1947.[1] They investigated 170 surgical cases from the files of a large national compensation carrier and found that only 17 percent of the patients had good results; 45 percent were judged to have poor or bad results. Discs were removed at levels that did not correlate with the neurologic examination or myelographic findings, and complications such as postoperative foot drop or paralysis of the quadriceps muscles occurred in 5 percent of the group.

Fortunately, with adherence to strict criteria, the results of spine surgery have become much better. In a recent review of 800 patients selected for lumbar spine surgery using the algorithmic indications for surgery, 90 to 95 percent had good results.[4] It cannot be overemphasized that objective criteria for surgery must be present. However, if appropriate conservative management has failed and the patient demonstrates pathology that lends itself to surgical intervention, the operation should not be delayed too long. Surgery to relieve a ruptured disc becomes less effective when delayed more than 3 months and has little benefit over nonoperative management after a year or two. There is an optimal time for surgical intervention, and this must be clearly defined and understood.[11,12] The appropriate timing of surgery for spinal stenosis is less clear.

The final objective should be to devise a treatment format that will make therapy available at an acceptable cost to society. With the enormous economic impact of low back pain, it is vital that the individual, and society, can afford the diagnostic tests and treatment. In this day of the $900 body scan and the $8000 surgical procedure, one must be careful to avoid unnecessary and cost-ineffective measures.

DIAGNOSTIC AND TREATMENT PROTOCOL

The physician's task is to integrate the patient's complaints into an accurate diagnosis and to prescribe appropriate therapy. Achieving this goal in a cost-effective fashion depends on the accuracy of the physician's assessment. To standardize and organize the decision-making process, a systematized approach to patients presenting with low back pain has been developed in the form of an algorithm.

The aim of the algorithm is to select the correct diagnostic category and proper treatment avenues for each patient with low back pain. A specific patient may fall outside the limits of the algorithm and require a different approach, and the physician must constantly be on the alert for these exceptions. The algorithm can be followed in sequence in Fig. 11–1 and is also presented in tabular form in Table 11–1.

The information necessary to use the algorithm is initially obtained through the history and physical examination, described in detail in Chapter 9. The key points in the history are differentiation of back pain that is mechanical in nature from nonmechanical pain that is present at rest, detecting changes in bowel or bladder function, and defining the precise location and quality of the pain. The physical examination must be oriented toward ruling out other medical causes of low back pain, assessing neurologic function, and evaluating for the presence of nerve root tension signs.

Following the low back pain algorithm, the first major decision is to make a ruling on the presence or absence of cauda equina syndrome. Mechanical compression of the cauda equina, with truly progressive motor weakness, is the only surgical emergency in lumbar spine disease.[3] This usually is due to pressure on the caudal sac, which contains the nerves to the lower extremities, bowel, and bladder. The signs and symptoms are a complex mixture of low back pain, bilateral motor weakness of the lower extremities, bilateral sciatica, saddle anesthesia, and even frank paraplegia with bowel and bladder incontinence. Cauda equina syndrome can be caused by either bone or soft tissue pressure, the latter generally from a ruptured or herniated disc in the midline. These patients should undergo an immediate definitive diagnostic test, and if it is positive,

LOW BACK PAIN ALGORITHM

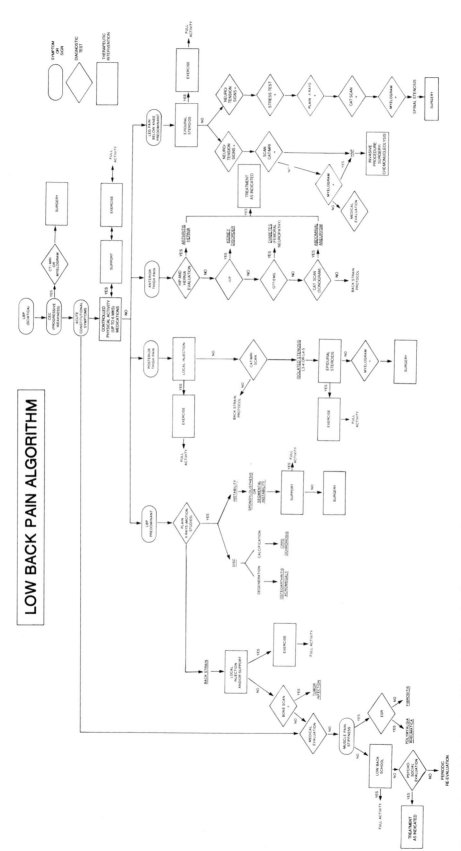

Figure 11–1. Algorithm for the differential diagnosis of low back pain.

Table 11–1. DIFFERENTIAL DIAGNOSIS OF LOW BACK PAIN*

Evaluation	Back Strain	Herniated Nucleus Pulposus	Spinal Stenosis	Spondylolisthesis/ Instability	Spondyloarthropathy	Infection	Tumor	Metabolic	Hematologic	Visceral
Predominant pain (back vs. leg)	Back	Leg (below knee)	Back/leg	Back	Back	Back	Back	Back	Back	Back (buttock, thigh)
Constitutional symptoms					+	+	+	+	+	
Tension sign		+	+/–							
Neurologic exam		+/–	+/– after stress							
Plain x-rays			+	+	+	+/–	+/–	+	+	
Lateral motion x-rays				+						
CT/MRI		+	+			+	+			+
Myelogram		+	+							
Bone scan					+	+	+	+	+	
ESR†					+	+	+		+	+
Serum chemistries							+	+	+	+

*From Borenstein DG, Wiesel SW: Low Back Pain: Medical Diagnosis and Comprehensive Management. Philadelphia, W.B. Saunders, 1989.
†Erythrocyte sedimentation rate.

emergency surgical decompression. Historically, the myelogram was the study used in this setting; however, the development of MRI has facilitated the noninvasive diagnosis of cauda equina syndrome. The principal reason for prompt surgical intervention is to arrest the progression of neurologic loss; the chance of actual return of lost neurologic function following surgery is small. Although the incidence of cauda equina syndrome in the entire back pain population is very low, it is the only entity that requires immediate operative intervention; if its diagnosis is missed, the consequences can be devastating.

The remaining patients, who comprise the overwhelming majority, should be started on a course of conservative (nonoperative) therapy regardless of the diagnosis. At this stage the specific diagnosis, whether that of a herniated disc or simple back strain, is not important to the therapy because the entire population is treated the same way. A few of these patients will eventually need an invasive procedure, but at this point there is no way to predict which individuals will respond to conservative therapy and which will not.

The vast majority in this initial group have nonradiating low back pain, termed lumbago or back strain. The etiology of lumbago is not clear. There are several possibilities, including ligamentous or muscular strain, continuous mechanical stress from poor posture, facet joint irritation, or a small tear in the annulus fibrosus. Patients usually complain of pain in the low back, often localized to a single area. On physical examination they demonstrate a decreased range and smoothness of lumbar spine motion, tenderness to palpation over the involved area, and paraspinal muscle spasm. Their roentgenographic examinations usually are normal, but if therapy is not rapidly successful, films should be obtained to rule out other possible etiologic factors such as infection, inflammatory arthritis, or tumor. Two exceptions to this rule are patients younger than 20 years of age and patients over age 50: roentgenograms are important early in the diagnostic process because these patients are more likely to have a diagnosis other than back strain (i.e., tumor or infection). Other situations warranting radiography sooner rather than later include a history of serious trauma, known cancer, unexplained weight loss, or fever.

The early stage of the treatment of low back pain, with or without leg pain, requires patience. The passage of time, anti-inflammatory medication, and controlled physical activity are the modalities proven safest and most effective.[13] The vast majority of these patients will respond to this approach within the first 10 days. Radiculopathy in and of itself is not a contraindication to nonoperative management.[10] In today's society with its emphasis on quick solutions and "high technology," many patients are pushed too rapidly toward more complex (i.e., invasive) management. This "quick fix" approach has no place in the treatment of low back pain. In most cases, surgical treatment does not return people to heavy work. In the long run, the best chance of getting a patient back to full duty is the nonoperative approach. Furthermore, many older individuals have other medical problems and are greater anesthetic risks.

The physician should treat the patient conservatively and wait up to 6 weeks for a response. As already stated, most patients will improve within 10 days. For the remainder, the problem arises in distinguishing those who have a true back problem from malingerers. If objective findings to substantiate the subjective complaints are lacking, the patient should be strongly encouraged to return to some type of work or to daily activities as quickly as possible, no later than the 2-week mark. In spite of this, some patients will complain of continued pain and inability to perform work or daily activities. The primary treating physician is in a precarious situation: on the one hand, as the patient's representative he accepts what the patient tells him (analogous to a lawyer representing a client who may not be telling the complete truth); on the other hand, he has a responsibility to society to keep medical costs down, to return people to work as quickly as possible, and to avoid unnecessary treatments such as long periods of physical therapy.

The solution for the primary physician in a litigation or workers' compensation case with claims of continued symptoms in the absence of objective physical findings is to recommend an independent medical examiner (IME). This does not destroy the patient-physician relationship. If the IME concurs with the primary physician that no serious pathology exists, the primary physician—with reinforcement from the "expert" IME—can recommend that the patient return to work as soon as possible. It cannot be overemphasized that the sooner an IME is consulted the more effective this is; if there are no objective findings at 10 days but the patient continues to complain of pain, an IME should be obtained. If 2 or 3 months pass before this is done, the patient will have the pain pattern firmly fixed in his mind and it will be difficult to convince him that there is nothing seriously wrong.

Continuing with the overall treatment plan, once the patient has achieved approximately 80 percent relief he should be mobilized. Use of a lightweight, flexible corset may be helpful. After he is more comfortable and has increased his activity level, he should begin a program of isometric lumbar exercises and return to his normal lifestyle.[2,7] The pathway along this section of the algorithm is reversible: should regression occur with exacerbation of symptoms, the physician can resort to more stringent conservative measures. The patient may require further bedrest. Most acute low back pain patients will proceed along this pathway, returning to their normal life patterns within 2 months of onset of symptoms.

If the initial conservative treatment regimen fails and 6 weeks have passed, symptomatic patients are sorted into four groups. The first group comprises people with low back pain predominating. The second group complains mainly of leg pain, defined as pain radiating below the knee and commonly referred to as sciatica. The third group has posterior thigh pain, and the fourth group, anterior thigh pain. Each group follows a separate diagnostic pathway.

Low Back Pain

Those patients who continue to complain predominantly of low back pain for 6 weeks should have their plain films carefully examined for abnormalities. Spondylolysis with or without spondylolisthesis is the most common structural abnormality causing significant low back pain. Spondylolysis can be defined as a break in the continuity of the pars interarticularis in the lamina. Approximately 5 percent of the population has this defect, thought to be caused by a combination of genetics and environmental stress.[9] If the defect permits displacement of one vertebra on another, it is termed spondylolisthesis. Most people with this defect are able to perform their activities of daily living with little or no discomfort. When symptoms are present, these patients usually will respond to nonoperative measures, including a thorough explanation of the problem, a back support, and exercises. In a small percentage of cases, conservative treatment fails and a fusion of the involved spinal segments becomes necessary.[8] This is one of the few situations in which primary fusion of the lumbar spine is indicated, and it must be stressed that it is a relatively infrequent occurrence. Most patients with spondylolisthesis do not require surgery.

The vast majority of patients with pain predominantly in the low back will have normal plain films. The diagnosis at this point is back strain. Before there is any additional work-up, a local injection of steroids and lidocaine can be tried at the point of maximum tenderness. This can be quite successful, and if there is a good response the patient is begun on exercises with gradual resumption of normal activity. In some instances, if there are no objective findings, a trigger-point injection can be considered as early as the third week after onset of symptoms. Aternatively, if the physical examination is suggestive of facet joint pain, a selective facet block (lidocaine/steroid) injection may prove diagnostic and palliative.

Should the patient not respond to controlled physical activity, nonsteroidal anti-inflammatory agents, and a local injection, other pathology must be seriously considered. A bone scan, along with a general medical evaluation, should be obtained. The bone scan is an excellent screening tool, often identifying early bone tumors or infections not visible on routine radiographic examinations. It is particularly important to obtain this study in the patient with nonmechanical back pain. If the pain is constant, unremitting, and unrelieved by postural adjustments, more often than not the correct diagnosis will be one of an occult neoplasm or metabolic disorder not readily apparent from other testing.

Approximately 3 percent of cases of apparent low back pain that present at orthopedic clinics are attributable to extraspinal causes.[14] The major diagnostic categories are distinguished in Table 11-1. A thorough medical search also frequently reveals problems missed earlier, such as a posterior penetrating ulcer, pancreatitis, renal disease, or an abdominal aneurysm.

Those patients who have no abnormality on their bone scans and do not show other medical disease as a cause of their back pain may be suffering from discogenic or facet joint pain syndromes.[6,15] Persistent nonradiating low back pain that is mechanical in nature presents a difficult problem. Evaluation of these patients with a discogram, in an attempt to reproduce their pain, or with a gadolinium-enhanced MRI scan, is still under investigation. Even when the pain syndrome can be attributed to disc degeneration, spine fusion has not achieved consistent results. Now that surgical treatment of properly selected patients with herniated discs yields reliable results, the remaining challenge is the identification and treatment of patients with refractory discogenic pain.

Patients with persistent low back pain and no evidence of extraspinal disease are referred for another type of therapy—the low back school.[16] The low back school concept has as its basis the belief that patients with low back pain, given proper education and understanding of their disease, often can return to a productive and functional life. Ergonomics, the proper and efficient use of the spine in work and recreation, is stressed. Back school need not be an expensive proposition. It can be a one-time classroom session with a review of back problems and a demonstration of exercises with patient participation. This type of educational process has proved very effective. It is most important, however, that patients be thoroughly screened before being referred to this type of program. One does not want to be in the position of treating a metastatic tumor in a classroom.

If low back school is not successful, the patient should undergo a thorough psychosocial evaluation in an attempt to explain the failure of the previous treatments. This is predicated on the knowledge that a patient's disability is related not only to pathologic anatomy but also to pain perception and psychosocial stability. It is quite common to see a stable patient with a frank herniated disc continue working—regarding his disability as only a minor problem—while a hysterical patient takes to his bed at the slightest twinge of low back discomfort.

Psychologically distressed patients often complain of symptoms that are vague, poorly localized, and lack a normal relationship to time, physical activity, and anatomy. The seven symptoms that have the highest degree of association with this category of patients are tailbone pain, whole leg pain, whole leg numbness, whole leg giving way, no pain-free intervals, intolerance of or inappropriate reaction to treatment, and a past history of emergency hospital admission for low back pain.

Drug habituation, depression, alcoholism, and other psychiatric problems are seen frequently in association with back pain. If the evaluation suggests any of these problems, proper measures should be instituted to overcome the disability. A surprising number of ambulatory patients addicted to commonly prescribed medications use complaints of back pain as an excuse to obtain these drugs. Percodan and diazepam, alone or in combination, are the two most popular offenders. Percodan is truly addictive; diazepam is both habituating and depressing. Since the complaint of low back pain may be a common manifestation of depression, it is counterproductive to treat such patients with diazepam.

Approximately 2 percent of patients who initially present with low back pain will fail treatment and elude any diagnosis.[14] There will be no evidence of any structural problem in the back, underlying medical disease, or psychiatric disorder. This is a very difficult group to manage. The author's strategy has been to discontinue narcotics, reassure the patient, and periodically reevaluate him. Over time, one third of these patients will be found to have an underlying medical disease; thus, one cannot abandon this group and discontinue treatment. For the rest, as much physical activity as possible should be encouraged.

Sciatica

The next group of patients consists of those with sciatica, which is pain radiating below the knee. These people usually experience symptoms secondary to mechanical pressure and inflammation of the lower lumbar nerve roots. The mechanical pressure can be of soft tissue (herniated disc) or bony origin or a combination of the two.

At this point in the algorithm, the patient has already had up to 6 weeks of controlled physical activity and medication but still has persistent leg pain. The next therapeutic step is an epidural steroid injection given on an outpatient basis. An epidural injection is worth trying; the chance of success is about 40 percent and morbidity is low, particularly compared with the next treatment step—surgery. The maximum benefit from a single injection is achieved at 2 weeks. The injection may have to be repeated once or twice, and 4 to 6 weeks should pass before its success or failure is judged.

If epidural steroids are effective in alleviating the patient's leg pain or sciatica, he is begun on a program of back exercises and encouraged to return promptly to as normal a lifestyle as possible. In most cases, heavy work (lifting more than 50 lb repetitively) is not recommended since these patients are prone to recurrences. Physical laborers who have sustained a disc herniation should be placed on some type of permanent light duty. Employee-patients who are told from the beginning that a permanent light duty job is available and that the only reason to undergo surgery is to relieve pain will generally respond to nonoperative therapy. Surgery does not return people to heavy work, it only controls acute pain. This conservative treatment pathway usually will be complete in less than 3 months, and most patients with sciatica will not have to undergo any major invasive treatment.

Should the epidural steroids prove ineffective, and if 3 months have passed since the initial injury without relief of pain, some type of invasive treatment should be considered. The patient group is then divided into those with probable herniated discs and those with symptoms secondary to spinal stenosis.

Patients with herniated discs have symptoms secondary to the nucleus pulposus escaping through the annulus fibrosus and causing pressure and inflammation of an individual nerve root. The fifth lumbar and first sacral nerve roots are those most commonly involved. The pain will radiate along the anatomic pathway of the nerves that travel below the knee and into the foot. Disc herniation is most common in the fourth decade of life, but it can also be seen in older patients.

The physician must now carefully reevaluate the patient for a neurologic deficit and for a positive tension sign or straight leg raising test. For those who have either a neurologic deficit or a positive tension sign along with continued leg pain, a computed tomographic (CT) or magnetic resonance imaging (MRI) scan should be obtained. The authors' preference is to use MRI as the initial study in patients younger than age 50 and to use CT in patients over 50 because of the increased likelihood of bony rather than soft tissue encroachment in the older patients. If either the CT or MR scan is clearly positive and correlates with the clinical findings, myelography no longer need be performed since it is invasive. If there is any question about the findings, one should proceed with the other noninvasive study not yet done (CT or MRI) or a metrizamide myelogram.

There is repeated documentation that for surgery to be effective in the treatment of a herniated disc, the surgeon must find unequivocal operative evidence of nerve root compression.[5] Accordingly, nerve root compression must be firmly substantiated preoperatively, not only by neurologic examination but also by radiography. There is no place for "exploratory" back surgery. Many asymptomatic patients have been found to have abnormal myelograms, electromyograms, and CT/MRI scans. If the patient has neither a neurologic deficit nor a positive straight leg raising test, then regardless of radiographic findings, there is not enough evidence of root compression to proceed with successful surgery. It is the surgeons who operate on patients without objective findings who have poor results and who have given back surgery a bad name.

If there are no objective findings, the physician should avoid surgery and proceed to the psychosocial evaluation. Exceptions should be few and far between. When sympathy for the patient's complaints outweighs the objective evaluation, treatment is fraught with difficulties. Of those who meet these specific criteria for lumbar laminectomy, 95 percent can expect good to excellent results.

The second group of patients whose symptoms are based on mechanical pressure on the neural elements are those with spinal stenosis. This narrowing of the spinal canal secondary to increased bone formation and intervertebral joint degeneration is a natural occurrence with age. Patients over 60 years of age are most affected by spinal stenosis. If the spinal canal is narrow to start with and then decreases further, pressure and irritation on the nerves can develop and cause radiation of pain into the legs. These patients may or may not have a positive neurologic examination or straight leg raising test. Ambulation may result in mechanical irritation, poor excursion of the spinal nerves due to entrapment, edema, and neural ischemia. Accordingly, if these patients ambulate until their symptoms are reproduced, such a "stress test" can cause the initially negative neurologic and tension signs to become positive.

The clinical diagnosis of spinal stenosis can usually be confirmed with plain films, which will demonstrate facet degeneration, disc degeneration, and decreased interpedicular and sagittal canal diameters.

CT will better define the involved areas and the myelogram is useful to delineate the extent of surgery required. With advances in technology, MRI may replace the myelogram in this setting. If symptoms are severe and there is radiographic evidence of spinal stenosis, surgery is appropriate. Age alone is not a deterrent to surgery; many elderly people who are in good health except for a narrow spinal canal will benefit greatly from adequate decompression of the lumbar spine.

Anterior Thigh Pain

A small percentage of patients will have pain that radiates from the back into the anterior thigh. This usually is relieved by rest and anti-inflammatory medication, but if the discomfort persists after 6 weeks of treatment, a work-up should be initiated to search for underlying extraspinal pathology. Several entities must be considered.

A hip problem or hernia can be ruled out with a thorough physical examination. If the hip examination is positive, radiographs should be obtained. An intravenous pyelogram is useful to evaluate the urinary tract, because kidney stones often can present as anterior thigh pain. Peripheral neuropathy, most commonly secondary to diabetes, also can present initially with anterior thigh pain; a glucose tolerance test as well as an electromyogram (EMG) will reveal this underlying problem. Finally, a retroperitoneal tumor can cause symptoms by pressing on the nerves that innervate the anterior thigh. A CT or MRI scan of the retroperitoneal area will eliminate or confirm this possibility.

On diagnosis of any of these disorders, appropriate treatment is begun. If no physical cause can be found for the anterior thigh pain, the patient is treated for recalcitrant back strain as outlined earlier.

Posterior Thigh Pain

This final group of patients complains of back pain with radiation into the buttocks and posterior thigh. Most will be relieved of their symptoms with 6 weeks of conservative therapy. However, if pain persists after the initial treatment period, they can be considered to have back strain and given a trigger-point injection of steroids and lidocaine in the area of maximum tenderness. If the injection is unsuccessful, it is necessary to distinguish between referred and radicular pain.

Referred pain is pain in mesodermal tissues of the same embryologic origin. The muscles, tendons, and ligaments of the buttocks and posterior thighs have the same embryologic origin as those of the low back. When the low back is injured, pain may be referred to the posterior thigh where it is perceived by the patient. Referred pain from irritated soft tissues cannot be cured with a surgical procedure.

Radicular pain is caused by compression of an inflamed nerve root along the anatomic course of the nerve. A herniated disc or spinal stenosis in the high lumbar area (e.g., at the L2-3 or L3-4 interspace) can cause radiation of pain into the posterior thigh. MRI or CT along with EMG can be used to differentiate radicular pain from referred pain or a peripheral nerve lesion. If the studies are within normal limits, the patient is considered to have back strain and is treated according to the algorithm. If a radicular abnormality is found, the patient is diagnosed as having mechanical compression on the neural elements either from a herniated disc or spinal stenosis. Epidural steroid injections should be attempted first; if these do not provide adequate relief, surgery should be contemplated.

Patients with unexplained posterior thigh pain are difficult to treat. The biggest mistake made is the performance of surgery on people thought to have radicular pain who actually have referred pain. Again, referred pain in this setting is not responsive to surgery.

Summary

In most instances the treatment of low back pain is no longer a mystery. The algorithm shown in Figure 11–1 presents a series of easy-to-follow and clearly defined decision-making processes. Use of this algorithm provides patients with the most helpful diagnostic and therapeutic measures at the optimal time. It neither denies them helpful surgery nor subjects them to procedures that are useless technical exercises.

References

1. Aitken AP, Bradford CH: End results of ruptured intervertebral discs in industry. Am J Surg 73:365–380, 1947.
2. DePalma A, Rothman RH: Surgery of the lumbar spine. Clin Orthop 63:162–170, 1969.
3. Floman Y, Wiesel SW, Rothman RH: Cauda equina syndrome presenting as a herniated lumbar disk. Clin Orthop 147:234–237, 1980.
4. Garfin SK, Glover M, Booth RE, et al: Laminectomy: A review of the Pennsylvania Hospital experience. J Spinal Dis 1:116–133, 1988.
5. Hakelius A: Long term follow-up in sciatica. Acta Orthop Scand (Suppl) 129:33–41, 1972.
6. Lippitt AB: The facet joint and its role in spine pain. Spine 9:746–750, 1984.
7. Nachemson A: The lumbar spine. An orthopaedic challenge. Spine 1:59–71, 1976.
8. Rothman RH: Indications for lumbar fusion. Clin Neurosurg 71:215–219, 1973.
9. Rothman RH, Simeone FA: The Spine, 2nd ed. Philadelphia, W.B. Saunders, 1982.
10. Saal JA, Saal JS: Nonoperative treatment of herniated lumbar intervertebral disc with radiculopathy. An outcome study. Spine 14:431–437, 1989.
11. Weber H: An evaluation of conservative and surgical treatment of lumbar disc protrusion. J Oslo City Hosp 20:81–93, 1970.
12. Weber H: The effect of delayed disc surgery on muscular paresis. Acta Orthop Scand 46:631–642, 1975.
13. Wiesel SW, Cuckler JM, DeLuca F, et al: Acute low back pain: An objective analysis of conservative therapy. Spine 5:324–330, 1980.
14. Wiesel SW, Feffer HL, Borenstein DG: Evaluation and outcome of low-back pain of unknown etiology. Spine 13:679–680, 1988.
15. Yang KH, King AI: Mechanism of facet load transmission as a hypothesis for low-back pain. Spine 9:557–565, 1984.
16. Zachrissen M: The Low Back Pain School. Danderyd, Sweden, Danderyd's Hospital, 1972.

CHAPTER 12

Nonoperative Treatment Modalities for the Lumbar Spine

As the algorithm featured in Chapter 11 indicates, all low back pain patients (except those with cauda equina syndrome) require an initial period of conservative therapy. At present there are many treatment modalities available; unfortunately, most of them are based on empiricism and tradition. Few are scientifically valid because of the difficulty in performing prospective double-blind studies in this field. Each treatment plan in popular use today is surrounded by conflicting claims for its indication and efficacy.

The purpose of this section is to discuss the rationale behind the use of some of the more common therapeutic measures. Each treatment modality will be described and the available scientific evidence for or against its use presented.

BEDREST (CONTROLLED PHYSICAL ACTIVITY)

Bedrest has evolved over the years as one of the most important elements in the treatment of low back pain. Patients should be asked to remain in bed, except for going to the bathroom, preferably at home. There is no real need to admit these people to a hospital unless they have no family or supportive friends to help them. The patient's position in bed should be one of comfort. For most people this means lying on the back with the hips and knees flexed to a moderate degree; several pillows can be placed under the knees to help maintain this position comfortably. Lying on either side, with the legs drawn up in the "fetal position" also can be quite comfortable. The only position to avoid is lying prone (face down), which will cause hyperextension of the lumbar spine; this can be uncomfortable for the patient and, theoretically, can lead to further extrusion of an already herniated disc.

The amount of bedrest prescribed varies for each patient; mobilization should not begin until the patient is reasonably comfortable. The type of pathology will determine the duration of bedrest required. Most patients with acute back strain will need only 2 to 7 days of bedrest before they can ambulate. However, a patient with an acute herniated disc may require up to 2 weeks of complete bedrest with a further 10 days of gradual mobilization. Complete bedrest for long periods (more than 2 weeks) has a deleterious effect on the body in general and should be closely monitored. As the discomfort eases, the patient should be strongly encouraged to take short walks but to do as little sitting as possible. Each patient should be followed carefully and not allowed complete mobility until the objective signs, such as a list or paravertebral muscle spasm, disappear. The patient's physical activity is tailored to increase movement without a recurrence of symptoms (Table 12–1).

The purpose of controlled physical activity is to allow any inflammatory reaction that is present to subside. Bedrest will not result in the disc's return to its original position. However, as the disc herniates, it causes a secondary inflammatory process responsible for the patient's

TABLE 12–1. GENERAL GUIDELINES FOR LOW BACK PAIN PATIENTS

Posture
    Active posture: standing pelvic tilt
    Passive posture: rest one leg higher than the other
    Never perform an activity that forces you to arch your back
    Avoid excessive bending, stooping, or twisting

Sitting
    Sit no longer than one-half hour at a time
    Keep one or both legs elevated
    Keep back supported
    Avoid leaning forward and arching back

Lifting
    Bend knees while lifting
    Always hold object close to your body: do not lift above chest level
    Try to maintain the pelvic tilt while lifting and carrying objects
    Keep knees bent while carrying objects
    While pushing or pulling, maintain the pelvic tilt and use hips and legs to do the work
    Do not arch your back while reaching—use a stool

Sleeping
    Sleep on your side with knees pulled up or on your back with a pillow under your knees. If you must sleep on your stomach, place pillow under hips.

Driving
    Pull seat close to the pedals

pain, and if this reaction can be brought under control, the patient's symptoms will disappear. This relief may or may not be permanent.

Scientific evidence that bedrest is effective is available. Biomechanically, Nachemson has demonstrated that the supine position significantly reduces the pressure on the intervertebral discs, compared with sitting or standing positions.[36,37] Assuming that increased pressure on the structures in the low back will increase symptoms, bedrest is a rational approach.

Clinically, Wiesel and colleagues compared bedrest with ambulation for treatment of low back strain in Army recruits.[48] Patients treated with strict bedrest experienced less pain and returned to duty sooner than those required to remain ambulatory. In another randomized study of 189 patients, Deyo and associates concluded that 2 days of bedrest was as effective as 7 days in low back pain patients with no neurologic deficit.[13] This investigation, however, was conducted with a highly selected group of patients—predominantly indigent patients from a primary care (nonspecialized) clinic setting with compensation cases excluded. Another difficulty with this study was compliance: the group assigned to 7 days of bedrest reported a mean of only 3.9 days in bed.

From the evidence available, controlled physical activity appears to be a most effective conservative treatment for low back pain. However, the optimal duration of bedrest remains in question. Two to seven days is reasonable for back strain, with the severity of symptoms at presentation serving as the guiding factor. Patients given prescriptions for longer periods of bedrest will have more days lost from work regardless of their compliance with bedrest,[13] and this must be minimized by customizing the recommended length of bedrest to the patient's symptoms and physical findings.

DRUG THERAPY

The judicious use of drug therapy is an important adjunct in the treatment of low back pain. There are three main categories of drugs in common use: anti-inflammatories, analgesics, and muscle relaxants.

Anti-inflammatory agents are employed because of the belief that inflammation within the affected tissues is a major cause of pain in the low back. This is especially true for those patients with symptoms secondary to a herniated disc. The leg pain these patients experience is due not only to the mechanical pressure from the ruptured disc but also to the inflammation around the involved nerve roots.[31] If the inflammatory component can be dispelled, the patient's pain usually will subside.

There are a variety of nonsteroidal anti-inflammatory agents available, but several scientific studies have shown none to be superior.[25,44,48] It should be noted that all these studies looked at the various agents in combination with bedrest. A double-blind placebo-controlled trial of proxicam (Feldene) showed that a greater amount of pain relief in the anti-inflammatory treated group was evident only during the first few days of back pain; however, after 2 weeks, more of the untreated group had returned to work.[2] Anti-inflammatory drugs should be considered only an adjunctive and not a primary treatment.

Oral corticosteroids are excellent anti-inflammatory agents and may be administered for a short period with rapidly tapering doses.[43] Unfortunately, avascular necrosis in the hips is an infrequent but serious side effect.[16] The effects of oral steroids in back pain relief have not been studied in a prospective, double-blinded fashion.

The authors' preference is to begin the patient on adequate doses of aspirin, which is effective and inexpensive. If the response is not satisfactory, nonsteroidal anti-inflammatory drugs (NSAIDs) such as naproxen (Naprosyn), ibuprofen (Motrin, Advil, Nuprin), or indomethacin (Indocin) can be tried. Most patients will get significant relief from one of these agents. Again, all anti-inflammatory medications are utilized in conjunction with controlled physical activity to relieve pain; they do not replace adequate rest. Occasionally, after an initial recovery, a patient will experience intermittent recurrent attacks or complain of a chronic low backache; in some instances these patients will be helped by a maintenance dose of an anti-inflammatory drug.

The most common side effects of NSAIDs are gastrointestinal and renal toxicities. Aspirin and other NSAIDs have been associated with acute gastrointestinal bleeding.[22,24,27] A small number of patients develop reversible renal failure from decreased renal prostaglandin production, and less frequently, an idiosyncratic interstitial nephritis. Other NSAID toxic effects produce neurologic, hepatic, or hematologic abnormalities.[9] Phenylbutazone is associated with a rare and severe bone marrow toxicity. Gastrointestinal effects can be minimized by taking the medications after meals, adding histamine-receptor blocking agents or antacids, or reducing alcohol, caffeine, and tobacco consumption. In addition, geriatric patients may require decreased dosages due to poorer metabolism and byproduct clearance.

Analgesic medication is very important during the acute phase of low back pain.[48] The goal is to keep the patient comfortable while in bed. Most of the anti-inflammatory agents also have analgesic properties. In more severe cases, most patients will respond to the addition of 30 to 60 mg of codeine to aspirin or acetaminophen every 4 to 6 hours. If stronger medication is necessary, it is the authors' feeling that the patient should be admitted to the hospital and given parenteral narcotics as required. As the pain decreases, non-narcotic analgesics may be substituted for the more potent drugs.

The biggest mistake seen is treatment with very strong narcotics such as meperidine (Demerol) or oxycodone (Percodan, Tylox) on an outpatient basis. Many of these patients become addicted to the medication. In other cases, patients try to shortcut the restrictions on physical activity and use analgesic medication instead. This, of course, will not work, and when the patient stops the drug, the back pain returns.

Analgesic medication must be prescribed with great care for the low back pain patient. The treating physician must maintain control of the patient's drug use at all times; there are too many instances of patients taking undue advantage of the situation. Finally, addicting narcotics have no place in the treatment regimen of patients with chronic low back problems.

Muscle relaxants are not routinely recommended for the treatment of low back pain. In most cases the muscle spasm is secondary to a primary problem such as a herniated disc. If the pain from the ruptured disc can be controlled, the muscle spasm will usually subside.

Occasionally, muscle spasm will be so severe that some type of treatment is required. Carisoprodol (Soma), methocarbamol (Robaxin), and cyclobenzaprine (Flexeril) are the drugs recommended to be taken with an anti-inflammatory agent.[4] Although baclofen (Lioresal) was shown to be minimally effective in the relief of lumbar pain, the relatively high frequency of adverse reactions is prohibitive.[11] Most patients will experience a sedative effect from these medications. Other side effects include headache, nausea, dry mouth, dizziness, and blurred vision. Diazepam (Valium) should be discouraged since it is actually a physiologic depressant, and depression is often an integral feature of back pain syndromes.[34] Administration of diazepam to depressed patients only increases their problems. If anxiety is prominent and a sedative is needed, phenobarbital will alleviate the symptoms. In patients with chronic low back pain without objective physical findings, antidepressant therapy may help alleviate some complaints.[1,40] Clinical studies have shown the tricyclic antidepressants amitriptyline, imipramine, and doxepin to yield superior pain relief compared to placebo.[45]

In summary, drug therapy for low back pain should be viewed as an adjunct to adequately controlled physical activity. Anti-inflammatory medication should be the primary agent employed. Analgesic medication should be used selectively in a controlled environment and not for extended periods. Muscle relaxants are generally not recommended, and if employed should be carefully monitored.

TRIGGER-POINT INJECTION

Trigger-point therapy is indicated for nonradiating low back pain when a point of maximal tenderness can be identified. This procedure involves the injection of steroids and a local anesthetic such as lidocaine (Xylocaine) at an area of maximal tenderness in the low back. The precise mechanism of action is not clear but may be related to modulation of peripheral nerve stimulation as it affects the afferent input perceived as pain.

Although anecdotal reports claim effectiveness for this technique, it has not been well studied in the setting of acute low back pain syndrome. A prospective randomized double-blinded evaluation of trigger-point injection in 51 acute low back pain patients was conducted by Garvey and colleagues.[19] Although not statistically significant, their data suggested that the medication injected is not the critical factor, since the patients treated with a needlestick and nothing injected (acupuncture) had a greater rate of improvement in symptoms (61%) than the patients injected with lidocaine alone (40%) or with steroids (45%). Their intended control group received vapocoolant spray followed by pressure from a plastic needle guard and had the highest frequency of improvement (66%) and the greatest average subjective decrease in pain. Unfortunately, no patients were randomized to a "watch and wait" control group to evaluate for the placebo effect.

Trigger-point therapy is easy to perform, has a negligible risk, and may help certain patients. Further controlled research is required to delineate the true value of this modality in the treatment of acute low back pain.

EPIDURAL STEROID INJECTION

Epidural steroid injections are indicated for severe lumbar radiculopathy but not for nonradiating low back pain. This has generally been viewed as an intermediate step between conservative treatment and surgical management. It is a more aggressive attempt at pain relief after conservative therapy has failed, yet it avoids the disadvantages of surgery. The rationale for this therapy is that lumbar radiculopathy (in the early phase) involves a significant inflammatory component, evoked by chemical or mechanical irritation or an autoimmune response—all of which should be amenable to treatment with corticosteroid drugs in the early stages.[31]

Unfortunately, few studies have systematically and accurately studied the efficacy of this treatment modality.[30] Poorly controlled, nonrandomized investigations have yielded controversial results with a success rate ranging from 25 to 75 percent.[6,41] Another problem is that some studies have attempted to determine the efficacy of epidural steroids compared to epidural saline injection, while others have compared their results to a true placebo (i.e., interspinous ligament injection). It is unclear whether the steroids themselves have a clinical effect or if just the mechanical violation of the epidural space is important.[42] Cuckler and colleagues concluded that the addition of steroids to epidural injections of procaine (Novocain) worked no better than procaine alone in relieving symptoms.[7] Problems with this particular study were that the authors did not compare their results to a group with no epidural injection and the questionable timing of efficacy assessment: 24 hours after injection was probably too soon to see beneficial effects in many patients.

Despite the lack of optimally designed investigations, upon review of the literature, certain trends seem to be evident.[5] Epidural steroids appear to be more beneficial in acute than in chronic radiculopathy, especially when no neurologic deficit is present. Improvement may not be noted until 3 to 6 days after injection and may be only temporary. No neurotoxicity has been reported in humans or animal models; complications stem from the technique of epidural injection and are rare.[6] Suppression of the plasma corticosteroid concentration can occur up to 3 weeks following the injection.[5]

The authors maintain that epidural steroids may be helpful in relieving an irritative component of radicular pain in 40 percent of patients. Until controlled investigations indicate otherwise, this is a treatment worth trying in patients who have failed 6 weeks of conservative management in an effort to avoid a major invasive procedure.

TRACTION

The application of traction to the lumbar spine is a popular treatment for patients with herniated discs. The theory is that stretching the lumbar spine distracts the vertebrae so that the protruded disc is allowed to return to a more normal anatomic position. In fact, the disc material probably does not change position at all. Scientific evidence indicates that a distraction force equal to 60 percent of body weight is needed just to reduce the intradiscal pressure at the third lumbar vertebra by 25 percent.[38] Such force could not practically be applied to a patient. Furthermore, there has never been any proof that disc material returns to its normal position following herniation.

Traction can be applied as gravity lumbar traction, autotraction, and through motorized techniques, using light weights for several hours or heavier weights for shorter periods. None of these methods has been proven to be more effective than the others.[14] While a few studies have shown traction to have a short-lived benefit on sciatica patients,[17] most double-blinded studies have not demonstrated any positive effect.[46,47] Weber studied two groups of patients with herniated discs (proven by myelogram) and applied a traction apparatus to each group, using weights in the traction bags for one group but not the other. There was no statistically significant difference between the two groups in terms of relief of symptoms. Traction had no effect on spinal mobility, tension signs, deep tendon reflexes, paresis, or sensory deficit, and while it usually was well tolerated, it did make some patients worse.[6]

In spite of the lack of concrete evidence of its effectiveness, traction is used frequently as an excuse for admitting patients to the hospital. Thousands of health care dollars are spent each year for this treatment modality. It is the authors' feeling that traction may benefit a patient by limiting his activity and creating a positive psychological effect on his expectations for recovery. It is recommended that patients be given a home traction unit rather than being admitted to the hospital.

MANIPULATION

Spinal manipulation is another popular nonoperative modality for the treatment of low back pain. In the United States it is somewhat controversial because it is performed mostly by chiropractors. The principle involved is that any malalignment of the spinal structures can be corrected by manipulation; the assumption is that the malalignment is the etiology of the patient's pain. Unfortunately, there is "no scientific proof for or against either the efficacy of this spinal manipulation therapy or the pathophysiological foundation from which it is derived."[3]

There have been several clinical randomized trials studying the efficacy of manipulation. A few studies demonstrated that patients felt some immediate relief of pain but had no long-term benefit.[15,20,23] In a study that randomized 54 subjects to spinal manipulation or spinal mobilization, there was no difference in benefit perceived between the two treatment modalities.[21] However, those subjects who had suffered a backache for 2 to 4 weeks prior to treatment experienced more rapid improvement after spinal manipulation; this response rate difference was not seen in the group with less than 2 weeks of symptoms prior to treatment.

The efficacy of spinal manipulation is neither scientifically proven nor disproven.[8] The majority of previous studies are flawed in one or more of these areas: (1) entry criteria too broad, too narrow, or undefined; (2) poor uniformity or standardization of manipulative technique used among multiple manipulators; (3) measurements of outcome vary from work return (affected by other factors) to subjective questionnaires; and (4) invalid control maneuvers that do not account for the personal contact of manipulation (placebo effect).

The authors' experience is that some patients do have short periods of symptomatic relief after manipulation but must keep returning for repeat sessions to maintain it, substantially increasing the cost of treatment. Patients with pathologic bone disease such as a tumor or osteopenia can be harmed by manipulation. At present it is felt that manipulation is not indicated for the routine treatment of low back pain. There is not adequate scientific evidence to justify its routine use, and it can result in serious complications.[10,18]

BRACES AND CORSETS

External support of the lumbar spine with a corset or brace is indicated for only a short period in the average patient's recovery process, and not every patient requires it. As the acute symptoms subside, a properly fitted corset or brace will aid the patient in regaining mobility sooner.[35] As recovery progresses, the patient usually should abandon the brace in favor of an exercise program. With continued long-term use of a brace, soft tissue contractures and muscle atrophy will occur. The young patient should rely on the brace only to hasten ambulation. In theory, strong, flexible lumbar and abdominal muscles function as an excellent "internal brace" because they are adjacent to the structures (vertebrae) that they are supporting.

There are no convincing data supporting benefits from lumbar corsets and braces, and these devices may cause increased movements of the lumbar spine.[17] One study has shown some relief of symptoms with a rigid plastic delordosating brace in patients with spondylolisthesis or spinal stenosis but no benefit in chronic low back pain of unknown etiology.[49]

Despite a paucity of clinical data, there are two situations in which the authors believe long-term bracing is a reasonable approach. One is for the obese patient with weak abdominal muscles. A firm corset with flexible metal stays will reinforce the abdominal muscles.[35] It has been demonstrated that if a lumbosacral corset is properly applied, the intradiscal pressure in the lumbar area will decrease by approximately 30 percent.[39] Long-term bracing may also benefit the aging patient with multilevel degenerative disease of the lumbar spine. These older people do not tolerate exercise very well, and in some cases exercise will aggravate their back condition. They can attain significant relief of pain with a well-fitted brace.

Most compensation patients are young, and long-term bracing is not indicated for them. However, a corset can be of great benefit to a patient who is returning to heavy work; it keeps the worker aware of his back and prevents him from applying maximum stress to this area as he resumes his normal activities. As soon as he can perform a regular set of exercises comfortably, he should be weaned quickly from the support.

EXERCISES

Some form of exercise is probably the most commonly prescribed therapy for patients recovering from low back pain. Two regimens are commonly advocated: isometric flexion exercises and hyperextension exercises. These programs are purported to reduce the frequency and intensity of low back pain episodes, although there is no scientific evidence to support this contention.

The isometric flexion exercises are the most popular.[12,26,28] They are based on Williams' theory that by reducing the lumbar lordosis, back pain is decreased. This goal is achieved by strengthening both the abdominal and the lumbar muscles, thereby creating a corset of muscles to support the lumbar spine.

Hyperextension exercises strengthen the paravertebral muscles and generally are used after a patient has satisfactorily performed a course of isometric flexion exercises. The goal is to have the paravertebral muscles act as an internal support for the lumbar spine. McKenzie also feels that extending the spine will move the nucleus pulposus anteriorly.[32] The-

Low Back Exercises

1. Pelvic Tilt: Lie on back with knees bent and feet flat on the floor. Squeeze buttocks together and pull stomach in, flattening low back against floor. Hold to count of 5; relax to count of 5.

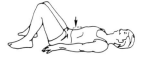

2. Pelvic Tilt: Lie on back with knees straight. Squeeze buttocks together and pull stomach in, flattening low back against floor. Hold to count of 5, relax to count of 5.

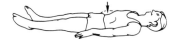

3. To Increase Back Flexibility: **a)** Bring right knee to chest and give a gentle stretch with arms. **b)** Bring left knee to chest and give a gentle stretch with arms. **c)** Bring right knee to chest; then, while holding that position, bring left knee to chest also. Give both a gentle stretch. Then lower one leg at a time.

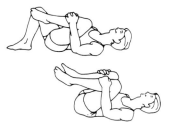

4. To Strengthen Abdominal Muscles: **a)** Lie on floor with knees bent; tuck chin in and raise upper body slowly until shoulder blades clear the floor; hold to count of 5. **b)** Same position as before; raise upper body, reaching hands toward right side of knees; hold to count of 5. **c)** Same position; reach hands to left sides of knees; hold to count of 5. Progression: Grade I — arms held straight out. Grade II — arms crossed in front of chest. Grade III — hands behind head.

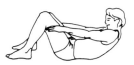

Figure 12–1. Low back exercises are begun with only the flexion routines (1–6). The extension exercises are added only when the flexion exercises can be performed comfortably. The number of repetitions and rate of increase are tailored to the individual patient. (From Wiesel SW, Feffer HL, Borenstein DG, and Rothman RH: Low Back Pain, 2nd ed. Charlottesville, VA, The Michie Co., 1989.)

Illustration continued on opposite page

oretically, these exercises can be used to keep the discs in anatomic position, but unfortunately, again there is no proof that this occurs. The McKenzie program also uses lateral bending and rotation in a regimen individualized to the patient's symptoms and abilities.

The authors feel that an exercise regimen (Fig. 12–1) is very important for the rehabilitation of low back patients. An exercise regimen should not be instituted while the patient is experiencing acute pain but may be started after symptoms have subsided to the point where no list or paravertebral spasm is present. The number of repetitions is increased gradually; if the patient has any recurrence of acute symptoms, the exercises are stopped. The patient is then closely monitored, and when symptoms again decrease, the exercises can be resumed. The authors' preference is for isometric flexion exercises. It should be stressed that there is no proof that exercises decrease recovery time or reduce the frequency of

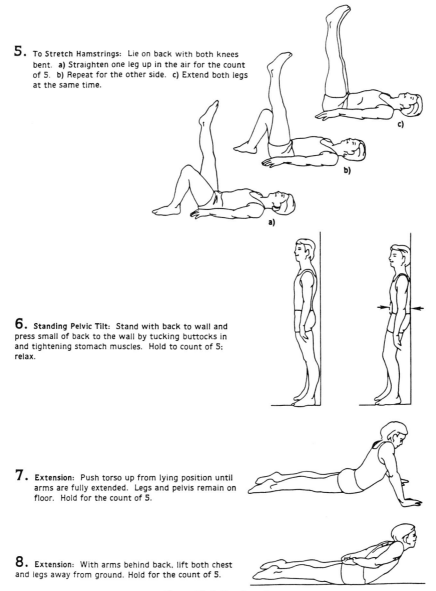

5. To Stretch Hamstrings: Lie on back with both knees bent. **a)** Straighten one leg up in the air for the count of 5. **b)** Repeat for the other side. **c)** Extend both legs at the same time.

6. Standing Pelvic Tilt: Stand with back to wall and press small of back to the wall by tucking buttocks in and tightening stomach muscles. Hold to count of 5; relax.

7. Extension: Push torso up from lying position until arms are fully extended. Legs and pelvis remain on floor. Hold for the count of 5.

8. Extension: With arms behind back, lift both chest and legs away from ground. Hold for the count of 5.

Figure 12–1 *Continued*

recurrences. Empirically, they appear to have a positive psychological effect and allow the patient to play an active part in his treatment program.

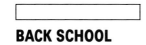

BACK SCHOOL

The concept of a back school was originated in 1970 by Zachrissen and Forsell in Sweden.[50] The theory is that patients who understand the anatomic, epidemiologic, and biomechanical factors that give rise to low back pain can more effectively participate in treatment and prevent recurrences.

An audiovisual approach to teaching this material was developed. After the patient is introduced to the goals of the program, the basic anatomy and physiology of various back disorders are presented in a classroom setting so each patient realizes his problem is not unique. Next the patient is taught the biomechanical principles of spinal movement and function and how to apply these to his daily activities to reduce the forces applied to his spine. Finally, an exercise program is outlined. This multifaceted approach has been quite successful and has yielded more encouraging results than routine physiotherapeutic modalities.[17]

There have been many variations on the program outlined above. Some of these back school programs are complex and costly, involving as much as 15 hours of classroom time. The authors feel that the simpler the program, the better accepted it will be by the patient.

Few well-controlled studies exist validating the use of low back schools for patients with chronic low back pain.[29] Moffett and associates recently compared the results of a low back school group with an exercise-only group of chronic low back pain patients.[33] Initially both groups improved, but after 16 weeks the back school group tended to improve further, while the exercise-only group returned to their baseline activity level. At longer follow-up, however, the only significant difference between groups was an increased knowledge of low back principles in the back school group. Use of the back school concept with acute low back pain has yielded more positive results. Unfortunately, no final conclusions can be reached concerning the effectiveness of low back school; further research must first examine patient compliance, test information retention, and assess subsequent behavioral modifications.

PHYSICAL THERAPY

Other treatment modalities used for low back pain include hot packs, cold packs, light massage, ultrasound, transcutaneous electrical nerve stimulation (TENS), and diathermy.[14,37] They are all well tolerated and pleasant. Most patients experience some immediate relief of symptoms but unfortunately, there is not a long-lasting impact on the disease process. There is no evidence that any of these treatment modalities offers any long-term benefit or even adds to the efficacy of bedrest alone.

References

1. Alcoff J, Jones E, Rust P, et al: Controlled trial of imipramine for chronic low back pain. J Fam Pract 14:841–846, 1982.
2. Amlie E, Weber H, Holme I: Treatment of acute low-back pain with piroxicam: Results of a double-blind placebo-controlled trial. Spine 12:473–476, 1987.
3. Anonymous: The scientific status of the fundamentals of chiropractic analysis and recommendations. National Institute of Neurological and Communicative Disorders and Stroke, April 8, 1975.

4. Basmajian JV: Acute back pain and spasm. A controlled multicenter trial of combined analgesic and antispasm agents. Spine 14:438–439, 1989.
5. Benzon HT: Epidural steroid injections for low back pain and lumbosacral radiculopathy. Pain 24:277–295, 1986.
6. Bogduk N, Cherry D: Epidural corticosteroid agents for sciatica. Med J Aust 143:402–406, 1985.
7. Cuckler JM, Bernini PA, Wiesel SW, et al: The use of epidural steroids in the treatment of lumbar radicular pain: A prospective, randomized, double-blind study. J Bone Joint Surg 67A:63–66, 1985.
8. Curtis P: Spinal manipulation: Does it work? Occup Med: State Art Rev 3(1):31–44, Jan–Mar 1988.
9. Dahl SL: Nonsteroidal anti-inflammatory agents: Clinical pharmacology/adverse effects/usage guidelines. In Wilkens RF, Dahl SL, (eds): Therapeutic Controversies in the Rheumatic Diseases. Orlando, Grune & Stratton, 1987, pp. 27–68.
10. Dan NG, Saccasan PA: Serious complications of lumbar spinal manipulation. Med J Aust 2:672–673, 1983.
11. Dapas F, Hartman SF, Martinez L, et al: Baclofen for the treatment of acute low-back syndrome: A double-blind comparison with placebo. Spine 10:345–349, 1985.
12. Davies JE, Gibson T, Tester L: The value of exercises in the treatment of low back pain. Rheumatol Rehabil 18:243–247, 1979.
13. Deyo RA, Diehl AK, Rosenthal M: How many days of bed rest for acute low back pain? N Engl J Med 315:1065–1070, 1986.
14. Dimaggio A, Mooney V: Conservative care for low back pain: What works? J Musculoskel Med 4:27–34, 1987.
15. Doran DM, Newell DJ: Manipulation in treatment of low back pain: A multi-center study. Br Med J 7:161–164, 1975.
16. Fast A, Alon M, Weiss S, et al: Avascular necrosis of bone following short-term dexamethasone therapy for brain edema. J Neurosurg 61:983–985, 1984.
17. Frymoyer JW: Back pain and sciatica. N Engl J Med 318:291–300, 1988.
18. Gallinaro P, Cartesegna M: Three cases of lumbar disc rupture and one of cauda equina associated with spinal manipulation (chiroprosis). Lancet 1:411, 1983.
19. Garvey TA, Marks MR, Wiesel SW: A prospective randomized double-blind evaluation of trigger-point injection therapy in low back pain. Spine 14:962–964, 1989.
20. Glover JR, Morris JG, Khosla T: Back pain: a randomized clinical trial of rotational manipulation of the trunk. Br J Ind Med 31:59–64, 1974.
21. Hadler NM, Curtis P, Gillings DB, et al: A benefit of spinal manipulation as adjunctive therapy for acute low-back pain: A stratified controlled trial. Spine 12:703–706, 1987.
22. Hart FD: Naproxen and gastrointestinal hemorrhage. Br Med J 2:51–52, 1974.
23. Hoehler FK, Tobis JS, Buerger AA: Spinal manipulation for low back pain. JAMA 245:1835–1838, 1981.
24. Holdstock DJ: Gastrointestinal bleeding: A possible association with ibuprofen. Lancet 1:541, 1972.
25. Jaffe G: A double blind multi-center comparison of naproxen and indomethacin in acute musculoskeletal disorders. Curr Med Res Opin 4:373–380, 1976.
26. Kendall PH, Jenkins JM: Exercises for backache: a double-blind controlled trial. Physiotherapy 54:154–157, 1968.
27. Lansa FL: Endoscopic studies of gastric and duodenal injury after the use of ibuprofen, aspirin, and other nonsteroidal anti-inflammatory agents. Am J Med 77:19–24, 1984.
28. Lidstrom A, Zachrissen M: Physical therapy on low back pain and sciatica: an attempt at evaluation. Scand J Rehab Med 2:37–42, 1970.
29. Linton SJ, Kamwendo K: Low back schools: A critical review. Phys Ther 67:1375–1383, 1987.
30. Mathews JA, Mills SB, Jenkins VM, et al: Back pain and sciatica: Controlled trials of manipulation, traction, sclerosant and epidural injections. Br J Rheumatol 26:416–423, 1987.
31. McCarron RF, Wimpee MW, Hudkins PG, et al: The inflammatory effect of nucleus pulposus. A possible element in the pathogenesis of low back pain. Spine 12:750–753, 1987.
32. McKenzie RA: The Lumbar Spine. New Zealand, Spinal Publications, 1981.
33. Moffett JA, Chase SM, Portek I, et al: A controlled, prospective study to evaluate the effectiveness of a back school in the relief of chronic low back pain. Spine 11:120–122, 1986.
34. Mooney V, Cairns D: Management of patients with chronic low back pain. Orthop Clin North Am 9:543–557, 1978.
35. Morris JM: Low back bracing. Clin Orthop 103:120–132, 1974.
36. Nachemson A: The load on lumbar disks in different positions of the body. Acta Orthop Scand 36:426–434, 1965.
37. Nachemson A: The lumbar spine—an orthopaedic challenge. Spine 1:59–71, 1976.
38. Nachemson A, Elfstrom G: Intravital dynamic pressure measurements in lumbar disc. Scand J Rehabil Med (Suppl) 7:5–40, 1970.
39. Nachemson A, Morris JM: In vivo measurements of intradiscal pressure: discometry, a method for determination of pressure in the lower lumbar disc. J Bone Joint Surg 46A:1077–1092, 1964.

40. Pheasant H, Bursk A, Goldfarb J, et al: Amitriptyline and low back pain: A randomized double-blind crossover study. Spine 8:552–557, 1983.
41. Rosen CD, Kahanovitz N, Bernstein R, et al: A retrospective analysis of the efficacy of epidural steroid injections. Clin Orthop 228:270–272, 1988.
42. Swerdlow M, Sayle-Creer W: A study of extradural medication in the relief of the lumbosciatic syndrome. Anaesthesia 25:341–345, 1970.
43. Tsairis P: Corticosteroid therapy in the management of lumbar radiculopathy. Contemp Orthop 17:53–57, 1988.
44. Vignon G: Comparative study of intravenous ketoprofen versus aspirin. Rheumatol Rehabil 15:83–84, 1976.
45. Ward NG: Tricyclic antidepressants for chronic low back pain: Mechanism of action and predictors of response. Spine 11:661–665, 1986.
46. Weber H: Traction therapy in sciatica due to disc prolapse. J Oslo City Hosp 23:167–179, 1973.
47. Weber H: Lumbar disc herniation: a prospective study of prognostic factors including a controlled trial. J Oslo City Hosp 28:36–61, 89–103, 1978.
48. Wiesel SW, Cuckler JM, DeLuca F, et al: Acute low back pain: An objective analysis of conservative therapy. Spine 5:324–330, 1980.
49. Willner S: Effect of a rigid brace on back pain. Acta Orthop Scand 56:40–42, 1985.
50. Zachrissen M: The back pain school. Spine 6:104–106, 1981.

CHAPTER 13

Operative/Invasive Management of the Aging Lumbar Spine

In 1934, Mixter and Barr presented their observations on the treatment of herniated intervertebral discs by laminectomy and disc excision.[23] Over 50 years later, we now have several invasive treatments for low back pain and sciatica that are extremely successful at acutely relieving symptoms in properly selected patients. However, since several studies have failed to demonstrate any benefit of surgical intervention over conservative management 4 years after treatment,[10,37] any invasive procedure for herniated nucleus pulposus must be considered palliative, not curative. While surgery may relieve neurogenic pain, it does not obliterate or prevent further degenerative spine disease. The purpose of this chapter is to present the general criteria for surgical intervention and to discuss the common invasive treatment modalities for low back and leg pain and the efficacy expected from each.

SURGERY FOR HERNIATED LUMBAR DISCS

A herniated disc requires immediate surgical intervention only when it presents as cauda equina syndrome. This classically includes low back pain, bilateral sciatica, saddle anesthesia, and motor weakness in the lower extremities that may progress to paraplegia and bowel/bladder incontinence. Other indications for surgical management of a herniated disc not responding to appropriate nonoperative management include documented progressive neurologic deficit, recurrent episodes of sciatica, and unrelenting sciatica. Failure to improve after 2 to 3 months of appropriate conservative therapy warrants surgical consideration if the diagnosis is certain, since further procrastination might adversely affect the end result. Surgical intervention has the greatest chance for success when there is correlation of the patient's pain and a positive tension sign or a neurologic deficit with confirmation of the lesion by an imaging study. A variety of procedures for herniated discs exist and each will be discussed.

Chemonucleolysis

Although chemonucleolysis was initially considered a noninvasive (conservative) treatment modality for sciatica, the associated complications and morbidity are comparable to and possibly exceed those of standard surgical techniques. Appropriately, it is considered here as an invasive procedure.

Chemonucleolysis, introduced by Lyman Smith in 1964, is the injection of a substance into the nucleus pulposus to dissolve it and relieve pressure on the neural elements. Two drugs, chymopapain and collagenase, are currently available; the majority of the published reports are concerned with the former. Each agent dissolves different material within the nucleus; chymopapain dissolves the proteoglycans, while collagenase works on the collagen. The mechanism of action is postulated to be reduction of the water-binding capacity of the disc, which results in decreased intradiscal pressure, or a decrease in disc height that may indirectly decrease the nerve root pressure.[24]

Clinical results with chemonucleolysis have been variable. In more recent studies, a 60 to 80 percent success rate has been reported.[3,24] In a prospective, double-blinded study, 77 percent of patients treated with chymopapain were assessed as moderately improved, compared with 47 percent of intradiscal saline-treated patients.[8] While some studies report 87 percent favorable results at 10-year follow-up,[2] it is important to analyze the selection criteria for treatment and to remember the favorable natural history of disc disease. Several nonrandomized retrospective studies have demonstrated comparable results at 10 years with chemonucleolysis and discectomy.[14,38,39] Other studies have shown that when strict clinical and radiographic indications are adhered to, conventional surgery approaches a 95 percent success rate with 90 percent of patients returning to work, while chymopapain achieves a 70 percent success rate at best[5]— better than placebo but worse than conventional surgery.

In addition to the questionable efficacy of chemonucleolysis, its use has declined since 1984 because of the increased frequency and severity of complications.[5] The incidence of anaphylaxis (and sometimes death) has diminished with the use of skin allergy testing and local rather than general anesthesia. However, paralysis (transverse myelitis or cauda equina syndrome) and cerebrovascular complications (subarachnoid and intracerebral hemorrhage) have been reported.[35] As a result of these potential complications (including the extended postoperative monitoring required to watch for them) and the relatively high incidence of failure, (therefore requiring another invasive procedure), chemonucleolysis is not the cost-effective treatment that it was once purported to be.[22,26]

There is no question that chemonucleolysis should be approached with the same seriousness as surgery. Every candidate for chemonucleolysis should meet all the criteria for conventional disc surgery; however, it has become clear that not all surgical candidates meet the criteria for chemonucleolysis. Many of the chymopapain failures have been attributed to sequestered or free disc fragments. Attempts at selecting patients who will benefit most from chymopapain injection have had limited success.[6,29] The role of computed tomography/discography in predicting the success of chemonucleolysis remains unclear.[12,15] At present, the exact indications for chemonucleolysis are not clear, and questions remain about its efficacy and safety, especially when compared with conventional surgical techniques.

Open (Conventional) Discectomy

Surgery has proved to be safe and efficient in treating patients with herniated discs who have failed to respond to appropriate conservative therapy. Conventional discectomy is commonly performed via an intralaminal approach (Fig. 13–1); more extensive laminectomies are necessary in patients who have lateral spinal canal stenosis. With proper pa-

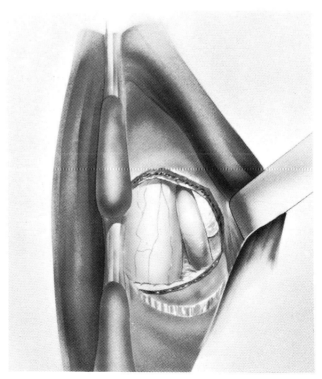

Figure 13–1. The extent of bone removal and ligamentum flavum removal prior to nerve root retraction is shown. The lateral border of the nerve root is well seen before the nerve is retracted. Note the extruded nucleus beneath the nerve root. (From Rothman RH, Simeone FA: The Spine, 2nd ed. Philadelphia, W.B. Saunders, 1982.)

tient selection, conventional discectomy can be expected to initially provide good to excellent results in 90 to 95 percent of cases,[11] but the long-term success rate in these patients may decrease to 70 percent over the subsequent decade due to recurrence or scarring.[10] It is estimated that conventional discectomy has a 0.03 percent mortality rate, with an incidence of neurologic complications of less than 0.5 percent and minor complications in 4.7 percent of cases.[14] Although acute lumbar disc herniation in the elderly is not a common problem, surgery yields a high rate of satisfactory results in selected patients over age 60.[19] With a high percentage of successful results and a low morbidity, this procedure has stood the test of time; other procedures must show definitive advantages before open discectomy can be abandoned in their favor.

Microsurgical Discectomy

Microsurgical discectomy involves the use of a small incision (2.5 to 3 cm), the operating microscope for high magnification, and intense illumination of the operative field. Its theoretical technical advantages are improved visualization of microanatomy, preservation of epidural fat, meticulous hemostasis, minimal nerve root trauma, and minimal dissection of paravertebral muscles.[21] An apparent economic advantage over conventional discectomy is the decreased hospital stay, although postoperative recovery time is similar.[16] At the extreme, ambulatory microsurgery for lumbar discs has also been reported.[1] However, retrospective studies have unfairly compared the length of hospitalization for microsurgical discectomies with that for open discectomies performed in the 1970s—a time when the average stay for all surgical procedures was much longer than today.[27,30]

Most reports claim at least a 90 percent success rate for microsurgical discectomy at relieving leg pain and somewhat less success at relieving back pain.[21,23,36] Concern with this technique includes the relatively high recurrence rate reported in some series[23] and an excessive number of dural tears.[7,30] A case of bowel perforation following microsurgical lumbar discectomy has also been reported.[34] In comparison with other techniques, the success rate of microsurgical discectomy appears to be superior to that of chemonucleolysis,[20,41] and comparable to that of conventional discectomy.[27,30,31,40] It should be noted, however, that no prospective, randomized investigations with standardized monitoring of postoperative pain have been conducted.

Many surgeons, including the authors, are not convinced that the theoretical technical advantages and apparent cost savings with microsurgical discectomy are worth compromising surgical exposure.[7] The microsurgical technique does not facilitate adequate assessment or treatment of stenosis of the nerve root canal (which may coexist with disc protrusion), nor does it ensure visualization of disc fragments that may be forced above or below the disc level—two common reasons for reoperation. The authors agree that a technique that decreases hospital stay and lost work days is attractive; however, these advantages must definitively be proven in a prospective, randomized study with long-term follow-up.

Percutaneous Discectomy

By mechanically decompressing the disc, percutaneous lumbar discectomy may have the beneficial effects of chymopapain without the associated complications. Various posterolateral and lateral approaches have been reported, usually with manual removal of disc material with forceps after confirmation of location with fluoroscopy. The reported complications included leg dysesthesia and paraspinal muscle spasm. Early trials indicated that this treatment was effective in 65 to 75 percent of patients.[4,9,17,18,32]

Onik and co-workers have described their experience with automated percutaneous discectomy.[28] The advantage of their technique is the introduction of a specially designed nucleotome through a narrow cannula (2.8 mm) to aspirate disc material without anterior perforation of the annulus. They reported an 86 percent success rate in 36 patients who met stringent clinical and radiographic criteria for surgery; those who had radiographic evidence of a free disc fragment or facet disease were excluded. When the procedure was performed under local anesthesia with fluoroscopic guidance, no neurologic complications occurred. As with chemonucleolysis, it is difficult to envision that removal of the nucleus pulposus will relieve pressure on neural elements caused by a large protrusion of disc material into the spinal canal. Regardless, these early results are promising and percutaneous discectomy may gain a place as a viable treatment option for some types of herniated discs pending larger studies with long-term follow-up.

SURGERY FOR SPINAL STENOSIS

The surgical indications in degenerative spinal stenosis are often less well-defined than in disc herniation. Because there frequently may be no objective physical findings, a careful history is essential. When leg pain constantly interferes with ambulation, surgery should be considered. Occasionally, symptoms may be reproduced after walking, and positive neurologic findings can be observed simultaneously. This "stress test" is helpful because of its objectivity. Confirmation of stenosis should be made with a metrizamide CT scan. Claudication due to peripheral vascular disease should always be ruled out prior to spinal surgery.

The goal of any operation for spinal stenosis is to completely remove all pressure from the neural elements. The type of pathology found will dictate the extent and nature of the decompression required. For example, if midline ridging is the only abnormality present and the nerve roots are free in the foramina, then a complete laminectomy of the affected levels, with preservation of the facet joints, will suffice (Fig. 13–2). If foraminal encroachment is present, a complete foraminotomy is indicated. If there is a narrow lateral recess, it should be unroofed completely out to the pedicle. When the operation is completed, there should be no residual mechanical pressure on the neural elements. Fusion is not usually required after decompression for lateral recess stenosis; however, patients with degenerative spinal stenosis requiring extensive decompression may benefit from simultaneous fusion.[25]

SURGERY FOR SPONDYLOLISTHESIS

Spondylolisthesis, the horizontal slippage of one vertebra upon another, usually does not require surgical intervention. Assuming the patient has low back pain due to instability, this disorder can often be treated by limiting stressful activities, a lumbosacral corset, and abdominal exercises. If the patient's symptoms are back pain alone and are incapacitating, then spinal fusion is appropriate. Patients with back and leg pain may require both a spinal fusion and decompression of the neural elements; success is less certain than with the back pain alone patients.[13] Reduction of the olisthesis with degenerative spondylolisthesis is generally not necessary and may result in neurologic damage.

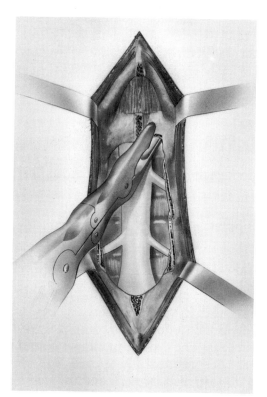

Figure 13–2. For decompression of spinal stenosis the lamina and ligamentum flavum are completely removed. The lateral portions of the facet joints are preserved if possible to retain the structural integrity and stability of the spine. With removal of the fifth and fourth laminae, and a portion of the third lamina, the surgeon should be able to inspect the L4, L5, and S1 nerve roots bilaterally without difficulty. (From Rothman RH, Simeone FA: The Spine, 2nd ed. Philadelphia, W.B. Saunders, 1982.)

SPINAL FUSION/INSTRUMENTATION

Precise indications for a spinal fusion with or without instrumentation have not been established. Fusion should be strongly considered for the following indications: (1) the presence of surgical instability created during decompression with removal of more than 50 percent of each facet joint at any level; (2) the presence of neural arch defects (spondylolysis); and (3) the presence of symptomatic and radiographically demonstrable segmental instability identified on weight-bearing lateral flexion-extension radiographs. In general, the number of levels included in a fusion should be minimized, since preservation of motion segments is desirable and since the incidence of nonunion increases substantially with each additional level fused.

Spinal fusion can be accomplished through the anterior, the posterior, or both approaches. Generally, corticocancellous bone from the patient's own iliac crest yields the best fusion results. There are a host of appliances available to reduce spinal deformity or to add immediate stability to the unstable spine as bony fusion progresses. The specific indications for augmentative instrumentation are controversial; they include reoperation in the multiply operated back, pseudarthrosis of a prior fusion, and previous failed instrumentation.

COMPLICATIONS

Trauma to the great vessels, as well as other visceral structures, can occur from penetration of the anterior portion of the annulus fibrosus by a surgical instrument during disc excision. Tears of the dura may occur during laminectomy, especially with tight spinal stenosis. Nerve roots may be injured from excessive retraction, laceration, or thermal burns from cautery. Damage to the cauda equina and nerve roots may occur if the surgery involves reduction of a deformity, as is sometimes done with severe spondylolisthesis.

Postoperative complications include pulmonary atelectasis, intestinal ileus, urinary retention, wound infection, thrombophlebitis, and cauda equina syndrome. Technical complications resulting in persistent symptoms may be related to inadequate nerve root decompression, fibrosis around the nerve roots and dura, disc space infection, or subarachnoid cysts. When instrumentation is used, hook/screw pull-out or breakage can result in loss of position and subsequent neurologic injury.

The frequency of these complications can be minimized by meticulous surgical technique, careful attention to anatomy, and awareness of early signs in the postoperative period. When they do occur, many of these problems constitute the genesis of the multiply operated low back, which is discussed in Chapter 14. Since no surgery is without the risk of complications, we cannot overstress the importance of proper surgical indications. There is nothing worse than surgical complications from a procedure that was not clearly indicated.

References

1. Cares HL, Steinberg RS, Robertson ET, et al: Ambulatory microsurgery for ruptured lumbar discs: Report of ten cases. Neurosurgery 22:523–526, 1988.
2. Dabezies EJ, Beck C, Shoji H: Chymopapain in perspective. Clin Orthop 206:10–14, 1986.
3. Dabezies EJ, Langford K, Morris J, et al: Safety and efficacy of chymopapain (Discase) in the treatment of sciatica due to a herniated nucleus pulposus: Results of a randomized, double-blind study. Spine 13:561–565, 1988.
4. Davis GW, Onik G: Clinical experience with automated percutaneous lumbar discectomy. Clin Orthop 238:98–103, 1989.
5. Day AL, Savage DF, Friedman WA, et al: Chemonucleolysis versus open discectomy: The case against chymopapain. Clin Neurosurg 33:385–397, 1986.
6. Edwards WC, Orme TJ, Orr-Edwards G: CT discography: Prognostic value in the selection of patients for chemonucleolysis. Spine 12:792–795, 1987.
7. Fager CA: Lumbar microdiscectomy: A contrary opinion. Clin Neurosurg 33:419–456, 1986.
8. Fraser RD: Chymopapain for the treatment of intervertebral disc herniation: The final report of a double-blind study. Spine 9:815–818, 1984.
9. Friedman WA: Percutaneous discectomy: An alternative to chemonucleolysis? Neurosurgery 13:542–547, 1983.
10. Frymoyer JW: Back pain and sciatica. N Engl J Med 318:291–300, 1988.
11. Garfin SK, Glover M, Booth RE, et al: Laminectomy: A review of the Pennsylvania Hospital experience. J Spinal Dis 1:116–133, 1988.
12. Ghelman B, Muari TM, Jacobs B: The role of CT/discography in chemonucleolysis. Contemp Orthop 6:43–49, 1988.
13. Hanley EN, Levy JA: Surgical treatment of isthmic lumbosacral spondylolisthesis. Analysis of variables influencing results. Spine 14:48–50, 1989.
14. Hill GM, Ellis EA: Chemonucleolysis as an alternative to laminectomy for the herniated lumbar disc: Experience with patients in a private orthopedic practice. Clin Orthop 225:229–233, 1987.
15. Kahanovitz N, Dorsky S, Verderame R: The role of discography as a prognostic indicator of chemonucleolysis. Contemp Orthop 17:37–40, 1988.
16. Kahanovitz N, Viola K, Muculloch J: Limited surgical discectomy and microdiscectomy. A clinical comparison. Spine 14:79–81, 1989.
17. Kambin P, Gellman H: Percutaneous lateral discectomy of the lumbar spine: A preliminary report. Clin Orthop 174:127–132, 1983.
18. Kambin P, Schaffer JL: Percutaneous lumbar discectomy. Review of 100 patients and current practice. Clin Orthop 238:24–34, 1989.
19. Maistrelli GL, Vaughn PA, Evans DC, et al: Lumbar disc herniation in the elderly. Spine 12:63–66, 1987.
20. Maroon JC, Abla A: Microdiscectomy versus chemonucleolysis. Neurosurgery 16:644–649, 1985.
21. Maroon JC, Abla A: Microlumbar discectomy. Clin Neurosurg 33:407–417, 1986.
22. Merz B: The honeymoon is over: Spinal surgeons begin to divorce themselves from chemonucleolysis. JAMA 256:317–318, 1986.
23. Mixter WJ, Barr JS: Rupture of the intervertebral disc with involvement of the spinal canal. N Engl J Med 211:210–214, 1934.
24. Nachemson AL, Rydevik B: Chemonucleolysis for sciatica: A critical review. Acta Orthop Scand 59:56–62, 1988.
25. Nasca RJ: Rationale for spinal fusion in lumbar spinal stenosis. Spine 14:451–454, 1989.
26. Norton WL: Chemonucleolysis versus surgical discectomy: Comparison of costs and results in workers' compensation claimants. Spine 11:440–443, 1986.
27. Nystrom B: Experience of microsurgical compared with conventional technique in lumbar disc operations. Acta Neurol Scand 76:129–141, 1987.
28. Onik G, Maroon J, Helms C, et al: Automated percutaneous diskectomy: Initial patient experience. Radiology 162:129–132, 1987.
29. Postacchini F, Lami R, Massobrio M: Chemonucleolysis versus surgery in lumbar disc herniations: Correlation of the results to preoperative clinical pattern and size of the herniation. Spine 12:87–96, 1987.
30. Rogers LA: Experience with limited versus extensive disc removal in patients undergoing microsurgical operations for ruptured lumbar discs. Neurosurgery 22:82–85, 1988.

31. Sachdev VF: Microsurgical lumbar discectomy: A personal series of 300 patients with at least 1 year of follow-up. Microsurgery 7:55–62, 1986.
32. Schreiber A, Suezawa Y, Leu H: Does percutaneous nucleotomy with discoscopy replace conventional discectomy? Eight years of experience and results in treatment of herniated lumbar disc. Clin Orthop 238:35–42, 1989.
33. Schutz H, Watson CP: Microsurgical discectomy: A prospective study of 200 patients. Can J Neurol Sci 14:81–83, 1987.
34. Schwartz AM, Brodkey JS: Bowel perforation following microsurgical lumbar discectomy. A case report. Spine 13:104–105, 1988.
35. Shields CB: In defense of chemonucleolysis. Clin Neurosurg 33:397–405, 1986.
36. Thomas AM, Afshar F: The microsurgical treatment of lumbar disc protrusion. J Bone Joint Surg 69B:696–698, 1987.
37. Weber H: Lumbar disc herniation: A controlled, prospective study with ten years of observation. Spine 8:131–140, 1983.
38. Weinstein JN, Lehmann TR, Hejna W, et al: Chemonucleolysis versus open discectomy: A ten-year follow-up study. Clin Orthop 206:50–55, 1986.
39. Weinstein J, Spratt KF, Lehmann T, et al: Lumbar disc herniation: A comparison of the results of chemonucleolysis and open discectomy after ten years. J Bone Joint Surg 68A:43–54, 1986.
40. Williams RW: Microlumbar discectomy: A 12-year statistical review. Spine 11:851–852, 1986.
41. Zieger HE: Comparison of chemonucleolysis and microsurgical discectomy for the treatment of herniated lumbar disc. Spine 12:796–799, 1987.

CHAPTER 14

The Multiply Operated Low Back Patient

Unfortunately, low back surgery is not always successful. The patient who has undergone one or more back operations and continues to have significant discomfort is becoming an ever-increasing problem. It is estimated that 300,000 new laminectomies are performed each year in the United States alone and that 15 percent of these patients will continue to be disabled.[38] The inherent complexity of these cases, especially when confounded by the degeneration of the aging spine, necessitates a method of problem solving that is precise and unambiguous.

The best possible solution for preventing recurrent symptoms after spine surgery is to prevent inappropriate surgery whenever possible.[15,34,39] It cannot be overstressed that proper surgical indications must be present before surgery is undertaken. The idea of "exploring" the low back when the necessary objective criteria are not met is no longer acceptable. In fact, even when there are objective findings, if the patient is psychologically unstable or there are compensation-litigation factors, the outcome of low back surgery is uncertain.[34] Thus, the initial decision to operate is the most important one. Once the situation of recurrent pain after surgery arises, the potential for a solution is limited at best.

In the evaluation of recurrent symptoms following surgery, the problem confronting the physician is to distinguish mechanical and nonmechanical causes. The types of mechanical lesions include recurrent herniated disc, spinal instability, and spinal stenosis. These three entities produce symptoms by causing direct pressure on the neural elements and are amenable to surgical intervention. The nonmechanical entities consist of scar tissue (either arachnoiditis or epidural fibrosis), psychosocial instability, or systemic medical disease. These problems will not be helped by any type of additional lumbar spine surgery.

The keystone of successful treatment is to obtain an accurate diagnosis. Although seemingly obvious, this essential step often is not taken. Consequently, the rehabilitation of this patient group has been fraught with difficulty. The goals of this chapter are to analyze the significant decision points in the evaluation of the multiply operated lumbar spine patient and to organize this information into a standardized approach for efficiently obtaining an accurate diagnosis.

PATIENT EVALUATION

When a multiply operated back patient first arrives for evaluation, it is important to obtain all the vital information in an organized manner. Use of a standardized approach may lessen the chance of missing significant details. This is important, for these patients are usually difficult to evaluate.

The evaluation of the multiply operated low back patient must begin with the history, which can be quite involved. Many patients want to relate their entire story to the evaluating physician, and it is best to let them do so. After the patient finishes talking, however, there are three specific historical points that must be elucidated.

The first is the number of previous lumbar spine operations that the patient has undergone. It has been shown that with every subsequent operation, regardless of the diagnosis, the likelihood of good results diminishes. Statistically, the second operation has a 50 percent chance of success, and beyond two operations, patients are more likely to be made worse than better.[11,39]

The next important historical point is the length of the pain-free interval following the patient's previous operation. If the patient awoke from surgery with pain still present, it is likely that the nerve root may not have been properly decompressed or the wrong level was explored. If the pain-free interval was at least 6 months, the patient's recent pain may be caused by recurrent disc herniation at the same or a different level. If the pain-free interval was between 1 and 6 months and recurrent symptoms had a gradual onset, the diagnosis most often is some type of scar tissue, either arachnoiditis or epidural fibrosis.[11]

Finally, the patient's pain pattern must be evaluated. If leg pain predominates, a herniated disc or spinal stenosis is most likely, although scar tissue is also a possibility. If back pain is the major component, instability, tumor, infection, and scar tissue are the major considerations. If both back and leg pain are present, spinal stenosis and/or scar tissue are the likely possibilities. Nonmechanical pain, especially in older patients, may be the harbinger of an infectious, neoplastic, or referred process unrelated to the original low back pain.

Physical examination is the next major step in the evaluation of the multiply operated back patient. The neurologic findings and existence of a tension sign, such as a positive sitting straight leg raising test, must be noted. It is helpful to have the results of a dependable previous examination so a comparison between the preoperative and postoperative states can be made. If the neurologic picture is unchanged from before the previous surgery and the tension sign is negative, mechanical compression is unlikely. If, however, a new neurologic deficit has occurred since the last surgery or the tension sign is positive, pressure on the neural elements is possible. However, one must realize that epidural or perineural fibrosis can cause a positive tension sign; the tension sign is not pathognomonic of a mechanical lesion in these patients.

Roentgenographic studies are the last major part of the patient's work-up. It is most helpful to have the results of prior studies for comparison of the pre- and postoperative situations. Often, careful analysis may reveal that the initial operation was not indicated. Since the various imaging modalities were outlined in an earlier chapter, the following discussion will be limited to specific applications of these techniques in evaluating the multiply operated low back patient.

Imaging Modalities

The *plain radiographs* must be evaluated for the extent and level of previous laminectomies and for any evidence of spinal stenosis. It should not be taken for granted that the correct level was decompressed; the laminectomy level on the plain film must correspond to the level on the preoperative radiographic studies, to the level described in the operative report, and to the neurologic findings demonstrated by the patient. The standing (weight-bearing) lateral flexion-extension films must be assessed for any evidence of abnormal motion; this will be discussed in detail in the section on Lumbar Instability.

Metrizamide myelography is of limited value in the multiply operated back patient with chronic back pain.[14] While this test can identify extradural compressions, myelography cannot distinguish between disc material and epidural scar.[6] The major remaining use of myelography in these patients is for confirmation of arachnoiditis when the diagnosis is otherwise uncertain. Computed tomographic (CT) scanning with metrizamide in the subarachnoid space is also a sensitive test for demonstrating the changes of arachnoiditis.[6]

Computed tomography (CT) is perhaps the most valuable procedure for evaluating the multiply operated back patient.[6] The size of the spinal canal, surgical deficits, and hypertrophied bony changes causing stenosis are visualized.[35] Intravenous contrast enhancement has significantly increased the diagnostic accuracy of CT differentiation of recurrent disc herniation and postoperative scar from 43 to 74 percent.[2,33] A herniated disc is avascular and will not enhance (light up) immediately after the injection of intravenous contrast material; scar tissue, on the other hand, is vascular and will enhance on the scan.[2,32] On delayed scans, there may be some enhancement of the discs, which appears to be a normal finding. CT may also be effective in the early diagnosis of discitis; hypodensity of the affected disc space may be detected as early as 10 days postoperatively.[21] With intravenous contrast enhancement, discitis will cause intense enhancement of the entire disc.[36] Finally, it has been reported that postoperative arachnoiditis may appear as a localized thickening of the dural sac on the CT scan. The exact sensitivity and specificity of CT for diagnosis of these entities remain unknown.

Magnetic resonance imaging (MRI) is just beginning to emerge as a useful diagnostic tool in these complicated multiply operated patients.[16,28] To distinguish recurrent disc herniation from epidural scar, MRI has been shown to have 100 percent sensitivity, 71 percent specificity, and 89 percent accuracy.[3,18] With the administration of an intravenous paramagnetic contrast material (gadolinium-diethylenetriaminopenta-acetic acid/dimeglutamine [Gd-DTPA]), the diagnostic accuracy increased to 100 percent in a surgically and histologically confirmed series.[18] In a study of the diagnosis of lumbar arachnoiditis verified by myelography and CT myelography, MRI demonstrated excellent sensitivity and specificity (92 and 100 percent, respectively).[29] MRI is also extremely sensitive in identifying inflammatory processes such as discitis, which demonstrates a decreased signal intensity on T1-weighted images.[45]

One potential drawback of MRI in postoperative patients is the problem of artifacts created by metal shards from suction devices used during surgery; the use of plastic suction tips could avoid this complication. As further experience with MRI is acquired, this imaging modality will likely be the most accurate diagnostic tool for differentiating the various postoperative soft tissue lesions. However, its sensitivity for bony encroachment must be evaluated further before it can obviate the need for CT scanning.

DIAGNOSTIC ALGORITHM

The primary goal of the evaluation of the multiply operated back patient is to efficiently arrive at the correct diagnosis. The most common lesions accounting for failed back surgery syndrome include recurrent or persistent disc herniation (12 to 16%), lateral (58%) or central (7 to 14%) stenosis, arachnoiditis (6 to 16%), epidural fibrosis (6 to 8%), and instability (<5%).[5] The various pathologic entities with their associated signs, symptoms, and radiographic findings are summarized in Table 14–1. A graphic display of the same data is presented in Figure 14–1 in the form of an algorithm. As new technology is introduced and more knowledge is gained, many of the decision-making steps in the algorithm may change.

The first step in the algorithm is to determine if the patient's complaint is based on a nonorthopedic cause such as pancreatitis, diabetes, or an abdominal aneurysm. Thus, a thorough general medical examination should be obtained routinely. In addition, if there is any indication of psychosocial instability, evidenced by alcoholism, drug dependence, depression, or of compensation/litigation involvement, a thorough psychiatric evaluation is necessary. It has been clearly demonstrated that persons with profound emotional disturbances and those involved in litigation rarely derive any observable benefit from additional surgery.[31] Even if an orthopedic diagnosis is made, the psychosocial problem should be addressed first. In many cases, once a patient's underlying psychosocial problem has been treated successfully, the somatic back complaints and disability will disappear.

Once the patients with medical and psychosocial problems are identified and separated, the physician is left with a group that has back and/or leg pain. The goal is then to separate those patients with specific mechanical problems from those whose symptoms are secondary to some form of scar tissue or inflammation. The former may benefit from additional surgery; the latter will not. It must be stressed that the incidence of surgically correctable problems is much lower than that of scar tissue.

Herniated Intervertebral Disc

Three possibilities exist if the patient's pain is caused by a herniated disc. First, the disc that caused the original symptoms may not have been satisfactorily removed. This can happen if the wrong level was decompressed; the laminectomy performed was not adequate to free the neural elements; or a fragment of disc material was left behind. Such patients will continue to have pain because of mechanical pressure on and irritation of the same nerve root that caused their initial symptoms. They will complain predominantly of leg pain, and their neurologic findings, tension signs, and radiographic patterns will remain unchanged from the preoperative state. The distinguishing feature is that they will report no pain-free interval; they will have awakened from the operation complaining of the same preoperative pain. Patients in this group will be aided by a technically correct laminectomy.

A second possibility is that there is a recurrent herniated intervertebral disc at the previously decompressed level. These patients complain of sciatica and have unchanged neurologic findings, tension signs, and radiographic studies. The distinguishing characteristic here is a pain-free interval of greater than 6 months. Another operative procedure is indicated in these patients provided that contrast-enhanced CT or MRI can demonstrate herniated disc material rather than just scar tissue.

Finally, a herniated disc can occur at a completely different level. Such patients generally will suffer sudden onset of recurrent pain after a pain-free interval of more than 6 months. Sciatica predominates and tension signs are positive. However, a neurologic deficit, if present, and the radiographic signs will be seen at a different level than on the original studies. A repeat operation for these patients will be beneficial.

Table 14–1. DIFFERENTIAL DIAGNOSIS OF THE MULTIPLY OPERATED BACK

History, Physical, Radiographs	Original Disc Not Removed	Recurrent Disc at Same Level	Recurrent Disc at Different Level	Spinal Instability	Spinal Stenosis	Arachnoiditis	Epidural Scar Tissue	Discitis
Pain-free interval	None	>6 months	>6 months			>1 month but <6 months	>1 month, gradual onset	
Predominant pain leg vs. back	Leg pain	Leg pain	Leg pain	Back pain	Back and leg pain	Back and leg pain	Back and/or leg pain	Back pain
Tension sign	+	+	+			May be positive	May be positive	
Neurologic examination	+Same pattern	+Same pattern	+Different level		+After stress			
Plain films	+Wrong level				+			±
Lateral motion films				+				
Metrizamide myelogram	+But unchanged	+Same level	+Different level		+	+	+	
CT scan	+	+	+		+	+	+ (IV contrast)	+ (IV contrast)
MRI	+	+	+		+	+	+ (Gadolinium contrast)	+

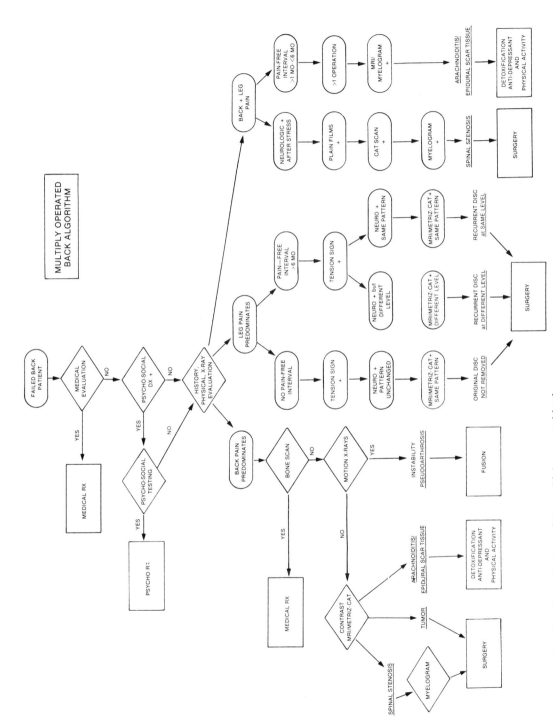

Figure 14-1. Algorithm for evaluation of the multiply operated back.

Lumbar Instability

Lumbar instability is another condition causing pain on a mechanical basis in the multiply operated back patient. Instability is the abnormal or excessive movement of one vertebra on another causing pain. The etiology may be the patient's intrinsic back disease or an excessively wide bilateral laminectomy.[17,19] Pseudarthrosis resulting from a failed spinal fusion is included in this category, since the pain is caused by the instability created by the failed fusion.

Patients with instability will complain predominantly of back pain and their physical examinations may be negative. Sometimes, the key to diagnosis of these patients is the weight-bearing lateral flexion-extension film; however, it is often difficult to precisely define the anatomic origin of back pain in the presence of radiographic instability. Relative flexion-sagittal plane translation of more than 8 percent of the anteroposterior diameter of the vertebral body, or a relative flexion-sagittal plane rotation of more than 9° between segments, are the most commonly cited guidelines for instability of the lumbar spine.[26,40] At the lumbosacral junction the criteria are slightly different: relative translation of more than 6 percent or rotation of more than −1° is significant. These criteria are based on maximum displacements on a single flexion or extension view; however, calculation of relative dynamic translation and rotation from flexion to extension may prove to be a more reliable indication of true instability.[1]

Unfortunately, there is little information to explain why some patients with segmental instability develop back pain while others do not. If there is radiographic evidence of instability in symptomatic patients, spinal fusion (or repair of the pseudarthrosis) may be considered.[20] Additional confirmatory evidence to determine the precise level of origin of the patient's symptoms may be gathered from facet injections and discography; however, these tests have a substantial rate of false positive results.[14]

Spinal Stenosis

Spinal stenosis in the multiply operated back patient can mechanically produce both back and leg pain. The etiology may be secondary to progression of the patient's inherent degenerative spine disease, a previous inadequate decompression, or overgrowth of a previous posterior fusion. The physical examination is often inconclusive, although a neurologic deficit may occur following exercise; with reproduction of the patient's symptoms this phenomenon is termed a positive stress test.

The plain films can be suggestive and may display facet degeneration, decreased interpedicular distance, decreased sagittal canal diameter, or disc degeneration. A CT scan will demonstrate bony encroachment upon the neural elements; this is especially helpful in evaluating the lateral recesses and neural foraminae. A metrizamide myelogram or MRI will show compression of the dural sac at the involved levels. It should be appreciated that spinal stenosis and scar tissue can co-exist.[10] Good results can be expected from surgery in at least 70 percent of properly selected cases, but if there has been a previous laminectomy and spinal fusion, surgery will be less successful.[24] If there is definite evidence of bony compression, a laminectomy is indicated; however, if substantial scar tissue is present, the degree of pain relief the patient can anticipate is uncertain.

Arachnoiditis, Epidural Scar Tissue, and Discitis

Scar tissue (arachnoiditis or epidural fibrosis) and discitis are nonmechanical causes of recurrent pain in the multiply operated back patient. While the etiologies and specific locations of these lesions are different, they are discussed in the same section because none of them will respond to another surgical procedure.

Postoperative scar tissue can be divided into two main types based on anatomic location. Scar tissue that occurs beneath the dura is commonly referred to as arachnoiditis. Scar tissue can also form extradurally, either directly on the cauda equina or around a nerve root.

Arachnoiditis is strictly defined as an inflammation of the pia-arachnoid membrane surrounding the spinal cord or cauda equina.[4] The condition may be present in varying degrees of severity, from mild thickening of the membranes to solid adhesions. The scarring may be severe enough to obliterate the subarachnoid space and block the flow of contrast agents.

This condition has been attributed to many factors: lumbar spine surgery and previous injections of contrast material seem to be the most frequent precipitating factors.[27] Postoperative infection may also play a role in the pathogenesis. The exact mechanism by which arachnoiditis develops from these events is not clear.[7,10]

There is no uniform clinical presentation for arachnoiditis. Statistically, the history will reveal more than one previous operation and a pain-free interval of between 1 and 6 months. Often these patients will complain of back and leg pain. Physical examination is not conclusive; alterations in neurologic status may be due to a previous operation. As mentioned earlier, myelography, CT, and MRI can be helpful in confirming the diagnosis.

At present there is no effective treatment for arachnoiditis. Surgical intervention has not proven effective in eliminating the scar tissue or significantly reducing the pain. Along with much needed encouragement, there are various nonoperative measures which can be employed.[4,7,9,13,23,25,30,37] Epidural steroids, transcutaneous nerve stimulation, spinal cord stimulation, operant conditioning, bracing, and patient education have all been tried. None of these will lead to a complete cure, but when used judiciously they can provide symptomatic relief for varying periods of time. Patients should be detoxified from all narcotics, placed on amitriptyline (Elavil), and encouraged to do as much physical activity as possible. Treating these patients is a challenge, and the physician must be willing to devote time and patience to achieve optimal results.

Formation of scar tissue outside the dura on the cauda equina or directly on nerve roots is a relatively common occurrence.[31] This *epidural scar tissue* acts as a constrictive force about the neural elements and frequently can cause postoperative pain. However, although most patients have some epidural scar tissue, only an unpredictable few become symptomatic.

Patients with epidural scarring may present with symptoms from several months to a year or two after surgery. They may complain of back pain, leg pain, or both. Commonly there are no new neurologic findings, but there may be a positive tension sign purely on the basis of scar formation around a nerve root. Epidural fibrosis is best differentiated from a recurrent herniated disc using contrast-enhanced CT or gadolinium-enhanced MRI.

As with arachnoiditis, there is no definitive treatment for epidural scar tissue. Prevention may be the best answer, and a free fat graft is sometimes used as an interposition membrane to minimize epidural scar tissue following laminectomy.[22] Use of too thick a fat graft may result in absorption of blood and swelling of the graft; there have been anecdotal reports of postoperative cauda equina syndrome associated with large fat grafts. Once scar has formed, surgery is not successful because scarring will often re-form in greater quantity. The treatment program should be similar to that already described for arachnoiditis.

Discitis is an uncommon but debilitating complication of lumbar disc surgery. Its pathogenesis is postulated to be direct inoculation of the avascular disc space but is not completely understood.[8] The onset of symptoms usually occurs about 1 month following surgery, and most patients will complain of severe back pain. Physical examination will sometimes reveal fever, a positive tension sign, and, occasionally, a superficial abscess.

If discitis is suspected from the history and physical examination, an erythrocyte sedimentation rate, blood cultures, and plain radiographs should be obtained. Plain films may not demonstrate the changes of disc space narrowing and end-plate erosion in the early stages. Contrast-enhanced CT or MRI should confirm the diagnosis.

Effective treatment has been controversial.[8] The authors recommend placing the patient at bedrest acutely with immobilization of the lumbar spine using a brace or corset. If the patient experiences progressive pain after adequate immobilization or has constitutional symptoms, a needle aspiration biopsy should be performed. If a bacterial organism is identified, 6 weeks of intravenous antibiotics is indicated. There is no need for open disc space biopsy provided the patient responds to conservative therapy. With improvement of symptoms and laboratory findings the patient may ambulate as tolerated.

Summary

In conclusion, it should be stressed that the physician must take an organized approach to evaluation of the multiply operated low back patient. The origin of the problem in many cases is the faulty decision to perform the original surgical procedure. Further surgery on an "exploratory" basis is not warranted and will lead only to further disability. Another operative procedure is indicated only when there are objective findings.

The etiology of each patient's complaint must be accurately localized and identified. In addition to the orthopedic evaluation, the patient's psychosocial and general medical status need thorough investigation. Once the spine is identified as the source of the patient's symptoms, specific findings should be sought in the patient's clinical history, physical examination, and radiographic studies. The number of previous operations, length of the pain-free interval, and predominance of leg pain versus back pain are the major historical points. The most important aspects of the physical examination are the neurologic findings and the presence of a tension sign. Plain radiographs, motion films, CT, and MRI all have specific roles in the work-up. When all of the information is integrated, the physician usually can separate the patients with arachnoiditis, epidural scarring, and discitis from those with mechanical problems of the spine.

Those involved with treatment of the multiply operated low back patient must realize that the likelihood of returning these patients to any kind of heavy work or activity is low. Almost all patients will have some permanent disability, the extent depending on the type of previous surgery and the patient's active complaints. Those patients still working need job retraining as quickly as possible, and the remainder must be strongly encouraged to resume a functional role in society.

References

1. Boden SD, Wiesel SW: Lumbosacral segmental motion in normal individuals. Spine 15:571–576, 1990.
2. Braun IF, Hoffman JC, Davis PC, et al: Contrast enhancement in CT differentiation between recurrent disk herniation and postoperative scar: A prospective study. AJNR 6:607–612, 1985.
3. Bundschuh CV, Modic MT, Ross JS, et al: Epidural fibrosis and recurrent disk herniation in the lumbar spine: MR imaging assessment. AJR 150:923–932, 1988.
4. Burton CV: Lumbosacral arachnoiditis. Spine 3:24–30, 1978.
5. Burton CV, Kirkaldy-Willis WH, Yong-Hing K, et al: Causes of failure of surgery on the lumbar spine. Clin Orthop 157:191–199, 1981.
6. Byrd SE, Cohn ML, Biggers SL, et al: The radiographic evaluation of the symptomatic postoperative lumbar spine patient. Spine 10:652–661, 1985.
7. Coventry MB, Stauffer RN: The multiply operated back. In American Academy of Orthopaedic Surgeons: Symposium on the Spine. St. Louis, C.V. Mosby, 1969, pp. 132–142.
8. Dall BE, Rowe DE, Odette WG, et al: Postoperative discitis: Diagnosis and management. Clin Orthop 224:138–148, 1987.
9. De La Porte C, Siegfried J: Lumbosacral spinal fibrosis (spinal arachnoiditis): Its diagnosis and treatment by spinal cord stimulation. Spine 8:593–603, 1983.
10. Epstein BS: The Spine. Philadelphia, Lea & Febiger, 1962.
11. Finnegan WJ, Tenlin JM, Marvel JP, et al: Results of surgical intervention in the symptomatic multiply-operated back patient. J Bone Joint Surg 61A:1077–1082, 1979.
12. Gabriel KR, Crawford AH: Magnetic resonance imaging in a child who had clinical signs of discitis. J Bone Joint Surg 70A:938–941, 1988.

13. Ghormley RK: The problem of multiple operations on the back. In American Academy of Orthopaedic Surgeons Instructional Course Lectures, Vol. XIV. Ann Arbor, MI, J.W. Edwards, 1957, p. 56.
14. Grubb SA, Lipscomb HJ, Gilford WB: The relative value of lumbar roentgenograms, metrizamide myelography, and discography in the assessment of patients with chronic low-back syndrome. Spine 12:282–286, 1987.
15. Hirsch C: Efficiency of surgery in low back disorders. J Bone Joint Surg 47A:991–1004, 1965.
16. Hochhauser L, Kieffer SA, Cacayorin ED, et al: Recurrent postdiskectomy low back pain: MR-surgical correlation. AJNR 9:769–774, 1988.
17. Hopp E, Tsou PM: Postdecompression lumbar instability. Clin Orthop 227:143–151, 1988.
18. Hueftle MG, Modic MT, Ross JS, et al: Lumbar spine: Postoperative MR imaging with Gd-DTPA. Radiology 167:817–824, 1988.
19. Johnsson KE, Willner S, Johnsson K: Postoperative instability after decompression for lumbar spinal stenosis. Spine 11:107–110, 1986.
20. Laasonen EM, Soini J: Low-back pain after lumbar fusion. Surgical and computed tomographic analysis. Spine 14:210–213, 1989.
21. Lahde S, Puranen J: Disk-space hypodensity in CT: The first radiological signs of postoperative diskitis. Europ J Radiol 5:190–192, 1985.
22. Langenskydd A, Kiviluoto O: Prevention of epidural scar formation after operations on the lumbar spine by means of free fat transplants. Clin Orthop 115:92–95, 1976.
23. Mooney V: Innovative approaches to chronic back disability. American Academy of Orthopaedic Surgeons Instructional Course Lecture. Dallas, 1974.
24. Nasca RJ: Surgical management of lumbar spinal stenosis. Spine 12:809–816, 1987.
25. Oudenhover RC: The role of laminectomy, facet rhizotomy and epidural steroids. Spine 4:145–147, 1979.
26. Posner I, White AA, Edwards WT, et al: A biomechanical analysis of the clinical stability of the lumbar and lumbosacral spine. Spine 7:374–389, 1982.
27. Quiles M, Marchisello PJ, Tsairis P: Lumbar adhesive arachnoiditis: Etiologic and pathologic aspects. Spine 3:45–50, 1978.
28. Ross JS, Masaryk TJ, Modic MT, et al: Lumbar spine: Postoperative assessment with surface-coil MR imaging. Radiology 164:851–860, 1987.
29. Ross JS, Masaryk TJ, Modic MT, et al: MR imaging of lumbar arachnoiditis. AJNR 8:885–892, 1987.
30. Rothman RH: Indications for lumbar fusion. Clin Neurosurg 71:215–219, 1973.
31. Rothman RH, Simeone FA: The Spine, 2nd ed. Philadelphia, W.B. Saunders, 1982.
32. Schubiger O, Valavanis A: CT differentiation between recurrent disc herniation and postoperative scar formation: The value of contrast enhancement. Neuroradiology 22:251–254, 1982.
33. Sotiropoulos S, Chafetz NI, Lang P, et al: Differentiation between postoperative scar and recurrent disk herniation: Prospective comparison of MR, CT, and contrast-enhanced CT. Am J Neuroradiol 10:639–643, 1989.
34. Spengler DM, Freeman DW: Patient selection for lumbar discectomy: An objective approach. Spine 4:129–134, 1979.
35. Teplick JG, Haskin ME: CT of the postoperative lumbar spine. Radiol Clin North Am 21:395–420, 1983.
36. Teplick JG, Haskin ME: Intravenous contrast-enhanced CT of the postoperative lumbar spine: Improved identification of recurrent disk herniation, scar, arachnoiditis, and diskitis. AJR 143:845–855, 1984.
37. Tibodeau AA: Management of the problem postoperative back. J Bone Joint Surg 55A:1766, 1973.
38. Waddell G: Failures of disc surgery and repeat surgery. Acta Orthop Belg 53:300–302, 1987.
39. Waddell G, Kummel EG, Lotto WN, et al: Failed lumbar disc surgery and repeat surgery following industrial injuries. J Bone Joint Surg 61A:201–207, 1979.
40. White AA, Panjabi MM, Posner I, et al: Spinal stability: Evaluation and treatment. American Academy of Orthopaedic Surgeons Instructional Course Lectures, Vol. XXX. St. Louis, C.V. Mosby, 1981, pp. 457–483.

Infectious, Neoplastic, Metabolic, and Rheumatologic Disease

CHAPTER 15

Infections of the Spine

Spinal infections can lead to catastrophic complications if not promptly recognized. They are uncommon, but must be included in the differential diagnosis of the patient with back or neck pain. If they are recognized early and treated appropriately, the prognosis is generally excellent. However, should the diagnosis be overlooked, spinal deformity and spinal cord compression with associated paralysis can occur. This chapter briefly reviews the pertinent anatomy and then discusses intervertebral disc space infections, vertebral osteomyelitis, and tuberculosis of the spine.

ANATOMIC CONSIDERATIONS

Spine infections are most likely secondary to hematogenous spread.[2,37] The vascular anatomy is similar in the cervical, thoracic, and lumbar areas. Each vertebral body is supplied by multiple small arterial vessels that branch from the major segmental artery. In addition, at each foramen the posterior spinal artery divides into an ascending and a descending branch. These arteries anastomose with segments above, below, and from the other side to form a network on the posterior surface of each vertebral body. From this network three to four nutrient arteries enter the vertebral body through the central foramen.

The venous drainage of the vertebral body is centered posteriorly and is composed of valveless veins. There are three interconnected systems: direct veins from the vertebral body; veins between the spinal canal and dura; and external veins. Batson felt that this interconnecting system was responsible for the majority of infections. His observations are especially attractive for explaining the association of urinary tract and pelvic infections with vertebral osteomyelitis.[2]

While there are proponents of both the arterial system and the venous system as the major source of spinal infections, there is no conclusive proof for either explanation. All that can be stated at present is that the theory of infections being blood-borne, via either the arterial or venous system, is certainly plausible. Each route is probably involved under certain circumstances.

The blood supply to the intervertebral disc is limited.[8] Small arterial vessels penetrate the disc early in life, but by the third decade these vascular channels have disappeared. The venous drainage of the intervertebral disc is similar to that of the vertebral body. The most likely explanation for primary childhood disc space infections is the direct vascular supply to the disc.[3]

INTERVERTEBRAL DISC SPACE INFECTION

Individuals with primary infections of the disc space can be divided into two major groups based on etiology. One is composed of children, which will be discussed briefly for comparative purposes, and the other consists of patients who have undergone some type of invasive procedure to the disc space.

Disc Space Infections in Children

In children, the intervertebral disc has a generous blood supply, and infections occur as a result of hematogenous spread of organisms. Young children are first seen because of difficulty walking or standing, and frequently they have a history of a recent upper respiratory infection and low grade fever.[36] In contrast, children over 3 years of age may present with abdominal complaints from meningeal irritation or with back pain. Limitation of back motion, localized tenderness, and hamstring muscle tightness are often found. Fever may be present in less than half the cases.

The upper lumbar spine is most commonly involved in these infections.[18] Initial radiographic changes become evident after 3 to 4 weeks and include disc space narrowing, end plate irregularity, and sometimes cavitation. Later, the end plates may become sclerotic with partial restoration of the disc space, and eventually, interbody fusion may occur.

When positive blood culture findings or a biopsy specimen is obtained, *Staphylococcus aureus* is the organism most frequently isolated. Obtaining a positive culture is difficult, and some do not consider this entity to be an infectious process.[26] Biopsy is indicated if the patient fails to respond to treatment or if the diagnosis is uncertain.

Discitis in children is usually a self-limited process with a relatively benign course. The most important aspect of treatment is rest.[9] A body cast or plastic orthosis may supplement bed rest. Antistaphyloccocal antibiotics should be initiated after blood cultures are obtained. Treatment is continued until back pain has resolved. Surgical debridement is only necessary if a paravertebral abscess develops or if there is no response to nonoperative management.

Postoperative Disc Space Infection

Infection due to external violation of the disc is more commonly a complication of surgery, but it has also been reported following needle biopsy, discography, and chemonucleolysis. The incidence following surgery is thought to be between 1 and 3 percent.[23]

Clinical Findings

The patient will complain of severe back pain that may or may not radiate into the legs beginning as early as 5 days or as late as 10 weeks following surgery. Pain can be referred into the lower abdomen, groin, or testes. The pain is exacerbated by movement and relieved by absolute rest. Motion may initiate paroxysms of paravertebral muscle spasm, and the patients usually have great difficulty walking. The pain complaint is out of proportion to the physical findings.

Physical findings include localized tenderness on palpation, limitation of motion of the lumbar spine, and paravertebral muscle spasm. Sensory abnormalities or loss of motor strength suggests spinal cord compression. Temperature elevation is rarely present.

Radiographic Findings

Roentgenographic changes from disc space infections lag behind the onset of symptoms by 2 to 3 weeks.[17] The first change is a decrease in the disc space height (Fig. 15–1). As the disease process advances (beyond the second month), reactive sclerosis of subchondral bone appears in the adjoining vertebral bodies. Next, progressive irregularity of the vertebral end plate develops, indicating local extension of the inflammatory process into the vertebral bone. Attempted repair may occur at any stage of infection and is manifested by bony proliferation about the outside margin of the disc. This new bone may obliterate the disc space, resulting in a bony ankylosis.

As the X-ray may be negative, a bone scan is useful for early diagnosis. It identifies increased bone activity in areas contiguous to the in-

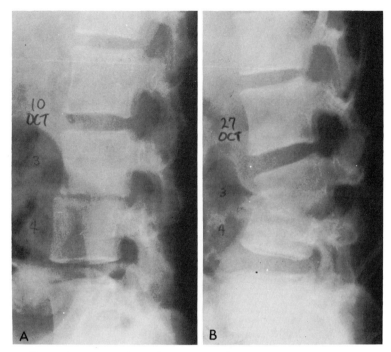

Figure 15–1. *A,* Six-weeks-postoperative patient presents with low back pain. *B.* Two weeks later there is collapse and destruction at L3-4 interspace with a proven staphylococcal infection. (From Wiesel SW, Bernini P, Rothman RH: The Aging Lumbar Spine. Philadelphia, W.B. Saunders, 1982.)

fected discs. In many instances, the bone scan may be positive when radiographs are normal.[19] Magnetic resonance imaging (MRI) will also be diagnostic early in the disease process.

Laboratory Findings

Although it is nonspecific, the erythrocyte sedimentation rate is the most commonly abnormal test, elevated in up to 75 percent of patients. A mild leukocytosis with a normal differential may also be seen. These findings usually follow the onset of clinical symptoms by several days.

Occasionally, blood cultures are positive during the acute phase of the illness. Cultures of needle aspiration samples or fluid obtained at surgery are usually positive. The most frequently cultured organism is *Staphylococcus aureus.* Gram-negative organisms (*Pseudomonas aeruginosa*) are frequently found in intravenous drug abusers.[29,30] Anaerobic organisms have also been found, as have fungal organisms.[21,22]

Differential Diagnosis

The diagnosis of an intervertebral disc infection is often missed because of the nonspecific symptoms and its relative infrequency as a cause of back pain. Physicians should consider this treatable entity in all cases of refractory low back pain. The definitive diagnosis of a disc infection depends upon aspiration or tissue biopsy of the infected site with subsequent confirmation by culture of the causative organism. A bone scan or MR scan may help to identify an infection in the patient who has normal radiographs.

Other disease processes that can demonstrate intervertebral disc narrowing accompanied by lysis or sclerosis of adjacent vertebrae include osteomyelitis of a vertebral body, degenerative disease, neuroarthropathy, and trauma. Primary or metastatic tumor in the spine does not lead to significant loss of intervertebral disc space. An intact disc space with adjacent vertebral body lysis is more characteristic of a tumor than of infection.

Treatment

Therapy of intervertebral disc infections includes antibiotics and immobilization by bedrest, casts, or bracing for a year or longer. Although some clinicians feel that rest is all that is required,[31] most patients receive a 4 to 6 week course of antibiotic therapy. The total treatment time usually is 8 to 10 weeks.[20] The response to treatment is measured by relief of pain, return of the sedimentation rate to normal, and radiographic evidence of disc space restoration or bony ankylosis of adjacent vertebral bodies.

Surgical drainage is not indicated unless there are signs of spinal cord compression or of a paravertebral abscess. An abscess should be considered when a patient's pain does not abate or the sedimentation rate remains elevated despite adequate therapy.

The majority of patients have a benign course and fully recover without disability. However, serious complications have been reported, including hemiplegia and paraplegia.[17]

VERTEBRAL OSTEOMYELITIS

Nontubercular vertebral osteomyelitis can lead to serious consequences for the patient such as paralysis, meningitis, or spinal instability. Thus, it is important to include pyogenic vertebral osteomyelitis in the differential diagnosis of spine lesions. The earlier a spinal infection is diagnosed and treatment is initiated, the better the outcome.

The aging lumbar spine appears to be the most vulnerable area as shown by Eismont and Bohlman's series.[10] In the lumbar spine, the first and second vertebral bodies are commonly affected. The thoracic spine has the second highest frequency of osteomyelitis, followed by the sacrum and cervical spine, in which the disorder occurs with equal frequency.[12] However, the majority of paravertebral abscesses are found in the cervical and thoracic areas.

Origin of Infection

The etiology of vertebral osteomyelitis can be determined in approximately half of the cases.[35] Vertebral body bone is most frequently infected by hematogenous spread. A urinary tract infection is the most common pre-existing focus. Other infectious sources include the skin, the upper respiratory tract, the female genital tract, and the bowel (especially after instrumentation). Iatrogenic infections can occur secondary to closed procedures such as discography or needle biopsy. Finally, any patient with a chronic disease that decreases host immunity such as diabetes mellitus, chronic alcoholism, malignancy, or sickle cell anemia is also at risk of developing vertebral osteomyelitis.

The infectious organisms gain entrance into the vertebral bodies in the subchondral area, which is richly supplied by nutrient arterioles on the anterior surface, and by the main nutrient artery entering through the posterior vertebral nutrient foramen. On occasion, the infection may spread across the periphery of the disc to involve the adjacent vertebra, or may rupture through the end plates into the disc. The infection then spreads through the disc material to reach the opposite end plate and vertebra. The disc material is quickly destroyed by bacterial enzymes. This is in marked contrast to tuberculous infection, which causes bony destruction but little damage to the intervertebral disc.[7]

An infection of a vertebral body may extend beyond the bone into the soft tissues. Infections in the lumbar spine can produce a psoas abscess. The infection may also drain into the spinal canal (causing an epidural abscess) or penetrate the dura (causing meningitis). In addition, bone destruction may cause instability of the spine, which may result in compression of the spinal cord or nerve roots.

Staphylococcus aureus is responsible for 60 percent of adult infections in which positive cultures are obtained. Other possible organisms include *Streptococcus, Escherichia coli, Pseudomonas,* and *Salmonella.* Certain clinical situations are associated with various bacteria. Heroin addicts are prone to infection with gram-negative organisms such as *Pseudomonas* and *E. coli.* Patients with sickle cell disease have a high incidence of *Salmonella* infection, and patients who are immunologically suppressed are more likely to acquire fungal infections.

Clinical Findings

The initial presentation in a patient with vertebral osteomyelitis may be quite varied. A history of a recent primary infection or an invasive diagnostic procedure is common. The two most frequent complaints are fever and the gradual onset of back pain.[27] The pain may be intermittent or constant; it may be present at rest, and is exacerbated by motion. Lower thoracic and lumbar involvement may present as an acute abdomen. In vertebral osteomyelitis secondary to a urinary tract infection, pain and fever may initially be ascribed to the primary infection. Neurologic symptoms including sciatica may be present if there is nerve root irritation.

On physical examination the patient will have a decreased range of motion of the involved spinal region, muscle spasm, and rigidity. Distinct percussion tenderness may be noted over the involved spinous processes. Patients with psoas muscle irritation may demonstrate decreased hip motion along with a flexion contracture. Those with thoracolumbar vertebral osteomyelitis may have abdominal tenderness on palpation. Neurologic abnormalities varying from the subjective complaint of sciatica to complete paraplegia have been reported in a number of series[17,27,29,31]; these may appear suddenly and progress rapidly. The treating physician must be aware of this possibility, since immediate surgical intervention is necessary.

It should be appreciated that many of these patients will have other significant illnesses. The major associated conditions include diabetes mellitus, chronic alcoholism, various forms of malignancy, and drug addiction. The possibility that there may be a combination of a chronic illness and a developing spinal infection should always be kept in mind.

Radiographic Findings

Radiographic changes in vertebral osteomyelitis follow the symptomatic onset of the disease by 2 to 8 weeks.[34] The earliest findings are narrowing of the disc space, superficial end-plate destruction, and paravertebral soft tissue swelling. As the disease progresses, active destruction of the end plate and disc space widening are appreciated (Fig. 15–2). Continued dissemination of infection may produce soft tissue swelling associated with paravertebral abscesses (loss of psoas shadow).

Once the lesion starts to heal, bony regeneration occurs and is characterized by osteosclerosis, which may result in bony fusion across the disc space within 6 to 24 months.

MRI has a high sensitivity for inflammatory processes in soft tissue or bone and can detect infection much earlier than plain films. Computerized tomography is also helpful in visualizing the extent of soft tissue abscesses and provides excellent bony detail. Finally a bone scan demonstrates abnormalities in the area of infection at an earlier stage of disease than does a plain radiograph. A bone scan may also demonstrate areas of involvement other than the one that is symptomatic. Currently the authors' choice, if infection is suspected, is to obtain an MR scan. If this is negative, but the treating physician still suspects that an infection is present, a bone scan should be obtained.

Laboratory Findings

The most consistent abnormal laboratory value is an increased erythrocyte sedimentation rate.[6] The white blood cell count is generally elevated in the young patient (under 20 years of age), but this is not a consistent finding in the older patient.

The best laboratory test for the diagnosis of vertebral osteomyelitis is the blood culture. Blood cultures may be positive in 50 percent of

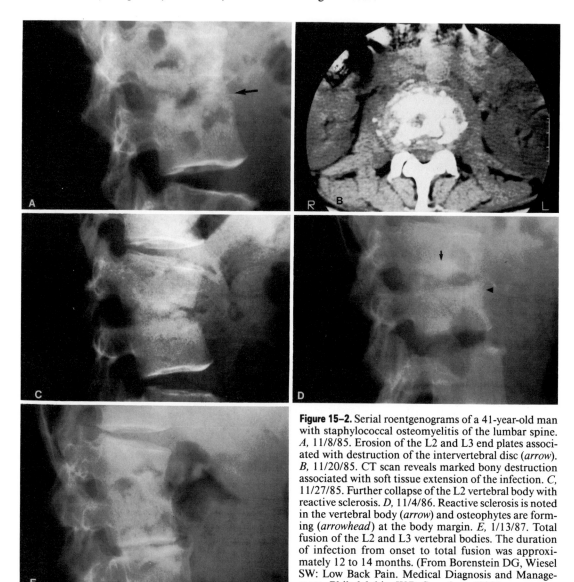

Figure 15–2. Serial roentgenograms of a 41-year-old man with staphylococcal osteomyelitis of the lumbar spine. *A,* 11/8/85. Erosion of the L2 and L3 end plates associated with destruction of the intervertebral disc (*arrow*). *B,* 11/20/85. CT scan reveals marked bony destruction associated with soft tissue extension of the infection. *C,* 11/27/85. Further collapse of the L2 vertebral body with reactive sclerosis. *D,* 11/4/86. Reactive sclerosis is noted in the vertebral body (*arrow*) and osteophytes are forming (*arrowhead*) at the body margin. *E,* 1/13/87. Total fusion of the L2 and L3 vertebral bodies. The duration of infection from onset to total fusion was approximately 12 to 14 months. (From Borenstein DG, Wiesel SW: Low Back Pain. Medical Diagnosis and Management. Philadelphia, W.B. Saunders, 1989.)

patients with acute osteomyelitis. A positive blood culture often obviates the need for bone biopsy. In patients with negative blood cultures, bone aspiration or surgical biopsy is strongly recommended. Percutaneous needle biopsy is safe and, if it produces a positive culture, definitive. If the culture is negative, an open procedure is suggested.

Differential Diagnosis

In any patient who has nonmechanical back pain, the diagnosis of vertebral osteomyelitis must be considered. Since these cases have a great potential for serious complications and the diagnosis can be very elusive, every effort should be made to confirm the presence of infection.

The definitive diagnosis of vertebral osteomyelitis is based upon the recovery and identification of the causative organism most often by needle aspiration or tissue biopsy. Findings on clinical history, physical examination, and laboratory investigation are too nonspecific to assure an accurate diagnosis. Conditions confused with vertebral osteomyelitis include metastatic tumors, multiple myeloma, eosinophilic granuloma, aneurysmal bone cyst, giant cell tumor of bone, and sarcoidosis. In addition, osteomyelitis can occur in bones in the pelvis and may be associated with severe low back pain, abdominal pain, or both.

The diagnosis of vertebral osteomyelitis is reached by careful review of biopsy material. If there is doubt, biopsy must be performed on any lesion of the vertebral body. Only after biopsy is it possible to differentiate osteomyelitis from entities such as myeloma, sarcoidosis, and other neoplasms.

Treatment

Immobilization of the spine is the principal treatment for vertebral osteomyelitis. Simple bedrest is usually adequate; however, some physicians advocate the addition of plaster casts or braces. A well-applied plaster jacket will allow a patient to move more comfortably during the initial treatment period. The main indication for using external immobilization is significant bone destruction or instability.

Appropriate antibiotic therapy is also necessary. It is recommended that patients be treated with parenteral antibiotics for 4 to 6 weeks followed by oral antibiotics for a total of 6 months. The absence of pain and fever and a decrease in the sedimentation rate are the parameters to follow.

Surgical intervention, which includes open biopsy, is indicated when the causative organism is not known, when a paravertebral abscess with any sign of spinal cord compression is present, or when nerve root deficit persists and there is a lack of response to medical treatment. For pyogenic vertebral osteomyelitis, the anterior approach is strongly recommended. A laminectomy is generally contraindicated for two reasons. Since the spinal cord must be manipulated to gain access to the anterior pathologic problem, the result may be further neurologic loss; and removal of the intact posterior vertebral elements may lead to instability. An anterior approach allows adequate debridement, abscess drainage, and decompression of the spinal cord with bone grafting when indicated.

Paraplegia is a disastrous sequel to vertebral osteomyelitis. Any patient with spinal cord involvement deserves a surgical decompression, as there is no clinical means at present to ascertain the degree of irreversible spinal cord damage that is present.

It should be emphasized that patients with vertebral osteomyelitis have a tremendous potential for developing serious complications. Awareness of the problem and a carefully considered approach to the diagnosis and treatment are necessary to properly handle these patients.

TUBERCULOSIS OF THE SPINE

The incidence of tuberculosis in the United States has steadily fallen as adequate housing, proper nutrition, and preventive medical measures have become generally available. Elderly patients, alcoholics, and drug abusers are at greatest risk of developing vertebral osteomyelitis secondary to infection with *Mycobacterium tuberculosis.* Prior to the antibiotic era, children were most frequently affected, but more recent data show that skeletal tuberculosis occurs more commonly in patients in the fifth and sixth decades of life.[4,11] Fifty to sixty percent of patients with skeletal tuberculosis have axial skeletal disease.[13]

Mycobacterium tuberculosis bacilli are strict aerobes, and they will flourish only in areas in which the oxygen tension is high. This is the probable explanation for involvement of the vertebral bodies, which are composed mainly of cancellous bone and have a relatively high oxygen tension. There is some controversy over the exact manner in which the bacilli travel to reach the vertebral bodies, although it is generally accepted that it is by hematogenous routes.

Pathogenesis

There are two forms of tuberculosis infection: primary infection, in which bacilli invade a host that has no specific immunity, and adult tuberculosis, in which bacilli produce disease in the face of specific acquired immunity.[28] Adult tuberculosis is often referred to as reinfection, and there is controversy over its pathogenesis. Two possibilities exist: (1) reactivation of foci implanted at the time of the primary infection, and (2) reinfection arising from an exogenous source.

Tuberculosis of the spine is always secondary to an active primary focus elsewhere in the body. Once the bacilli reach the vertebral body, metaphysitis (formation of granulation tissue with inflammation and caseation necrosis) occurs. If tissue destruction continues, a paraspinal abscess will form which is composed of necrotic bone and cartilage surrounded by a wall of granulation tissue and edema. The intervertebral disc is usually not involved and lies free within the pus.

The clinical consequences of a paraspinal abscess depend on its size and the anatomic structures it affects. With vertebral body destruction, kyphosis may occur, and if the structural loss is greater on one side than on the other, a scoliosis may result. If the mechanical integrity of the spinal canal is lost, neural compression will occur and some degree of paralysis may result.[14] If the abscess is in direct contact with the dura, pachymeningitis may result.

Clinical Findings

The clinical presentation of a patient with tuberculous spondylitis (Pott's disease) consists of pain over the involved vertebrae. The pain can vary in intensity and is aggravated by activity. The pain may be increased by percussion of the involved vertebrae or on longitudinal compression of the entire vertebral column. Patients may also have a low-grade fever and give a history of an unexplained weight loss, but often have no constitutional signs.

Patients with more advanced disease may present with neurologic findings. Paralysis secondary to tuberculosis was first described by Pott in 1779.[24,25] In active tuberculosis, paraplegia can result from external pressure on the spinal cord or tubercle bacilli actually penetrating the dura and involving the spinal cord.

External pressure on the spinal cord is probably the most common cause of paralysis.[15] The external compression can result from several sources. Pus within an abscess can cause direct pressure, and sequestra or intervertebral discs can likewise exert pressure. Granulation tissue, as it expands, can press upon the spinal cord. Finally, an involved vertebral body can collapse, resulting in a kyphosis with anterior tenting of the spinal cord. When two or more vertebral bodies have been destroyed, instability can occur, with subluxations and dislocations. This is common in the thoracolumbar region, and if the cord is subjected to any pressure paralysis will result.

Penetration of the dura by the tubercle bacilli can occur without paraplegia. However, when the spinal cord is involved, tuberculous meningomyelitis results. This is a very grave condition, and the prognosis for any neurologic return is poor.

The most common physical finding in the spine is some degree of kyphosis.[1] This is a result of anterior collapse of one or more vertebral bodies. Kyphosis will be most pronounced in the thoracic spine. With lumbar disease, there will be approximation of the ribs to the iliac crests, with a prominent abdomen.

An abscess may develop with sinus formation. The drainage should always be cultured, for the sinus tract may become secondarily infected. The site of the sinus depends on the level of the disease. An extensive abscess can be present even when the patient has no pain and few if any systemic signs of infection. This is commonly referred to as a cold abscess.

Radiographic and Laboratory Findings

In tuberculous spondylitis, the vertebral body is more commonly affected than are posterior elements, which are involved in only 2 percent of spinal tuberculous cases.[5] Pott's disease is much more common in the lower half of the spine between T6 and L4. The infection causes erosion of the subchondral bone and invades the disc space (Fig. 15–3). These changes occur much less rapidly with tuberculous spondylitis than with pyogenic spondylitis. Patients who have back pain secondary to tuberculous spondylitis will usually present with readily identifiable destruction of vertebral bodies. In other words, the radiographic changes are usually far advanced in the spine by the time the disease is clinically appreciated. This is in marked contrast to patients with pyogenic spondylitis, who de-

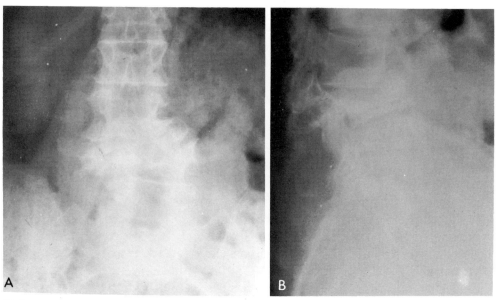

Figure 15–3. *A*, Anteroposterior radiograph of a patient with proven tuberculosis of L4. *B*, The lateral view shows that there is significant destruction with collapse. (From Wiesel SW, Bernini P, Rothman RH: The Aging Lumbar Spine. Philadelphia, W.B. Saunders, 1982.)

velop back pain before roentgenographic alterations are noted in the vertebral elements.

The infection can also spread to soft tissue, forming paraspinal abscesses. In this form, the anterior cortex of the vertebral body is destroyed. Severe angular deformities occur with marked destruction of vertebral bodies; these may appear wedge-shaped, while the disc spaces are preserved. The lesion may look like a vertebra plana and may be confused with eosinophilic granuloma. The reactive sclerosis characteristic of healing pyogenic vertebral osteomyelitis does not occur with tuberculous spondylitis. In many patients the disease is limited to two contiguous vertebrae, although four, five, or more segments may be involved.

The tuberculin (PPD) test is usually positive for patients with tuberculous spondylitis unless they are anergic. Anergy is most commonly seen in patients with miliary disease, advanced age, malnutrition, or immunodeficiency states. The number of organisms in an infected spine is less than 1 million; therefore, it is appropriate to culture both purulent material and biopsy specimens in order to improve the potential for a positive culture. Histologic evidence of granulomas suggests tuberculous.

Treatment

The goal in the therapy of tuberculosis is to eradicate the active infection and provide stability for the spine. Three different approaches exist today in treating spinal tuberculosis, all of which include 18 months of chemotherapy. The traditional treatment is nonsurgical, utilizing prolonged bed rest with a plaster jacket. At the opposite end of the spectrum is the belief that every vertebral lesion should be surgically treated. The authors' believe that a "middle-path" regime should be followed, as advocated by Tuli in India and Riska in Finland.[32,33]

Rest and chemotherapy are the initial treatment modalities. Rest is enforced and a plaster jacket is used for comfort if necessary. Once the diagnosis is made, drugs are administered. The exact chemotherapy regimen varies from institution to institution, and it is suggested that an infectious disease consultation be obtained. Tuberculous spondylitis usually requires a three-drug regimen for 2 to 3 months, and two drugs are usually continued for a total of 18 months. Progressive ambulation is begun at 6 to 9 months if the pain has disappeared and the radiographs are satisfactory. A spinal orthosis will be most helpful to the patient in the initial stages of mobilization. Spontaneous spinal fusion often does not occur for five years following the onset of disease.

Surgical intervention is recommended for patients who do not respond to antibiotics and rest. The failure of nonoperative treatment is denoted by continued pain with at least 3 months of treatment and an increasing sedimentation rate. Patients who present with a neurologic loss and fail to respond to conservative therapy or patients who develop paraplegia while under adequate treatment are definite surgical candidates. Patients who have an unstable spine (progressive kyphosis) or a paravertebral abscess need surgical intervention. Abscesses, however, may be superficial and palpable, in which case aspiration and instillation of antibiotics may be attempted. If the abscess is deep or does not respond to antibiotics, surgery is necessary. Finally, surgery is required in some cases to confirm the diagnosis.

The first goal of surgery is to remove all of the infected tissue, which can include pus, sequestrated intervertebral discs, bony sequestra, and granulation tissue. The second aim is to leave the patient with a stable spine, which is best accomplished by a fusion. Since the infection is usually anterior, an anterior approach is recommended.[16] This will allow the surgeon, under excellent exposure, to eradicate the infection, decompress the neural elements, and perform a solid fusion.

Summary

Spinal infections are uncommon but must be included in the differential diagnosis of the patient with atypical back or neck pain. Although intervertebral disc space infections occur more commonly in children, discitis may be seen in adults after surgery or after violation of the disc space during a diagnostic procedure. Laboratory findings are not consistently abnormal, and therefore a strong clinical suspicion is imperative. MRI is a helpful confirmatory test. The majority of disc space infections are treated with antibiotics, bed rest, and casting/bracing. Surgery is only required when there is no response to therapy or if a paravertebral abscess is present. In the majority of patients, the disease has a benign course and results in a full recovery.

In contrast, vertebral osteomyelitis can lead to serious complications, including neurologic compromise, meningitis, kyphosis, and spinal instability. Early diagnosis is beneficial. Immobilization of the spine is the principal treatment. Nontubercular osteomyelitis is also treated with antibiotics, whereas tubercular infections require the appropriate chemotherapy. Open biopsy is indicated when the causative organism is not known and there is no response to medical therapy. Surgical decompression is necessary with spinal cord compression, when a paravertebral abscess is present, or when a nerve root deficit persists after appropriate medical therapy. The vast majority of these infections eventually lead to intervertebral fusion, which may take over a year to occur. If progressive kyphosis or instability occurs, surgical stabilization may be required.

References

1. Bailey HL, Gabriel M, Hodgson AR, et al: Tuberculosis of the spine. J Bone Joint Surg 54A:1633–1657, 1972.
2. Batson OV: The function of the vertebral veins and their role in the spread of metastases. Ann Surg 112:138–149, 1940.
3. Boston HC, Bianco AJ, Rhodes KH: Disc space infections in children. Orthop Clin North Am 6:953–964, 1975.
4. Brashear HR Jr, Rendleman DA: Pott's paraplegia. South Med J 71:1379–1382, 1978.
5. Chapman M, Murray RO, Stoker DJ: Tuberculosis of the bones and joints. Semin Roentgenol 14:266–282, 1979.
6. Collert S: Osteomyelitis of the spine. Acta Orthop Scand 48:283–290, 1977.
7. Compere EL, Garrison M: Correlation of pathologic and roentgenologic findings in tuberculosis and pyogenic infections of the vertebrae. Ann Surg 104:1038–1067, 1936.
8. Coventry MB, Ghormley RK, Kernohan JW: The intervertebral disc: Its microscopic anatomy and pathology. I. Anatomy, development and physiology J Bone Joint Surg 27:105–112, 1945.
9. Dich VQ, Nelson JD, Haltalin KC: Osteomyelitis in infants and children—review of 163 cases. Am J Dis Child 129:1273–1278, 1975.
10. Eismont FJ, Bohlman HH: Pyogenic and fungal vertebral osteomyelitis—a review of sixty-five cases. Annual Meeting of the American Academy of Orthopaedic Surgeons, Las Vegas, 1977.
11. Friedman B: Chemotherapy of tuberculosis of the spine. J Bone Joint Surg 48A:451–474, 1966.
12. Garcia A, Grantham SA: Hematogenous pyogenic vertebral osteomyelitis. J Bone Joint Surg 42A:429–436, 1960.
13. Goldblatt M, Cremin BJ: Osteoarticular tuberculosis. Its presentation in the coloured races. Clin Radiol 29:669–677, 1978.
14. Gorse GJ, Pais MJ, Kusske JA, et al: Tuberculous spondylitis: A report of six cases and a review of the literature. Medicine 62:178–193, 1983.
15. Griffith DLL, Seddon HJ, Roaf R: Pott's Paraplegia. London, Oxford University Press, 1956.
16. Hodgson AR, Stock FE: Anterior spine fusion for the treatment of tuberculosis of the spine. J Bone Joint Surg 42A:295–310, 1960.
17. Kemp HBS, Jackson JW, Jeremiah JD, et al: Pyogenic infections occurring primarily in intervertebral discs. J Bone Joint Surg 55B:698–714, 1973.
18. Milone FP, Bianco AJ Jr, Ivins JC: Infections of the intervertebral disc in children. JAMA 181:1029–1033, 1962.
19. Norris S, Ehrlich MG, Keim DE, et al: Early diagnosis of disc-space infection using gallium-67. J Nucl Med 19:384–386, 1978.
20. Onofrio BM: Intervertebral discitis: Incidence, diagnosis and management. Clin Neurosurg 27:481–516, 1980.
21. Pate D, Katz A: Clostridia discitis: A case report. Arthritis Rheum 22:1039–1040, 1979.
22. Pennisi AK, Davis DO, Wiesel S, et al: CT appearance of Candida diskitis. J Comput Assist Tomogr 9:1050–1054, 1985.
23. Pilgaard S: Discitis (closed space infection) following removal of lumbar intervertebral disc. J Bone Joint Surg 51A:713–716, 1969.
24. Pott P: Remarks on that Kind of Palsy of the Lower Limbs Which Is Frequently Found to Accompany a Curvature of the Spine and Is Supposed To Be Caused by It, Together with Its Method of Cure. London, 1779.
25. Pott P: Further Remarks on the Useless State of the Lower Limbs in Consequence of a Curvature of the Spine. London, 1782.

26. Rocco HD, Eyring EJ: Intervertebral disc infections in children. Am J Dis Child 123:448–451, 1972.
27. Ross PM, Fleming JL: Vertebral body osteomyelitis: Spectrum and natural history: A retrospective analysis of 37 cases. Clin Orthop 118:190–197, 1976.
28. Rothman RH, Simeone F: The Spine, 2nd ed. Philadelphia, W.B. Saunders, 1982.
29. Scherbel AL, Gardner JW: Infections involving the intervertebral discs: Diagnosis and management. JAMA 174:370–374, 1960.
30. Selby RC, Pillary KV: Osteomyelitis and disc infection secondary to Pseudomonas aeruginosa in heroin addiction: Case report. J Neurosurg 37:463–466, 1972.
31. Sullivan CR: Diagnosis and treatment of pyogenic infections of the intervertebral disc. Surg Clin North Am 41:1077–1086, 1961.
32. Tuli SM: Results of treatment of spinal tuberculosis by "middle-path" regime. J Bone Joint Surg 57B:13–23, 1975.
33. Tuli SM, Srivastava TP, Varma BP, et al: Tuberculosis of spine. Acta Orthop Scand 38:445–458, 1967.
34. Waldvogel FA, Medoff G, Swartz MN: Osteomyelitis: A review of clinical features, therapeutic considerations and unusual aspects. N Engl J Med 283:821–822, 1970.
35. Waldvogel FA, Vasey H: Osteomyelitis: The past decade. N Engl J Med 303:360–370, 1980.
36. Wenger DR, Bobechko WP, Cilday DL: The spectrum of intervertebral disc-space infection in children. J Bone Joint Surg 60A:100–108, 1978.
37. Wiley AM, Trueta J: The vascular anatomy of the spine and its relationship to pyogenic vertebral osteomyelitis. J Bone Joint Surg 41B:796–809, 1959.

CHAPTER 16

Tumors of the Spine

Tumors involving the spine are relatively uncommon. However, the consequences of a neoplastic spinal lesion are so disastrous that the physician should keep the possibility of its existence in mind when dealing with back or neck pain of unclear etiology. The purpose of this chapter is to first present a general overview of the evaluation of a patient with a suspected tumor and then discuss the more common benign and malignant lesions. Although many of the benign lesions are most commonly seen in the young, recurrence, late presentation, and sequelae may affect older patients.

EVALUATION

Diagnosis of spine tumors must follow a logical sequence beginning with the history and physical examination. Pain originating from a tumor in the spine is nonmechanical; in other words, it is not related to activity and, in fact, tumor pain may increase with recumbency. Thus patients may complain of pain that is often worse at night, a phenomenon that may be related to vascular engorgement of the tumor. In addition, the level of pain is usually much higher and more consistent than that experienced with mechanical problems (such as a herniated disc).

Physical examination may demonstrate localized tenderness at the site of the lesion or deformity. For example, the development of a thoracic gibbus may indicate vertebral collapse; or torticollis may be a sign of an intraspinal cervical lesion. Finally, a careful neurologic examination is essential. Painless radiculopathy may be the first sign of an intraspinal neoplasm, and objective neurologic dysfunction will occur as the spinal cord is compressed.

Laboratory examination for screening purposes consists of a broad group of basic tests—complete blood count, sedimentation rate, SMA-20 blood chemistry tests, and urinalysis. If abnormalities are noted on any of these tests, then more specific studies can be ordered, such as serum and/or urine protein electrophoresis. It should be noted that only 20 percent of patients with multiple myeloma will have an abnormal urine protein electrophoresis. The acid phosphatase is helpful for prostatic cancer. The alkaline phosphatase may be elevated with metastatic disease, Paget's disease, or gastrointestinal abnormalities. The sedimentation rate, although nonspecific, will rise with many cancerous entities, especially multiple myeloma. While the sedimentation rate is quite sensitive, it is often elevated in the normal population, especially in older individuals. Calcium and phosphorus abnormalities suggest parathyroid disease, osteomalacia, and other metabolic bone abnormalities.

Radiographic examination begins with the plain films. It should be remembered that approximately 30 percent of the bone must be involved by tumor before a change is visible on the plain film. Therefore, a normal film does not necessarily exclude the presence of a bone tumor. For lesions in the lumbar spine, it is important to always have a film of the pelvis, since with tumors about the hip the patient may complain of thigh pain, with lesions about the greater sciatic notch, there may be leg pain, and with lesions in the pubis the patient may present with radiating back pain.

The *technetium phosphate bone scan* is useful in several situations. First, it is ideal for screening purposes when there is a high index of suspicion (e.g., osteoid osteoma or a sacral lesion with bowel gas obstructing the sacrum). It is also helpful in evaluating bone metastases with skip lesions and can be used to evaluate patients with persistent nonmechanical back pain in whom the plain film was unremarkable. It must be remembered that the bone scan does have a 5 percent false-negative rate because it depends on new bone formation or vascularity for uptake of radiosotope. Lesions most likely to give a false negative scan are multiple myeloma, nasopharyngeal carcinoma, lung and breast carcinoma, and hypernephroma.

Myelography is indicated to quantitate the extent of neural compression in those cases in which neurologic involvement is present and to assist in planning the surgical resection. Water-soluble dye is used routinely, except in those cases in which it is important to evaluate the response to treatment. One example is the need to assess the degree of reduction in epidural compression following radiation therapy. Pantopaque, an oil-based contrast agent, is employed in these situations so that further lumbar punctures will not be necessary.

High-resolution *computerized tomography* (CT) is helpful in a variety of situations. It can determine the amount of soft tissue extension of the lesion; evaluate the encroachment of the lesion on the spinal canal; assist in planning a surgical resection; better evaluate lesions about the pelvis and sacrum where bowel shadows restrict visualization; and, finally, localize the tumor to the specific anatomic area of the vertebra. In the cervical spine, CT scanning is routinely combined with a water-soluble dye myelogram to evaluate both the extent of the lesion and its relationship to the spinal cord. CT is also useful in evaluating the result of surgical resection and tumor recurrence following surgery.

Magnetic resonance imaging (MRI) is becoming extremely useful in the evaluation of spinal pathology. As its technology advances and its general availability increases, the MR scan is playing an increasingly significant role in tumor diagnosis. It appears that it will be equally useful in evaluating soft and bony tissues. It is hoped, and expected, that owing to its superior imaging of the spinal cord and dural sac, MR scanning will obviate the need for myelography before tumor surgery.

Arteriography is still helpful in a number of situations. The first is in evaluating vertebral artery compression from lesions about the foramen transversarium in the cervical spine. Additionally, arteriography can localize the feeder vessels of vascular tumors, which can then be embolized prior to surgery. Finally, for large anterior spinal resections, arteriography can identify the dominant feeder vessel to the spinal cord so that ligation can be avoided.

BENIGN TUMORS

Aneurysmal Bone Cyst

Prevalence and Pathogenesis

A benign, nonneoplastic, cystic vascular lesion of bone, aneurysmal bone cyst (ABC) represents about 1 to 2 percent of primary bone lesions.[14,35] The vast majority of affected patients are under the age of 30; however, some tumors may be asymptomatic and discovered later in life as an incidental finding. Unlike other primary bone tumors, there is a slight female predominance. Synonyms for aneurysmal bone cyst include edifying hematoma, plain bone cyst, and atypical giant cell tumor.[4,13]

The etiology of ABC is unclear, but the leading theory involves trauma with secondary formation of arteriovenous malformations (AVMs). These AVMs, which consist of abnormal vascular channels, lead to the development of an ABC.[2,17]

In a third of the cases, ABC is superimposed upon another pathologic process, which may be either a benign or a malignant tumor. The basic abnormality, in either circumstance, is a local change in interosseous blood flow.[7] The blood pools in bone, resulting in increased interosseous pressure, followed by resorption, expansion, and cyst formation. The recognition of an underlying process is necessary because the clinical course of the patient, especially if the lesion is malignant, will follow that for the primary process.

Although a majority of ABCs occur in the long bones of the extremities, 15 to 25 percent of cases occur in the spine.[12,28] The lumbosacral spine is affected in 36 percent of cases, the thoracic spine in 32 percent, and the cervical spine in 32 percent. As with most benign tumors, ABCs are usually located in the posterior elements (spinous and transverse processes or laminae).

Clinical History

Patients with ABCs generally present with symptoms of pain or swelling in the affected area. The pain is usually of acute onset and increases in severity over a short period of time. The duration of symptoms can range from months to several years.

The clinical manifestations vary with the location and size of the lesion. A lesion of the spinous or transverse process may be entirely asymptomatic. Neurologic symptoms and signs include a spectrum of abnormalities from sensory changes to paraplegia, depending on the location of the lesion.

Physical Examination

Physical examination may demonstrate tenderness to palpation over the site of involvement as well as limitation in the range of motion. The overlying skin may be erythematous and warm if the ABC is close to the skin surface. Neurologic findings correlate with the location of nerve root or spinal cord compression.

Laboratory Findings

All of the blood and urine tests are normal in patients with this benign lesion. Patients with secondary cysts will have abnormal results that correspond to their underlying lesion.

On gross inspection the cyst contains anastomosing cavernous spaces that compose the bulk of the lesion. The blood is unclotted and subperiosteal new bone that is eggshell-thin separates the lesion from surrounding tissue.

On histologic examination, the cystic cavities are composed of vascular channels filled with fibrous connective tissue, osteoid, granulation tissue, and multinucleated giant cells. Although fibrous, the solid portions of an ABC may contain a lacework of osteoid trabeculae.

Radiographic Findings

The radiographic features of an ABC consist of a solitary, eccentrically located, osteolytic, expansile lesion that is sharply demarcated by a thin subperiosteal shell of bone. The cyst cavity may be traversed by fine strands of bony cortex. A soft tissue mass may also be associated with the bony lesion (Fig. 16–1). ABCs occur most commonly in the posterior elements affecting pedicles, laminae, and spinous and transverse processes. Lesions can occur within the vertebral body, and may involve more than one vertebra by extension across the disc space. ABCs may attain considerable size.

Differential Diagnosis

In the posterior elements, the characteristic radiographic appearance of the ABC helps differentiate it from other benign and malignant lesions. On the other hand, a solitary lytic lesion of the anterior body of a vertebra is more likely to be a metastasis, infection, or giant cell tumor. Biopsy is necessary, but it is important to remember that some primary bone tumors, including chondroblastoma and giant cell tumor, may have areas that are histologically similar to ABCs. Careful evaluation of the entire specimen should alert the pathologist to the underlying lesion.

Treatment

Aneurysmal bone cysts can be treated by surgery, radiotherapy, or cryotherapy.[33,45] Although benign, they are highly prone to local recurrence after curettage. The addition of cryosurgery has been reported to halt expansion of the cyst and to minimize recurrence after curettage.

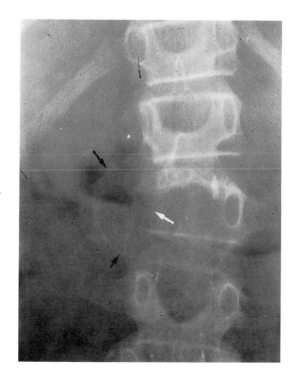

Figure 16–1. Aneurysmal bone cyst arising from the posterior elements of the second lumbar vertebra. Notice the loss of the pedicle (*white arrow*) and faint line of calcification lateral to the vertebral body (*black arrows*). (Courtesy of Anne Brower, M.D.) (From Borenstein DG, Wiesel SW: Low Back Pain: Medical Diagnosis and Management. Philadelphia, W.B. Saunders, 1989.)

If the location of an ABC allows removal of a section of bone without loss of function, en bloc resection is the treatment of choice. Lesions in the posterior elements of the spine may be treated with resection and the addition of bone grafting. Patients with lesions that are too large or that involve a vertebral body may be candidates for radiotherapy. However, the benefit of radiotherapy must be weighed against the potential for radiation-induced sarcoma many years later.

Prognosis

Aneurysmal bone cyst is a benign lesion but may cause severe dysfunction because of its expansile characteristics. If the lesion is diagnosed early and treated appropriately, dysfunction may be kept to a minimum. However, if it is located in the spine and is allowed to expand unchecked, serious neurologic deficits may result. In addition, an ABC weakens the bone and increases the risk of pathologic fracture.

Osteoid Osteoma

Prevalence and Pathogenesis

Osteoid osteomas constitute about 2.6 percent of all excised primary tumors of bone.[14,35] Adults between 20 and 30 years of age are at greatest risk; however, recurrent cases may be seen in older individuals. Between 7 and 18 percent of osteoid osteomas are located in the spine. The lumbar area is the most common location (lumbar 40%, thoracic 30%, cervical 30%).[8,21]

The pathogenesis of osteoid osteoma is unclear. Some feel that osteoid osteoma may represent a chronic infection or reparative process instead of being an actual neoplasm.[24] Factors favoring this hypothesis are its limited growth potential (less than 2 cm), a histologic appearance independent of the duration of the lesion, a mature osseous envelope surrounding an immature nidus, and marginal sclerosis. Others believe that osteoid osteoma is a benign bone neoplasm that has limited growth potential.

Clinical History

Pain at the area of the lesion is the characteristic feature of osteoid osteoma. Initially, the pain is intermittent and vague, but with time it becomes constant and aching with a boring quality. The pain is not relieved with rest and is frequently more severe at night. The pain from an osteoid osteoma may be relieved with small doses of aspirin or other nonsteroidal drugs. The mechanism of analgesia by nonsteroidals has been postulated to be inhibition of osteoma prostaglandin production. The concentration of prostaglandins is greatest at night, secondary to decreased blood flow, correlating with increased symptoms.[41] An alternative explanation for the pain is the irritation of nerve fibers situated near the center (nidus) of the osteoid osteoma. It should be appreciated that osteoid osteomas do not always respond to nonsteroidal medications. There are also osteoid osteomas that are entirely painless.

In the spine, osteoid osteomas are associated with nonstructural scoliosis.[26] The appearance of marked paravertebral muscle spasm with the sudden onset of scoliosis in a young adult requires an evaluation for this lesion. The tumor is usually located on the concave side of the curvature.

The pain associated with osteoid osteoma is slowly progressive over months. In some patients symptoms can exist for years before the correct diagnosis is made, and symptoms may be present for a considerable time before radiographic findings become evident.

Physical Examination

The most common physical finding is tenderness with palpation over the affected bone. Marked muscular spasm with associated scoliosis may be noted in a patient with an osteoid osteoma of the spine. The spine may be curved without rotation. Early in the course of the lesion, the scoliosis is reversible. However, with prolonged spasm, muscle atrophy may occur, along with structural abnormalities, and result in permanent deformity.

Laboratory Findings

Screening laboratory tests are normal. Pathologically, the nidus is usually less than 1 cm in diameter and contains areas of osteoid, irregular woven bone trabeculae, and vascular fibrous tissue surrounded by dense lamellar bone.

Radiographic Findings

The finding of a lucent nidus about 1 cm in diameter with a surrounding well-defined area of dense sclerotic bone is virtually pathognomonic of osteoid osteoma (Fig. 16-2). The amount of sclerosis is out of proportion to the small size of the nidus. Osteoid osteomas arise in the posterior elements of a vertebra. The neural arch is affected in about 75 percent of the cases and the vertebral body in only about 7 percent.[1] The size and location of these lesions make them difficult to detect with plain radiographs. Bone scans are the most helpful in localizing the lesion. Computerized tomography (CT) is also useful in localizing the nidus and in detecting encroachment of the tumor on the spinal canal or the neural foramen.

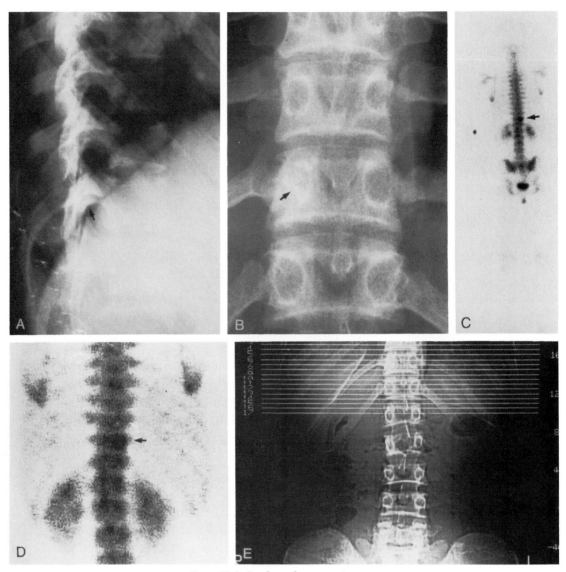

Figure 16–2. *See legend on opposite page.*

Differential Diagnosis

The diagnosis of an osteoid osteoma is suggested by characteristic clinical and radiographic features and is confirmed by the histologic examination of biopsy material. Despite its characteristic appearance, osteoid osteoma of the spine can remain an elusive diagnosis. Lumbosacral strain, psychogenic back pain, Scheuermann's disease, herniated nucleus pulposus, and nonspecific mechanical back pain are frequent prior diagnoses.[30] The physician's degree of suspicion should be raised when patients with nontraumatic back pain have associated paravertebral muscle spasm and recent onset of scoliosis.

Other diagnoses that need to be considered include osteoblastoma, osteosarcoma, osteomyelitis, Ewing's sarcoma, eosinophilic granu-

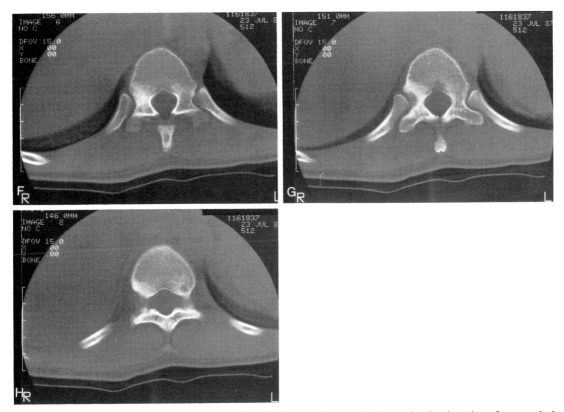

Figure 16–2. A 21-year-old woman gave a history of localized back pain over the thoracolumbar junction of one year's duration. The pain was increased at night and was responsive to salicylate therapy. *A*, Lateral view of the thoracolumbar junction reveals increased sclerosis in the pedicle of the T11 vertebra (arrow). B, Spot view of the lower thoracic vertebrae revealing an irregular border of the right pedicle (*arrow*). *C* and *D*, technetium-99m methylene diphosphonate bone scan. *C*. Posterior view shows increased traces of accumulation in T11 (*arrow*). *D*, Spot view detects increased uptake in the lateral compartment of T11 (*arrow*). *E* to *H*, CT scan of the thoracolumbar junction. AP view (*E*) and views of levels 6 (*F*), 7 (*G*), and 8 (*H*) through T11, demonstrating reactive sclerosis around an area of central clearing without soft tissue extension. The diagnosis of osteoid osteoma was made and the patient's pain responded to diflunisal. The patient is being followed and is asymptomatic on the nonsteroidal drug 12 months later. She will have a biopsy of the lesion if it increases in size. (From Borenstein DG, Wiesel SW: Low Back Pain: Medical Diagnosis and Management. Philadelphia, W.B. Saunders, 1989.)

loma, metastases, fracture, aseptic necrosis, osteochondritis, and aneurysmal bone cyst. Abnormalities in laboratory tests (elevated white blood cell count, abnormal erythrocyte sedimentation rate, bone chemistries) and characteristic histologic findings help differentiate these inflammatory, infectious, and malignant lesions from osteoid osteoma.

Treatment

The most effective treatment is to completely excise the lesion. One must remove the entire nidus to prevent recurrence,[36] but this may pose a difficult problem in poorly accessible areas of the spine. If the entire lesion is not removed, symptoms may be relieved by unroofing a cortical lesion with removal of some surrounding sclerotic bone; however, symptoms often persist when the nidus is not entirely removed. Medical therapy may alleviate symptoms, but never to the same degree as is achieved with surgical excision. It should be appreciated that osteoid osteomas can undergo spontaneous healing with reduction of symptoms.

Prognosis

Osteoid osteomas are benign. They may be a difficult diagnostic problem, however, because clinical symptoms may appear before the lesions are radiographically evident. Low back pain and associated limitation of activities may be inappropriately ascribed to malingering or psychoneurosis. When an adult presents with low back pain that is exacerbated at night, a high index of suspicion should be raised. Although it is not a malignant tumor, osteoid osteoma should not be considered an innocuous lesion. Persistent evaluation and appropriate surgery are necessary to prevent potential physical deformities and psychic stress in patients with this elusive neoplasm.

Osteoblastoma

Prevalence and Pathogenesis

A rare lesion, osteoblastoma accounts for only about 3 percent of all benign bone tumors.[14,35] A majority of the lesions appear during the second and third decades of life; thus, most patients diagnosed with an osteoblastoma are younger than 30 years of age. The tumor has a predilection for the spine, with about 40 percent located in the axial skeleton.[34]

Osteoblastoma has been referred to as an osteogenic fibroma, giant osteoid osteoma, spindle cell variant of giant cell tumor, and osteoblastic osteoid tissue–forming tumor. The pathogenesis is unknown.

Clinical History

The major clinical symptom is a dull aching pain localized over the involved bone. The pain usually has an insidious onset and may persist for many months to years before the diagnosis is reached. In contrast to osteoid osteoma, the pain of an osteoblastoma is less severe, is not nocturnal, and is not relieved by salicylates. Pain may be aggravated by activity, but this is not always the case.

Osteoblastoma located in the lumbar spine may be associated with pain radiating into the legs, which may be accompanied by muscle spasm and/or limitation of motion. Radicular pain and spinal cord compression are more likely to occur in osteoblastoma than in osteoid osteoma because of the former lesion's larger size and potential for occupying space. An osteoblastoma can also cause abdominal symptoms when it is located in the anterior part of the sacrum.

Physical Examination

The physical examination of a patient with osteoblastoma is nonspecific. There may be local tenderness on palpation, with mild swelling over the involved spinal area. Osteoblastoma associated with spinal cord compression will result in abnormalities on sensory and motor examination of the involved nerves, including abnormal reflexes, atrophy of the involved muscles, and muscle weakness.

Laboratory Findings

An osteoblastoma does not have any associated abnormal hematologic parameters. However, characteristic abnormalities are present on pathologic examination. On gross examination the tumors are well circumscribed and are composed of hemorrhagic granular tissue with variable calcification. The tumors range in size from 2 to 10 cm.

Histologically, an osteoblastoma contains cellular osteoblastic tissue with a large amount of osteoid material but no chondrocytes and cartilage. Multinucleate giant cells may be observed and mitotic figures may also be seen. However, atypical mitoses are not present. Vascular characteristics of the tumor are similar to those seen with an aneurysmal bone cyst. The borders of the tumor are well demarcated.

Radiographic Findings

Osteoblastomas in the spine are most commonly located in the posterior elements of the vertebra, including pedicles, laminae, and transverse and spinous processes (Fig. 16–3). The vertebral body is rarely involved. The lesion is located in the sacrum or lumbar spine in 40 percent of the cases, in the cervical spine in 36 percent, and in the thoracic spine in 24 percent.[14] Osteoblastomas are expansile and may grow rapidly. Characteristically, the lesion is well delineated and is covered by a thin layer of periosteal new bone. The extent of reactive new bone formation, however, is much less than that associated with osteoid osteoma. The center of the lesion may be radiolucent or radiopaque. A bone scan is helpful in localizing the lesion but the finding of localized high uptake is nonspecific.

A CT scan may provide better localization of the tumor, particularly when the lesion is obscured on plain radiographs. An MR scan should also prove extremely useful in localizing this lesion.

Differential Diagnosis

The diagnosis of osteoblastoma is made by a thorough histologic examination of the biopsy sample. Osteogenic sarcoma may be easily confused clinically, radiographically, and histologically with osteoblastoma.

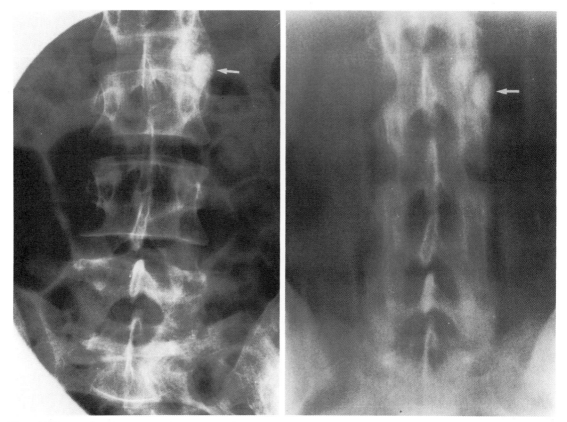

Figure 16–3. AP (*A*) and tomographic (*B*) views of the lumbar spine reveal an oval blastic lesion of the posterior elements of L2 (*arrows*). The size, location, and configuration are consistent with an osteoblastoma. (Courtesy of Anne Brower, M.D.) (From Borenstein DG, Wiesel SW: Low Back Pain: Medical Diagnosis and Management. Philadelphia, W.B. Saunders, 1989.)

The presence of an outer rim of bone on radiographic examination and the absence of cartilage and anaplastic cells on biopsy can differentiate osteoblastoma from a malignant process.

Mirra has suggested five histologic aids that help differentiate osteoblastoma from osteosarcoma:[35]

1. Osteoblastomas do not produce cartilage.

2. Osteoblastomas produce thick trabeculae of osteoid with prominent capillaries and osteoclasts. Osteosarcomas produce extensive areas of poorly calcified bone, with a paucity of prominent vessels.

3. The osteoid and woven bone of osteoblastomas are sharply delineated from surrounding lamellar bone. Osteosarcoma, on the other hand, infiltrates surrounding bone. This implies that when a biopsy is obtained a margin of normal bone should be secured.

4. Osteoblastomas are rimmed by osteoblasts.

5. Osteoblastomas do not include areas that contain cells with bizarre nuclei, abnormal chromatin distribution, abnormal nuclei, or atypical mitoses.

Osteoblastoma must also be differentiated from osteoid osteomas. The latter are associated with more intense and nocturnal pain, are of smaller size (<2 cm), have no associated soft tissue mass, and histologically demonstrate osteoid trabeculae with continuous and regular bone formation.

Treatment

Local excision of the entire lesion is the treatment of choice if bone can be sacrificed without loss of function or excessive risk of neurologic dysfunction. Osteoblastomas involving the posterior elements of the spine are often inaccessible for complete excision (in up to 40 percent of cases).[15] Partial curettage of these lesions may be associated with cessation of tumor growth and relief of symptoms for an extended period of time. Rapidly expanding recurrent osteoblastomas may be controlled with radiation therapy, but excision is certainly the treatment of choice.

Prognosis

The course of osteoblastomas is usually benign. The lesion is responsive to partial curettage and to low-dose radiation therapy. Less than 5 percent of osteoblastomas recur; however, repeated recurrences have been described.[25] Malignant changes occur in a very few lesions considered to have been correctly diagnosed as benign osteoblastomas.[43]

Hemangioma

Prevalence and Pathogenesis

Hemangiomas are benign vascular lesions, composed of cavernous, capillary, or venous blood vessels that may affect soft tissues or bone. They account for fewer than 1 percent of clinically symptomatic primary bone tumors.[14,35] Necropsy studies have demonstrated that asymptomatic vertebral body lesions are found in 12 percent of autopsies. The prevalence of hemangiomas increases with age, and it is estimated that 25 percent of adults have the lesion by the fifth decade of life. Men and women are affected equally.

The pathogenesis of hemangioma remains unknown. The lesions are considered congenital vascular malformations by some investigators and benign neoplasms by others.

Approximately 50 percent of patients with a hemangioma will have the lesion in the spine or skull. The thoracic spine is the site of 65 percent of spinal lesions, the cervical spine 25 percent, and the lumbar spine 10 percent.

Clinical History

The initial complaints of patients with symptomatic vertebral hemangiomas are localized pain and tenderness over the involved vertebra along with associated muscle spasms. The pain has an insidious onset, beginning as a vague nondescript ache that increases in intensity and duration until it becomes constant and throbbing. Neurologic manifestions of cord compression include sensory changes, motor weakness, radiculitis, and transverse myelitis.

Multiple hemangiomas may cause spinal cord compression resembling metastatic disease to the spine.[37] Neurologic symptoms tend to occur as the lesion expands into the epidural space or a pathologic fracture may occur, resulting in an extradural hematoma.

Physical Examination

The physical examination may demonstrate tenderness on palpation over the involved vertebral body. Limitation of motion and muscle spasm may also be present.

Hemangiomas that cause bone to expand can result in clinically apparent swelling. Increased weakening of the vertebral body can cause fractures, which will markedly increase tenderness and muscle spasm. Increased pain and spasm can also result in kyphoscoliosis.

Laboratory Findings

Screening blood tests are generally normal in hemangiomas, although on occasion, a consumptive coagulopathy with thrombocytopenia has been reported in patients with multiple vertebral hemangiomas.[29]

On gross examination, the well-demarcated lesion is reddish brown and either is confined to the vertebral body or extends into the surrounding soft tissue. The vertebral body is the preferential location of primary involvement with secondary extension into the arch or transverse process of the vertebra.

Microscopically, a hemangioma is composed of numerous capillary and larger vascular channels contained in a fibrous stroma. The trabeculae that are not affected by the tumor are thickened in comparison to the lesional thin osseous trabeculae.

Radiographic Findings

Vertebral hemangiomas primarily involve the vertebral bodies. In an affected vertebral body, the vertebral striations are prominent, but horizontal striations are absent because of absorption,[44] giving rise to a "corduroy" appearance (Fig. 16–4). This is most prominent on the lateral projection of the roentgenogram. The alteration of vertebral stria-

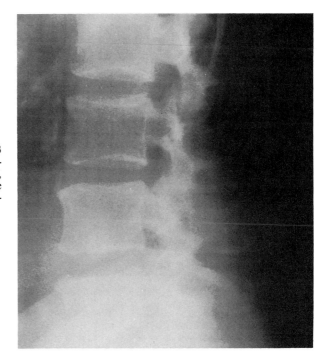

Figure 16–4. Hemangioma of L3 demonstrating prominent vertical striations. (From Wiesel SW, Bernini P, Rothman RH: The Aging Lumbar Spine. Philadelphia, W.B. Saunders, 1982.)

tions is diffuse and the vertebral body configuration is generally unchanged. Occasionally, vertebral body hemangiomas may extend from the body to the lamina, pedicles, or transverse or spinous processes. Symptomatic vertebral hemangiomas may have thinner and wider vertical striations. Vertebral hemangiomas may be associated with vertebral body collapse, hemorrhage, and soft tissue masses.[1]

Differential Diagnosis

Diagnosis of a vertebral hemangioma is uncomplicated when only the vertebral body is affected, owing to the characteristic radiographic changes. It becomes more difficult when portions of a vertebra other than the body are affected. Bony resorption of a pedicle may mimic the destructive changes of some form of metastatic cancer. A vertebral body fracture can occur with the hemangioma, but it is more frequently seen with metastatic tumor.

Skeletal lymphangiomatosis can affect vertebral bodies, causing increased striation, bony lysis with bone compression, and progressive scoliosis. Lymphangiography may be required to confirm this diagnosis. Histologically, lymph node tissue is present to an increased degree in the vascular channels of the bone.[40]

Coarse trabeculation of a vertebral body may also be seen in Paget's disease. Abnormal laboratory tests (elevated erythrocyte sedimentation rate, serum alkaline phosphatase) should differentiate Paget's disease from a hemangioma.

Treatment

The treatment of choice for symptomatic vertebral hemangiomas is radiation, since the lesions are radiosensitive. Radiation therapy effectively relieves symptoms even though the radiographic appearance of the lesion remains unchanged.[31] Because surgical intervention in the form of laminectomy has an excessive morbidity and mortality owing to profuse hemorrhage, it should be reserved for those patients with neurologic defects who require decompression of the spinal cord. If surgery is to be undertaken, preoperative embolization of feeder vessels may render the surgical decompression a safer procedure.

Prognosis

Vertebral hemangiomas are usually asymptomatic and have a benign course; however, when they become symptomatic they require therapy to prevent expansion of the lesion. The major complication of vertebral hemangioma is neural compression due to compression fracture, expansion of an involved vertebra, direct extension of the hemangioma into the extradural space, or extradural hemorrhage. Appropriate diagnosis and treatment may help prevent this potentially disabling complication of this benign vascular neoplasm.

MALIGNANT TUMORS

Multiple Myeloma

Prevalence and Pathogenesis

Multiple myeloma is a primary tumor of bone composed of malignant plasma cells. These cells, which produce immunoglobulins and antibodies, are located throughout the bone marrow. The multiplication of plasma cells in the bone marrow produces profuse bone destruction with associated bone pain, pathologic fractures, and increased serum calcium. Multiple myeloma is the most common primary malignant bone tumor in adults, accounting for 27 percent of bone tumors examined by biopsy and 45 percent of all malignant bone tumors.[14,35] The incidence is 3 cases per 1000 people in the United States. Most patients are between the ages of 50 and 70 years, although there have been reported cases in patients below the age of 40. There is a slight male predominance.[24]

The pathogenesis of multiple myeloma is unknown. Viral infections, chronic inflammation, and myeloproliferative disorders have been postulated as possible initiating factors. Although the symptoms of a fracture associated with trauma are frequently the reason for a patient's initial evaluation, trauma is not a factor in the etiology of multiple myeloma. A majority of patients have lesions in the axial skeleton; the thoracic spine is involved in 59 percent, the lumbar spine in 31 percent, and the cervical spine in 10 percent. Overall, the spine is affected in 30 to 50 percent of patients with multiple myeloma.

Clinical History

Pain is the most common initial complaint, occurring in 75 percent of patients, and low back pain is the presenting symptom in 35 percent of patients. Initially, the pain is mild, aching, and intermittent. The pain is aggravated by weightbearing and relieved by bedrest. Occasionally, patients will have radicular symptoms and are diagnosed as having a herniated intervertebral disc or some form of nonspecific arthritis. Twenty percent of patients give a history of trauma that results in a pathologic fracture of the vertebral body as the initial presenting event. Paraplegia more often occurs with solitary plasmacytoma than with multiple myeloma.[46] Involvement of the ribs, sternum, and thoracic spine may result in kyphosis and loss of height. Pain is not confined to the back, since bone pain can arise in any part of the skeleton secondary to a lesion.

Owing to widespread bone destruction, abnormal immunoglobulin production, and infiltration of bone marrow, patients with multiple myeloma develop a broad range of clinical symptoms. Hypercalcemia due to bone destruction is associated with easy fatigability, anorexia, nausea, vomiting, mental status changes, and kidney stones. Increased abnormal immunoglobulin concentrations cause progressive renal insufficiency, increased susceptibility to infection, and amyloidosis. Most patients with multiple myeloma have symptoms for less than 6 months before seeking medical attention. Patients who are subsequently diagnosed with solitary lesions may have had symptoms for several years.

Physical Examination

In the early stages of the illness, the physical findings may be unremarkable, but as the illness progresses and bone marrow infiltration increases, diffuse bone tenderness, fever, pallor, and purpura become permanent findings on examination. Neurologic examination can demonstrate signs of compression of the spinal cord or nerve routes if vertebral collapse has progressed to a significant degree.

Laboratory Findings

Laboratory examination can be significant, revealing many and major abnormalities. Abnormal serum chemistries include hypercalcemia, hyperuricemia, and elevated creatinine.[38] There is usually associated thrombocytopenia and anemia. While serum alkaline phosphatase is usually normal, characteristic serum protein abnormalities occur in the vast majority of patients with multiple myeloma. The total serum protein concentrations are increased secondary to an increase in the globulin fraction. The increase in globulins is due to the presence of abnormal immunoglobulins of the A, D, E, G, or M classes. Immunoglobulins are composed of light and heavy chains. Multiple myeloma has a single antibody, composed of a light and a heavy chain, that is produced to the exclusion of others. The balance between light and heavy chains may also be disturbed with excess light-chain production resulting in Bence-Jones proteinuria in the urine or excess heavy chain production resulting in heavy-chain disease. Serum protein electrophoresis demonstrates the elevation in globulin levels; there will be a spike in 76 percent of patients, hypogammaglobulinemia in 9 percent, and no abnormality in 15 percent. Urine protein electrophoresis will detect the presence of Bence-Jones proteinuria.

Examination of a bone marrow aspirate and biopsy material shows characteristic changes of multiple myeloma that are diagnostic. The bone marrow aspirate has increased numbers of plasma cells, at levels greater than 30 percent. Diffuse infiltration of bone marrow with plasma cells is evident on bone marrow biopsy. Gross pathologic examination of bone shows a soft, gray, fibril tumor that frequently expands beyond the confines of the bone into the soft tissue. In the spine, such pathologic fractures are commonly identified.

Radiographic Findings

The major radiographic finding in multiple myeloma is osteolysis with multiple "punched-out" bone lesions (Fig. 16–5). Diffuse osteolysis of the axial skeleton may resemble osteoporosis.[5] A characteristic finding in multiple myeloma is the absence of reactive sclerosis surrounding lytic lesions in the spine. Preferential destruction of vertebral bodies with sparing of posterior elements helps in differentiating multiple myeloma from osteolytic metastases, which affect the vertebral pedicles and body.

Benign solitary plasmacytoma may occur almost anywhere in the body, including bone and kidney. Bone plasmacytomas are the most common, affecting in order of decreasing frequency the vertebral body, pelvis, and long bones. Solitary plasmacytomas located in the spine will have variable radiographic features. A purely osteolytic area without expansion or an expansile lesion with thickened trabeculae may be observed. An involved vertebral body may fracture and disappear completely, or the lesion may extend across the inner vertebral disc space to invade an adjacent vertebral body, simulating an infection. The lesion may have coarse trabeculae with vertebral striations, simulating a vertebral angioma.

Bone scans are not helpful in multiple myeloma because the osteolytic lesions will not be visualized. Computerized tomography may demonstrate vertebral body involvement before it is evident on plain radiographs. This is due to the fact that radiographs are able to detect abnormalities in bone calcium only after 30 percent of the calcium is lost. Computed tomography is useful in demonstrating the extent of tumor,

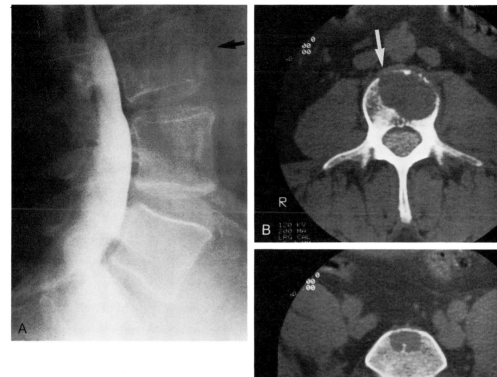

Figure16–5. A 48-year-old man with a 6-week history of acute-onset back pain with radiation to the pelvis and right thigh associated with left leg weakness. Tenderness was demonstrated over the L3 vertebral body, and there were decreased sensation in a left L2 dermatome and decreased strength in the left iliopsoas muscle. *A,* Myelogram revealing an expansile lesion of L3 (*arrow*). The spinal cord is normal. *B,* CT scan of L3 vertebral body demonstrating a sharply marginated hypodense area occupying the greater part of L3 associated with interruption of the anterior cortex (*arrow*). *C,* CT scan of L5 vertebral body revealing a similar, smaller lesion. A bone biopsy of the L3 vertebral body revealed collections of plasma cells consistent with multiple myeloma. Subsequently, lesions in the thoracic spine were noted and a monoclonal IgG kappa protein was identified. A diagnosis of multiple myeloma was made, and the patient was started on chemotherapy along with radiation therapy to the spine. (From Borenstein DG, Wiesel SW: Low Back Pain: Medical Diagnosis and Management. Philadelphia, W.B. Saunders, 1989.)

delineating the soft tissue component of an osseous lesion, and detecting an extramedullary plasmacytoma. MRI should prove to be useful in the early detection of multiple myeloma since it can demonstrate very early changes in the osseous architecture.

Differential Diagnosis

The diagnosis of multiple myeloma in its early stages requires a high index of suspicion. The diagnostic work-up should include information derived from the clinical, radiographic, and laboratory evaluations. Once a lesion is identified, a biopsy for histologic examination is necessary. Diagnosis is more difficult in the patient who presents with diffuse osteoporosis and no detectable myeloma protein in the serum or urine.

Low back pain in middle-aged to elderly patients with osteoporosis on radiographs must be evaluated thoroughly for possible myeloma.

Solitary plasmacytoma is also a difficult entity to diagnose. The diagnosis may be achieved if the character of the lesion is established by biopsy, if a bone survey is negative, if a bone marrow specimen is free of plasma cells, if hypogammaglobulinemia and Bence-Jones proteinuria are absent, and if the patient has been followed for a number of years.

The list of other diseases that must be considered in the differential diagnosis of multiple myeloma is quite broad, with metastatic tumors and malignant lymphoma at the top of the list. Focal osteolysis on a roentgenogram may be associated with hemangioma or infections. Hypoparathyroidism may be accompanied by generalized bone lesions and hypercalcemia. Results of blood tests and biopsy need to be carefully correlated so that the physician can make the appropriate diagnosis.

Treatment

Clinically active multiple myeloma requires systemic therapy with melphalan and prednisone over an extended course.[10] Approximately 70 percent of patients will respond to this type of therapy with a reduction in bone destruction and pain. There will also be a decreased concentration of abnormal proteins, as well as a normalization of hematocrit, urine nitrogen, creatinine, and calcium. Patients with more aggressive disease may benefit from the M-2 drug program, which combines vincristine, melphalan, cyclophosphamide, prednisone, and BCNU.[6] In patients with cord compression secondary to multiple myeloma, decompression laminectomy and/or radiotherapy is indicated. Radiotherapy may also be indicated for a solitary plasmacytoma.

Prognosis

The usual course of multiple myeloma is one of gradual progression. Therapy may improve clinical symptoms and reduce the amounts of myeloma protein, but the average survival remains approximately 5 years. Many patients may have more extensive disease than is clinically apparent. Over 50 percent of patients will have compression fractures at autopsy. In addition, the effects of myeloma may extend beyond the involvement of bone alone. Even in the absence of a marrow packed with plasma cells, erythropoiesis may be depressed by the proliferative plasma cells.

Chondrosarcoma

Prevalence and Pathogenesis

Chondrosarcoma is a malignant tumor that forms cartilaginous tissue. It is frequently located in the pelvis, sacrum, or lumbar spine. Since the tumor is extremely slow growing and usually painless, chondrosarcoma of the pelvis and/or spine may be present for a long time before it is discovered. Chondrosarcoma makes up 11 to 22 percent of primary bone tumors examined by biopsy. The usual age of onset is between 40 and 60 years and the ratio of men to women is three to two.[14,24]

The pathogenesis of chondrosarcoma is unknown. Primary chondrosarcomas arise de novo from previously normal bone, while secondary chondrosarcomas develop from other cartilaginous tumors, such as osteochondroma or enchondroma. Chondrosarcoma may be induced by radiation; such cases account for 9 percent of radiation-induced bone sarcomas.[18] It also develops in a small number of patients with Paget's disease, fibrous dysplasia, or Maffucci's syndrome (enchondromas with soft tissue hemangiomas).

Nine percent of patients with chondrosarcomas have lesions involving the spine. The lumbar sacral spine is the site of the tumor in 50 percent of patients; in 32 percent and 18 percent of patients, the tumor occurs in the thoracic and cervical portions of the spine, respectively.[22]

Clinical History

Chondrosarcoma may be symptomless or may present a palpable swelling with mild discomfort. Tumors in the pelvis are detected when they are palpable through the abdominal wall or cause nerve compression with radicular pain, mimicking symptoms of a herniated disc. Pain, when it occurs, is strongly suggestive of an actively growing tumor. This is particularly important in a patient who has had an osteochondroma for decades that suddenly becomes painful.

Physical Examination

Physical examination may demonstrate a nontender tumor mass or one that is mildly tender on palpation. Rectal examination may be helpful in detecting a mass originating in the pelvis or sacrum. Neurologic findings may be abnormal if neural elements are compressed by the tumor.

Laboratory Findings

Laboratory findings are nonspecific and may not be abnormal until late in the course of the tumor. Abnomalities correlate with the tumor size and extent of metastasis. The data to obtain include blood counts, serum chemistries, and sedimentation rates. Gross pathologic inspection of chondrosarcomas reveals a pearly, translucent tissue that is lobulated. Areas of calcification within the lesions are represented by yellow-white areas of speckling. The extent and the exact boundaries of the lesion are often hard to identify. More reactive new bone is seen with slow-growing tumors than with high-grade anaplastic chondrosarcomas.

According to microscopic appearance, chondrosarcomas are graded by the degree of abnormality in the nuclei of the cells: the higher the abnormality, the higher the grade.

Radiographic Findings

The characteristic radiographic findings of chondrosarcoma include a well-defined lesion with expansile contours (Fig. 16–6). The interior of the lesion may demonstrate lobular or fluffy calcification with scalloping of the inner cortex of bone. Periosteal and endosteal reactive bone formation can lead to a thickened cortex, which is typical of a slow-growing tumor.[3] Cortical destruction and soft tissue invasion are indicative of more aggressive lesions. In the spine, the vertebral body or posterior elements may be the site of origin. Plain radiographs are useful in detecting tumors that have calcified; however, soft tissue extension may not be appreciated on plain films. Computerized tomography may be useful in determining the extent of extraosseous involvement associated with a chondrosarcoma.

Differential Diagnosis

The diagnosis of chondrosarcoma must be based upon clinical, radiographic, and pathologic findings. The chondrosarcoma is the most difficult of the malignant tumors of bone for the histopathologist to diagnose. The histologic appearance of a low-grade chondrosarcoma may be similar to that of a cellular enchondroma, a benign lesion. Malignant tumors with similar histologic appearances may have different aggressive properties. Pain, rapid growth, cortical destruction, soft tissue extension, and anaplastic cells on biopsy are characteristic of higher grade chondrosarcoma.[35]

A wide range of benign and malignant processes can mimic the characteristics of chondrosarcomas. These lesions in the spine include giant cell tumor, chordoma, and osteogenic sarcoma. Careful attention to the clinical symptoms along with a thorough review of the biopsy material should give the pathologist adequate information to make the appropriate diagnosis.

Treatment

Surgery is the treatment of choice for chondrosarcomas. En bloc resection of the tumor with a margin of normal tissue, to prevent implantation of malignant cells in the surgical wound, offers the best chance of long-term survival. Tumors that are partially resected frequently recur with increased cytologic malignancy. Chondrosarcomas are radioresistant, and radiotherapy is reserved for tumors that are inaccessible to excision.

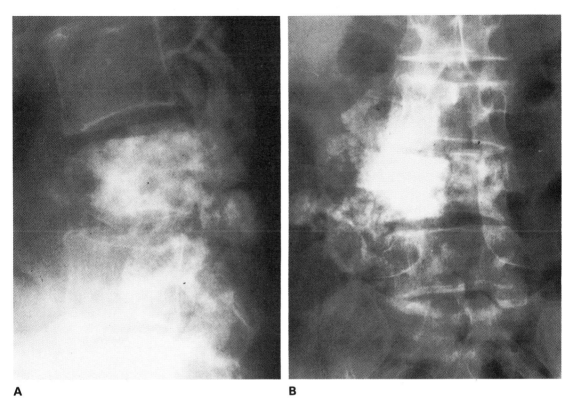

A   **B**

Figure 16–6. Chondrosarcoma. Lateral (*A*) and anterior (*B*) views of a vertebral body with soft tissue extension of the tumor associated with disorganized chondroid matrix calcification. Lateral view shows relative sparing of the disc spaces. (Courtesy of Anne Brower, M.D.) (From Borenstein DG, Wiesel SW: Low Back Pain: Medical Diagnosis and Management. Philadelphia, W.B. Saunders, 1989.)

Prognosis

The patients with chondrosarcoma who present with pain frequently have more malignant tumors. High-grade tumors grow rapidly and metastasize early. Chondrosarcomas with a low degree of malignancy grow slowly, recur locally, and metastasize late. Patients with low-grade, well-differentiated chondrosarcoma have a longer survival rate and a longer interval between treatment and recurrence than those with high-grade tumors. These facts hold true for chondrosarcomas of the pelvis, spine, and sacrum. The patients with the best outcomes are those with low-grade tumors and successful en bloc resection. The 5-year survival rates for grades 1, 2, and 3 pelvic chondrosarcomas after excisional surgery are 47, 38, and 15 percent, respectively.[32]

Chordoma

Prevalence and Pathogenesis

Chordoma is a malignant tumor that originates from the remnants of embryonic tissue of the notochord, a structure that develops into a portion of the vertebral bodies of the spine in the embryo. These tumors are slow growing and may be present for an extended period of time before symptoms appear.[35]

Chordomas account for 3 percent of primary tumors. The tumors usually become evident between the ages of 40 and 70. The ratio of men to women with sacrococcygeal chordomas is three to one, while the ratio is one to one for chordomas at other locations in the spine.[14]

The factors that initiate the regrowth of notochordal vestigial cells in the spine are unknown. Trauma has been suggested as a possible initiating factor, but whether trauma is a causative factor or a chance event in the pathogenesis of this lesion remains unknown.

All chordomas are located in the axial skeleton, ranging from the spheno-occipital area in the skull to the tip of the coccyx. The most common location is the sacrum, which is the site of 50 percent of the lesions. Thirty-eight percent of the tumors are located in the skull. The cervical, lumbar, and thoracic portions of the spine are unusual locations for this neoplasm, accounting for 6, 4, and 2 percent of lesions, respectively.[24]

Clinical History

The symptoms are dependent on the location and extent of the tumor. Patients with sacrococcygeal chordoma present with lower back pain that may be characterized as dull or sharp and intermittent or constant and is localized to the sacrum. It may be of long duration since the patient may not have thought it to be a significant problem. Some patients present with severe constipation, urinary frequency or hesitancy, dysuria, incontinence, or muscular weakness. Patients with chordomas in the spheno-occipital area can present with neurologic symptoms secondary to pressure on the neural elements.

Physical Examination

The neurologic examination is quite helpful in detecting the presence of a chordoma compressing neural elements. On some occasions when the chordoma is in the pelvis it can be palpated by rectal examination. Lesions in the pelvis and sacrum can cause flaccidity in the lower extremities, while lesions higher in the axial skeletal are associated with muscle spasticity.

Laboratory Findings

Laboratory findings may be unremarkable early in the course of this tumor. Abnormalities in hematologic and chemical parameters appear late.

Gross examination of the tumor reveals a soft lobulated grayish mass that is usually well encapsulated except in the region of direct bony invasion. Sacral chordomas have a presacral extension that is covered by periosteum. In the vertebral column, the chordoma originates in the vertebral body and spreads either along the posterior longitudinal ligament or through the intervertebral disc.

Histologically, chordomas are characterized by cells of notochordal origin, physaliphorous cells. These cells contain a large, clear area of cytoplasm with an eccentric, flat nucleus and form columns that are interspersed with fibrous tissue. The tumor is also characterized by the production of large amounts of mucin, and this histologic appearance bears a close resemblance to that of an adenocarcinoma.[9]

Radiographic Findings

Sacrococcygeal and vertebral chordomas produce lytic bone destruction with a calcified fossa and a soft tissue mass.[23] Sacral chordomas produce destruction of several sacral segments with a presacral soft tissue mass. Vertebral chordomas initially cause destruction of a vertebral body without intervertebral disc involvement. Subsequently, intervertebral discs become narrowed and opposing vertebral end plates are eroded. CT and MRI are both useful in accurately assessing the invasion and extent of the tumors (Fig. 16–7). If neural compression is present, myelography occasionally will give additional information.

Differential Diagnosis

The diagnosis of chordoma is suggested by its location and radiographic features, but the definitive diagnosis is dependent on examination of a biopsy specimen. Needle biopsy is usually adequate for a vertebral chordoma, but open biopsy is frequently required for sacral chordoma because of the tumor location.

A number of lesions need to be considered in the differential diagnosis of a chordoma. Giant cell tumor of bone frequently involves the sacrum. Other possibilities include osteochondroma, chondrosarcoma,

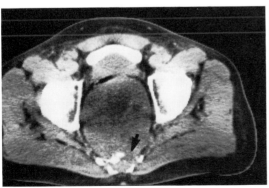 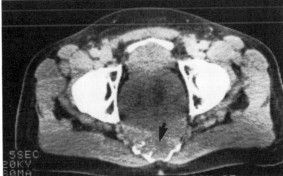

Figure 16–7. A 60-year-old man with minimal back discomfort with a mass detected on rectal examination. CT scan reveals a large mass anterior to the sacrum. The sacrum contains lytic lesions with destruction of the bony cortex (*arrows*). A biopsy of this lesion revealed a chordoma. (From Borenstein DG, Wiesel SW: Low Back Pain: Medical Diagnosis and Management. Philadelphia, W.B. Saunders, 1989.)

metastases, multiple myeloma, osteosarcoma, osteoblastoma, aneurysmal bone cyst, and intrasacral cyst.

Treatment

The definitive treatment for chordoma is en bloc excision. Unfortunately, because of the size of the tumor at the time of diagnosis and the approximation of the tumor to vital structures, partial resection may be the only surgical option. In patients with inaccessible chordomas, radical radiation therapy may slow tumor growth.[39] Vertebral chordomas are treated by decompression laminectomy with excision of accessible tumor located in bone. Depending on the location of the tumor an anterior and/or posterior approach may be indicated. Chemotherapy is usually ineffective.

Prognosis

Chordomas are slowly growing tumors that metastasize in 10 percent of patients late in the course of the illness.[47] The common locations for metastatic lesions are lung, bone, and lymph nodes. The 5-year survival rates for sacrococcygeal tumors and vertebral tumors are 60 percent and 50 percent, respectively, and the 10-year survival ranges between 10 and 40 percent. A few patients have survived with chordoma for 20 years. The prognosis for each patient must be determined by taking into account the location, pathologic characteristics, and invasiveness of the tumor.

SKELETAL METASTASES

Prevalence and Pathogenesis

Lesions caused by migration of tumor cells from the primary lesion are referred to as metastases and are found commonly in the skeletal system. Skeletal lesions result from either dissemination through the blood stream or direct extension. The axial skeleton and pelvis are common sites for metastatic disease.

Metastatic lesions in the skeleton are much more common with primary tumors of the bone than with extraskeletal neoplasms, with the overall ratio being 25:1.[20,35] The increasing prevalence of metastases with age follows from the increasing number of tumors in an older population. Patients who are over 50 years old are at greatest risk of developing metastatic disease. The ratio of males to females varies for each type of malignancy, but considering all neoplasms with a potential to metastasize, men and women are equally at risk of developing metastatic lesions.

Each tumor has a different propensity for metastasizing to bone, and the true incidence of skeletal metastases from each tumor is difficult to ascertain. Neoplasms that are frequently associated with skeletal metastasis include tumors of the prostate, breast, lung, kidney, thyroid, and colon. Data from autopsy material suggest that up to 70 percent of patients with a primary neoplasm will develop pathologic evidence of metastases to vertebral bodies in the thoracolumbar spine.[19,42]

Metastases occur more commonly in the axial skeleton than in the appendicular skeleton. In the axial skeleton, the lumbar and thoracic portions of the spine are affected in approximately 50 percent of cases, with the cervical spine involved in only 6 percent.

Clinical History

A high index of suspicion for the presence of metastases is important in the evaluation of patients with a prior history of malignancy, or of an adult over 50 years of age with pain that is not associated with trauma. Metastatic pain has a gradual onset and increases in intensity over time. It tends to be localized initially to the site of the metastasis but may radiate in a radicular pattern over time.

Patients with spinal cord or nerve root compression secondary to bony or epidural lesions develop neurologic dysfunction that correlates with the location of the lesion. Neurologic symptoms may include numbness, tingling, decreased steadiness of gait, weakness, and bladder or bowel incontinence.

Physical Examination

Physical examination may demonstrate pain on palpation over the affected bone. Muscle spasm and limitation of motion are also associated findings in the spine. Careful attention to neurologic deficits may help locate the lesion in the axial skeleton. Lesions that affect the T12 or L1 vertebra may compress the conus medullaris, which contains the S3 through coccygeal nerve segments. Nerves originating from these segments innervate the urinary bladder, the bladder and rectal sphincters, and the sensory fibers of the perineal region.

Laboratory Findings

Early in the course of metastasis, laboratory parameters are unremarkable. However, subsequent evaluation, although nonspecific, may demonstrate anemia, elevated erythrocyte count and sedimentation rate, abnormal urinalysis, and abnormal blood chemistries, including increased serum alkaline phosphatase concentration.

In patients without a known primary tumor, bone biopsy may provide the first evidence of a malignancy. On many occasions, the histologic features may be associated with a primary lesion in various organs. However, some lesions may be so undifferentiated that the pathologic findings offer no clue to the possible source of the tumor. Radiographic identification of the lesions may help localize the area for biopsy.

Radiographic Findings

Radiographic abnormalities associated with the axial skeleton include osteolytic, osteoblastic, and mixed lytic and blastic lesions.[48] Osteolytic lesions that affect a vertebral body or posterior element such as a pedicle are associated with carcinomas of the lung, kidney, breast, and thyroid (Fig. 16–8). Multiple osteoblastic lesions are seen with prostatic, breast, and colon carcinoma (Fig. 16–9). Involvement of a single blastic

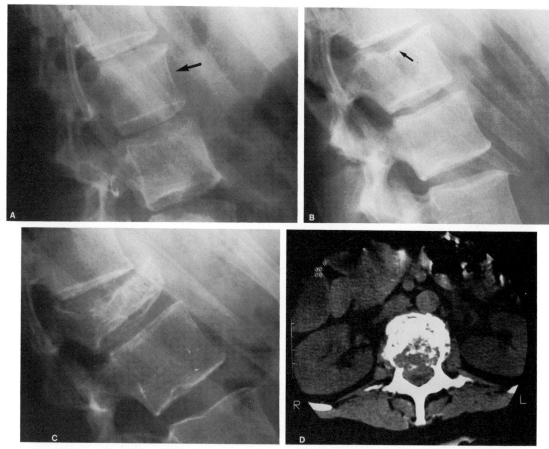

Figure 16–8. Serial views of L1 in a 43-year-old woman with metastatic breast cancer. *A,* 10/3/85. This patient developed radicular symptoms associated with an acute herniated lumbar disc. Her back pain resolved with conservative management. Calcification of bone is normal in L1 (*arrow*). *B,* 2/9/87. This patient developed acute-onset, localized back pain over the L1 vertebra. The lateral view reveals sclerosis of the superior end plate of L1 associated with a mild loss of vertebral body height. *C,* 4/17/87. The patient's pain persisted. Repeat roentgenogram demonstrates marked destruction of the L1 vertebral body. *D,* CT scan of L1 revealing marked destruction of the vertebral body and beginning encroachment of the tumor into the spinal canal. (From Borenstein DG, Wiesel SW: Low Back Pain: Medical Diagnosis and Management. Philadelphia, W.B. Saunders, 1989.)

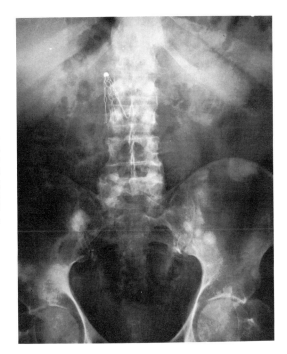

Figure 16–9. AP view of the lumbosacral spine and pelvis in a 66-year-old man with a 3-month history of back pain revealed multiple, discrete osteoblastic lesions, which proved to be metastatic prostatic carcinoma on biopsy. (From Borenstein DG, Wiesel SW: Low Back Pain: Medical Diagnosis and Management. Philadelphia, W.B. Saunders, 1989.)

vertebral body can occur in prostatic carcinoma but is more closely associated with Hodgkin's disease or Paget's disease. Vertebral lesions that contain both lytic and blastic metastases are associated with carcinoma of the breast, lung, prostate, or bladder. Kidney and thyroid carcinoma can cause an expansile lesion from periosteal growth without destruction. Osteolytic lesions are more frequently seen with vertebral body collapse than are osteoblastic lesions. Vertebral body destruction is not associated with changes in the invertebral disc, so the presence of vertebral body destruction and loss of intervertebral disc space height suggests infection.

Early in the course of metastasis plain roentgenograms will be unremarkable. However, a bone scan will detect areas of symptomatic and asymptomatic bone involvement in up to 85 percent of patients with metastases.[11] Computerized tomography can also be useful in localizing lesions that are difficult to identify on plain radiographs. However, CT should not be used as a screening technique because of the amount of radiation exposure. The role of MRI in visualizing metastatic disease of the axial skeleton holds much promise. There is no associated radiation and the specificity appears to be quite high. MRI also appears to show the extent of the tumor inside the cord, the extent of extraosseous spread, and bone marrow invasion quite adequately.

Differential Diagnosis

In the patient with a known primary tumor who develops low back pain, a destructive spinal lesion is associated with a primary neoplasm in the vast majority of cases. These patients may not require a biopsy of the spinal lesion for diagnosis. The problem is when there are destructive lesions of the spine with no known primary lesion. These cases require a biopsy for tissue diagnosis as well as a complete work-up to find the primary source of the tumor.

Other conditions can cause bony changes on plain films and hot spots on bone scans. Elevated alkaline phosphatase may be seen in osteomalacia, Paget's disease, hypoparathyroidism, and sarcoidosis. Only with careful review of all the data can the various diagnosis be eliminated. In some circumstances, tissue biopsy is the only way to obtain the information needed to make an accurate diagnosis.

Treatment

Treatment of metastatic disease of the spine is directed toward palliation of pain. A cure is rarely possible, since most solitary metastatic lesions are accompanied by a number of silent deposits in other bones or tissues that become evident only over time. The pain of the metastatic lesion of the spine may be secondary to bony destruction or a pathologic fracture. Therapy directed specifically at vertebral and spinal cord lesions can include radiation therapy, corticosteroids, and decompressive laminectomy.[16] Radiotherapy may be used alone as primary treatment to decrease pain and slow growth or as an adjunctive therapy after some type of surgical decompression.[27] Metastatic lesions from breast, thyroid, and lymphoid tumors are most sensitive to radiotherapy. Corticosteroids may help reduce edema and alleviate symptoms in patients with spinal cord compression. If spinal instability develops, patients may require instrumentation to control pain. Surgical decompression may remove the majority of tumor or may provide palliation in the case of an unresectable lesion.

Prognosis

The course of each patient with skeletal metastases is dependent on the general course of the primary tumor. Unfortunately, once a metastasis has occurred, the overall prognosis is poor. Neurologic involvement signals a downward trend.

Summary

The majority of tumors arising in the spine result in nonmechanical pain (unrelated to activity), which may often be worse at night and even awaken the patient from sleep. A high index of suspicion for the presence of spinal metastases is important in the evaluation of a patient with a history of a prior malignancy or an adult with pain that is not associated with trauma. Diagnostic evaluation must include a bone scan to assess the skeleton for other lesions, routine laboratory studies, and a CT or MR scan to as-

sess the spinal canal for impingement. In most cases, a biopsy for tissue diagnosis is essential. The required treatment is then dictated by the histologic diagnosis and the clinical symptoms. Unfortunately, many tumors in the spine are not amenable to en bloc resection, and some lesser treatment must be undertaken, such as partial resection or radiation therapy. Vascular lesions may first be controlled by selective embolization. Overall prognosis is influenced by the tumor type as well as the level and extent of neural element impingement when present.

References

1. Banna M: Clinical Radiology of the Spine and the Spinal Cord. Rockville, MD, Aspen Systems, 1985.
2. Barnes R: Aneurysmal bone cyst. J Bone Joint Surg 38B:301–311, 1956.
3. Barnes R, Catto M: Chondrosarcoma of bone. J Bone Joint Surg 48B:729–764, 1966.
4. Biesecker JL, Marcove RC, Juvos AG, et al: Aneurysmal bone cyst: A clinicopathologic study of 66 cases. Cancer 26:615–625, 1970.
5. Carson CP, Ackerman LV, Maltby JD: Plasma cell myeloma: A clinical, pathologic and roentgenologic review of 90 cases. Am J Clin Pathol 25:849–888, 1955.
6. Case DC Jr, Lee BJ III, Clarkson BD: Improved survival times in multiple myeloma treated with melphalan, prednisone, cyclophosphamide, vincristine, and BCNU—M-2 protocol. Am J Med 63:897–903, 1977.
7. Clough JR, Price CHG: Aneurysmal bone cyst: Pathogenesis and long term results of treatment. Clin Orthop 97:52–63, 1973.
8. Cohen MD, Harrington TM, Ginsburg WW: Osteoid osteoma: 95 cases and a review of the literature. Semin Arthritis Rheum 12:265–281, 1983.
9. Congdon CC: Benign and malignant chordomas: A clinicoanatomical study of twenty-two cases. Am J Pathol 28:793–822, 1952.
10. Costa G, Engle RL Jr, Schilling A, et al: Melphalan and prednisone—effective combination for the treatment of multiple myeloma. Am J Med 54:589–599, 1973.
11. Craig FS: Metastatic and primary lesions of bone. Clin Orthop 73:33–38, 1970.
12. Dabska M, Buraczewski J: Aneurysmal bone cyst: Pathology, clinical course and radiologic appearance. Cancer 23:371–389, 1969.
13. Dahlin DC, Besse BE, Pugh DG, et al: Aneurysmal bone cysts. Radiology 64:56–65, 1955.
14. Dahlin DC, Unni KK: Bone Tumors: General Aspects and Data on 8,542 Cases, 4th ed. Springfield, IL Charles C Thomas, 1986.
15. DeSouza-Dias L, Frost HM: Osteoblastoma of the spine: A review and report of eight new cases. Clin Orthop 91: 141–151, 1973.
16. Dewald RL, Bridwell KH, Brodromas C, et al: Reconstructive spinal surgery as palliation for metastatic malignancies of the spine. Spine 10:21–26, 1985.
17. Donaldson WF: Aneurysmal bone cyst. J Bone Joint Surg 44A:25–40, 1962.
18. Fitzwater JE, Caboud HE, Farr GH: Irradiation-induced chondrosarcoma: A case report. J Bone Joint Surg 58A:1037–1040, 1976.
19. Fornaiser VL, Jorne JG: Metastases to the vertebral column. Cancer 36:590–594, 1975.
20. Francis KC, Hutter RVP: Neoplasms of the spine in the aged. Clin Orthop 26:54–66, 1963.
21. Freiberger RH: Osteoid osteoma of the spine: A cause of backache and scoliosis in children and young adults. Radiology 75:232–235, 1960.
22. Henderson ED, Dahlin DC: Chondrosarcoma of bone—A study of 280 cases. J Bone Joint Surg 45A:1450–1458, 1963.
23. Higinbotham NL, Phillips RF, Farr HW, et al: Chordoma: Thirty-five year study at Memorial Hospital. Cancer 20:1841–1850, 1967.
24. Huvos AG: Bone Tumors. Diagnosis, Treatment and Prognosis. Philadelphia, W.B. Saunders, 1979.
25. Jackson RP: Recurrent osteoblastoma: A review. Clinic Orthop 131:229–233, 1978.
26. Keim HA, Reina EG: Osteoid osteoma as a cause of scoliosis. J Bone Joint Surg 57A:159–163, 1975.
27. Khan FR, Glickman AS, Chu FCH, et al: Treatment by radiotherapy of spinal cord compression due to extradural metastases. Radiology 89:495–500, 1967.
28. Lichtenstein L: Aneurysmal bone cyst: Observations on fifty cases. J Bone Joint Surg 39A:873–882, 1957.
29. Lozman J, Holmblad J: Cavernous hemangiomas associated with scoliosis and a localized consumptive coagulopathy: A case report. J Bone Joint Surg 58A:1021–1024, 1976.

30. MacLellan DF, Wilson FC Jr: Osteoid osteoma of the spine. J Bone Joint Surg 49A:111–121, 1967.
31. Manning JH: Symptomatic hemangioma of the spine. Radiology 56:58–65, 1951.
32. Marcove RC, Mike V, Hutter RVP, et al: Chondrosarcoma of the pelvis and upper end of the femur: An analysis of factors influencing survival time in 113 cases. J Bone Joint Surg 54A:561–572, 1972.
33. Marcove RC, Miller TR: The treatment of primary and metastatic bone localized tumors by cryosurgery. Surg Clin North Am 49:421–430, 1969.
34. Marsh BW, Bonfiglio M, Brady LP, et al: Benign osteoblastoma: Range of manifestations. J Bone Joint Surg 57A:1–9, 1975.
35. Mirra J: Bone Tumors: Diagnosis and Treatment. Philadelphia, J.B. Lippincott, 1980.
36. Moberg E: The natural course of osteoid osteoma. J Bone Joint Surg 33A:166–170, 1951.
37. Mohan V, Gupta SK, Tuli SM, et al: Symptomatic vertebral hemangiomas. Clin Radiol 31:575–579, 1980.
38. Paredes JM, Mitchell BS: Multiple myeloma: Current concepts in diagnosis and management. Med Clin North Am 64:729–742, 1980.
39. Pearlman AW, Friedman M: Radical radiation therapy of chordoma. AJR 108:333–341, 1970.
40. Reilly BJ, Davison JW, Bain H: Lymphangiectasis of the skeleton: A case report. Radiology 103:385–386, 1972.
41. Saville DP: A medical option for the treatment of osteoid osteoma. Arthritis Rheum 23:1409–1411, 1981.
42. Schaberg J, Gainor BJ: A profile of metastatic carcinoma of the spine. Spine 10:19–20, 1985.
43. Schajowicz F, Lemos C: Malignant osteoblastoma. J Bone Joint Surg 58B:202–211, 1976.
44. Sherman RS, Wliner D: The roentgen diagnosis of hemangioma of bone. AJR 86:1146–1159, 1961.
45. Slowick FA, Campbell CJ, Kettelkamp DB: Aneurysmal bone cyst. J Bone Joint Surg 50A:1142–1151, 1968.
46. Valderrama JAF, Bullough PG: Solitary myeloma of the spine. J Bone Joint Surg 50B:82–90, 1968.
47. Wang CC, James AE Jr: Chordoma: Brief review of the literature and report of a case with widespread metastases. Cancer 22:162–167, 1968.
48. Young JM, Fung FJ Jr: Incidence of tumor metastasis to the lumbar spine: A comparative study of roentgenographic changes and gross lesions. J Bone Joint Surg 35A:55–64, 1953.

CHAPTER 17

Metabolic Bone Disease and the Spine*

Metabolic bone diseases are generalized disorders of skeletal homeostasis. In many instances, the disease entity presents as back pain or deformity, especially in the older patient. Thus, it is important to include metabolic bone disease in the differential diagnosis of back pain.

The bony components of the spine, like those in all regions of the adult skeleton, consist of a unique anatomic arrangement of cortical and trabecular bone. Although both types of bone are composed of similar constituents, trabecular bone has a much larger surface area to volume ratio, resulting in an eight-fold higher rate of bone turnover than in cortical bone.[120] Since the vertebral bodies are predominantly trabecular bone, it is not surprising that the spine is often the earliest and most profoundly affected site in metabolic bone disorders.

The goal of this chapter is to present an organized diagnostic and therapeutic approach to the patient with a potential metabolic disorder. An overview of the various diagnostic tools as well as the basic pathophysiology of some of the major metabolic disorders affecting the spine is presented. An understanding of normal calcium homeostasis is a prerequisite to the knowledgeable evaluation of various pathologic conditions of bone metabolism.

---

*Written with Frederick S. Kaplan, M.D.

CALCIUM HOMEOSTASIS

Calcium homeostasis is imperative for neural transmission, enzyme activity, blood coagulation, and other functions critical to life. Calcium is the fifth most abundant element in the human body and the most abundant inorganic component of the skeleton. Ninety-nine percent of total body calcium is sequestered in the skeleton, with only 1 percent in soft tissue and circulating in extracellular fluids.[123] In contrast to calcium, a larger portion of the body's phosphorus, the other major skeletal mineral, is located intracellularly and in extracellular fluid. However, 80 to 85 percent of total body phosphorus is in the skeleton, where it plays an important role in the nucleation of crystals. Elaborate mechanisms have evolved to maintain this distribution of calcium and phosphorus in such a way that skeletal integrity and metabolic homeostasis are preserved.

The extracellular control of calcium and phosphorus is primarily modulated by three important hormones. Parathyroid hormone (PTH) acts directly on bone and kidney and indirectly on the intestine to restore a lowered serum calcium level to normal.[113] The signal for increased PTH synthesis and secretion is a decrease in the serum ionized calcium concentration and a decrease in serum levels of the active form of vitamin D $(1,25(OH)_2\text{-}D)$. Calcitonin inhibits bone resorption in pharmacologic doses and is produced in parafollicular cells of the thyroid.[8] A decrease in calcium decreases calcitonin production and release. The role of calcitonin in normal human physiology, however, remains in question. Finally, the biologically potent metabolite of vitamin D $(1,25(OH)_2\text{-}D)$ stimulates intestinal absorption of calcium and phosphorus.[44,116] It also probably plays a role in the orderly mineralization and resorption of bone and has some influence on renal resorption of filtered calcium and phosphorus. PTH is a major stimulus to the production of $1,25(OH)_2\text{-}D$ by proximal renal tubule cells, and the absence of PTH as well as high serum calcium and phosphate levels can reduce its synthesis and secretion. These three hormones (PTH; $1,25(OH)_2\text{-}D$; and calcitonin), along with other paracrine and autocrine factors, work in concert to maintain the normal calcium homeostasis. A disturbance at any level in this intricate regulatory network will result in a host of compensatory changes that may lead to clinically evident disease.

Although great progress has been made over the past decade in the understanding of disorders of skeletal homeostasis, great confusion often arises from the most basic matters. Some simple definitions are essential. Osteopenia is a generic term used to describe the radiographic picture of "washed-out bone" and conveys no information about the underlying etiology of the condition. Osteoporosis, on the other hand, is a more specific term referring to a state of decreased mass per unit volume (density) of normally mineralized bone matrix. The bone is qualitatively normal, but there is less of it when compared to normal age- and sex-matched controls. Osteomalacia (soft bone, or adult rickets) must be considered in the differential diagnosis of osteopenia. Osteomalacia is a qualitative disorder of bone metabolism and refers to an increased, normal, or decreased mass of insufficiently mineralized bone matrix.

The remainder of this chapter will focus on diagnosis, pathophysiology, and treatment of metabolic bone disease, with special attention to issues relevant to the aging spine.

PATIENT EVALUATION

History

The metabolic bone diseases do not have a unique or specific complex of back symptoms. Often the patient will be asymptomatic, with an incidental radiographic abnormality. Pain is the most frequent presenting complaint, and it often does not have a mechanical basis. However, with compression fractures of the vertebral bodies, the pain may have mechanical characteristics. Other symptoms seen with metabolic disorders include muscular weakness, fatigue, and vague localized pains, especially in peripheral joints.[42]

Considered as a symptom in the more common metabolic bone disorders, spinal pain is frequently reported in osteomalacia. Complete absence of pain is common in osteoporosis, except in the presence of an acute fracture, and is rare in osteitis fibrosa. Pain is usually more severe with walking and often is worse in the lower limbs. Frequently, pain may be referred bilaterally, which may help distinguish it from nerve root pain and from other mechanical causes such as degenerative intervertebral disc disease.

In addition to determining the time of onset, location, radiation, quality, and postural relationship of the pain, several other historical points are helpful in evaluating patients with suspected metabolic bone disease. It is necessary to assess possible etiologies including endocrine abnormalities, malabsorption, dietary deficiencies, and drug effects. A review of related symptoms includes malaise, recent weight loss or gain, loss of height; hypertension, goiter or neck swelling; change in voice, skin texture, or hair consistency; sensitivity to temperature changes; palpitations; epigastric pain or burning, changes in bowel habits, diarrhea, or foul-smelling stools; dysuria, flank pain, fever, renal colic, nephrolithiasis; joint pain or swelling, generalized bone pain, or muscle weakness. It is also important to note previous hospitalizations or surgery including thyroidectomy, pituitary surgery, ulcer or bowel surgery, surgery for malignancy, and surgery for scoliosis or fractures. Women should be questioned as to menstrual history, pregnancies, lactation, amenorrhea, hot flashes, and previous oophorectomy. A careful drug history should be obtained, including use of antacids, anticonvulsants, tranquilizers, vitamins, minerals, oral contraceptives, gonadal or corticosteroids, and thyroid hormone replacement. The history should also include daily intake of dairy products, protein, alcohol, and laxatives as well as an assessment of the patient's activity level and exposure to sunlight. Finally, the family history should be screened for osteoporosis, bone/joint problems, growth disturbances, fractures, and evidence of collagen disease (blue sclerae, deafness, scoliosis, childhood dental problems, and joint laxity).

Physical Examination

Spinal manifestations of the various metabolic bone diseases often will not be easily distinguished without a complete physical examination to rule out metastatic disease, renal failure, thyroid or parathyroid abnormalities, adrenal or gonadal abnormalities, malabsorption syndromes, and collagen disorders. Kyphoscoliosis is the most prevalent spinal deformity in the metabolic bone diseases. This problem may be progressive in osteopenic disorders and may be associated with vertebral body compression fractures. Usually there is no neurologic involvement, and thus the neurologic examination and nerve root tension signs will be normal. A paucity of objective physical findings in combination with nonspecific subjective complaints is the harbinger of an underlying metabolic disturbance involving the spine.

Laboratory Studies

An extensive history and physical examination should facilitate the selection of appropriate baseline tests. Routine laboratory tests should include a complete blood count and leukocyte differential; an erythrocyte sedimentation rate; a 24-hour urine collection to measure calcium and creatinine excretion; and determination of serum calcium, albumin, phosphorus, alkaline phosphatase, BUN, and creatinine.

Additional tests are ordered as necessary if bone loss secondary to conditions other than age-related and postmenopausal osteoporosis is suspected. For patients with suspected primary or iatrogenic hyperthyroidism, TSH (thyroid-stimulating hormone) and T_4 serum levels should be obtained. Serum and/or urine protein electrophoresis is done when multiple myeloma is suspected, especially in patients over age 50. In patients with hypercalcemia, C-terminal immunoreactive PTH levels are obtained. Osteomalacia should be considered, especially in a patient with generalized myopathy, bone pain or tenderness, and symmetric long bone fractures. Abnormalities in vitamin D absorption and metabolism often play a major role in the pathogenesis of the disease, and plasma levels of 25(OH)-D and 1,25(OH)$_2$-D should be measured when osteomalacia is suspected.

Imaging Studies

Radiographic studies of the spine and any other symptomatic areas are essential. Often radiographs of the skull or hands will hold clues to the specific diagnosis. A ^{99m}Tc methylene diphosphonate bone scan may be helpful in the patient with an isolated compression fracture or a history of malignancy to rule out skeletal metastases. In addition, the bone scan can document new fractures or involvement not apparent in osteopenic bone on plain films. Finally, in centers where the diagnostic techniques are available, noninvasive tests to monitor the progression of bone loss and the response to treatment may be desirable.

Noninvasive Bone Density Measurement

Plain radiographs are useful in the initial evaluation of osteopenia; however, they are the least accurate, least precise method of assessing bone density. It is estimated that at least a 30 percent decrease in bone mass is necessary to be detected on plain films.[31] Other noninvasive radiographic and radioisotope techniques have been developed to determine skeletal mass that are precise, sensitive, and safe.

Most noninvasive measurements of bone mineral density (BMD) provide information about the quantity of bone at the specific site being measured. The ability of a bone density measurement at one site to predict the density at other sites is highly variable.[89] Although BMD measurements at one site have only limited value in predicting future fractures at other sites, density measurements of the lumbar spine have correlated well with the incidence of spontaneous vertebral fractures.[24] However, a single noninvasive measurement does not provide information about current or past rates of bone remodeling, and offers no predictive information on future bone loss rates. In order to determine the concurrent status of bone remodeling, various indirect serum and urine biochemical determinations should be performed in conjunction with dynamic bone remodeling parameters from nondecalcified bone obtained at transiliac biopsy.

Although accuracy of BMD measurement is important, precisions, or reproducibility, is even more essential for clinical applications of these techniques. Since net trabecular bone loss associated with aging is well under 5 percent per year, extremely reproducible BMD measurement techniques are necessary to detect the small annual changes in density. Isolated bone mass determinations are not recommended as a general screening tool because of a large overlap between symptomatic and asymptomatic patients and the relatively high cost of such techniques.[59] Determination of baseline and serial bone density measurements is useful to monitor progress of therapeutic regimens. One must keep in mind that while bone mass is a major determinant of fracture threshold, other factors, including cardiovascular status, medications, neuromuscular disorders, body habitus, and falls, play an important role in the generation of fractures.[144]

Three methods are widely available at the present time for BMD measurement: single photon absorptiometry (SPA) for measurement of bone mineral in the appendicular skeleton, dual photon absorptiometry

(DPA) for assessment of integral (cortical and trabecular) bone mineral in the spine or hip, and quantitative computed tomography (QCT) for the assessment of trabecular bone mineral in the vertebral bodies.[48] The newest noninvasive modality is dual-energy X-ray absorptiometry (DEXA), which can measure bone density of the spine, hip, or peripheral sites. Total-body neutron activation analysis (TBNAA) uses high energy neutrons to convert calcium to a radioactive isotope that can be measured to assess total body bone mass. TBNAA is primarily a research tool and will not be discussed further.

Single Photon Absorptiometry (SPA)

In SPA, the radioisotope iodine-125 emits a monoenergetic beam of photons that pass through the forearm, which is surrounded by a soft tissue equivalent. A sodium iodide scintillation counter is moved systematically across the other side of the forearm to detect transmitted photons. With denser bone, more of the photon beam is attenuated, and fewer photons pass through to the counter. The difference in photon absorption in bone and in soft tissue allows measurement of the mineral content of the bone. The examination is most commonly performed to detect the bone mineral content of the radius at the middiaphysis, which is predominantly cortical bone, or at the distal metaphysis, which normally contains abundant trabecular bone. The distal site is irregular in shape, and reproducibility is more difficult. SPA of the midradius, however, is reproducible to within 4 percent, and provides an accurate determination (± 3 to 4%) of the density of cortical bone at that site.[48] Although the radiation dose is minimal (10 mrem), the cost is low, and patient acceptance is high, this method cannot be used to accurately predict changes in the axial skeleton. The two most useful techniques for assessing the mineral status of the axial skeleton are dual photon absorptiometry and quantitative computed tomography.

Dual Photon Absorptiometry (DPA)

In DPA, the use of gadolinium-153 abolishes the need for a soft tissue equivalent and enables the measurement of bone mineral content in the hip and spine. This radioisotope emits photons of two distinct energies that have different attenuation by soft tissue and bone. The vertebral bodies are composed of predominantly trabecular bone and are commonly scanned from L1 to L4. Precision (3 to 5%) and accuracy (2 to 4%) are both excellent, cost and patient acceptability are high, and radiation dose is more than in SPA but less than in QCT.[149] Since all mineral within the path of the photon beam is measured, potential sources of error with DPA include aortic calcification and degenerative spinal osteophytes. Although DPA has recently been applied to measurement of bone content in the hip, preliminary data have indicated a lack of correlation between spinal and proximal femoral bone density.[34]

Quantitative Computed Tomography (QCT)

With QCT, a cross-sectional image of the vertebral body is generated, allowing differential measurement of cortical and trabecular bone density.[49] Since the rate of turnover in trabecular bone is nearly eight times that in cortical bone, this technique (in theory) provides a uniquely sensitive indicator in a region of the skeleton that is highly vulnerable to early metabolic changes. This method, developed by Cann and Genant,[24] involves the simultaneous scanning of a phantom with tubes containing standard solutions of a bone mineral equivalent that is used to calculate a standard calibration curve from which the vertebral trabecular bone density can be extrapolated. Measurements are taken from the centers of vertebral bodies T12-L4 and averaged to yield a mean bone density. Since the central portion of the vertebral body (trabecular bone) can be selectively measured, osteophytes and aortic calcifications are not a problem. As with DPA, precision is within 3 to 5 percent, but may be reduced in severely osteopenic and kyphotic individuals, owing to difficulty in relocating the exact sites of previous measurements.[18,124] Accuracy is within 5 to 10 percent, although additional error is possible because of the variable fat content of the bone marrow, especially in older patients.[84,88] The radiation dose is higher than in the radioisotope techniques (300 to 1000 mrem), but attempts are being made to modify image acquisitions to reduce radiation exposure.[23,126]

The use of mineral phantoms external to the body for standardization of density measurements is associated with some degradation of precision, owing to various physical artifacts and phantom irregularities.[50] Research is under way to develop more reliable phantoms and even to eliminate the need for an external phantom by using the body's internal paraspinal tissues as calibration standards.[15] Such improvements may further increase the reproducibility of QCT.

QCT densitometry of cadaveric vertebral bodies has demonstrated a strong correlation between density and compressive strength.[83,91] Bone density measurements of the lumbar spine have also been shown to reflect vertebral fracture morbidity in osteopenic patients.[70] Research continues on QCT assessment of proximal femur bone content and the potential correlation with hip fracture risk.[128]

Dual-Energy X-ray Absorptiometry (DEXA)

In the last 5 years, an X-ray–based, rather than isotope-based, dual-energy projectional system has been developed. This technology, also known as quantitative dual-energy radiographic absorptiometry (DRA), was initially applied to bone density measurements in the proximal femur and has shown good correlation with DPA in the spine.[16,73] Preliminary results have demonstrated significant advantages over DPA, including superior precision, lower radiation dose, shorter examination time, higher image resolution, and greater technical ease.[106] In time, this technique is likely to replace DPA.

At present, the most useful noninvasive techniques for the quantitative assessment of osteopenia are DPA, DEXA, and QCT. Each may be applied to the spine or to the hip. Further refinements in technology that allow increased resolution, decreased radiation, and diminished costs promise to make these modalities important diagnostic tools in the initial screening and long-term management of patients with early osteopenia or symptomatic disease.

Transiliac Bone Biopsy

Information indicative of the rate of bone turnover and mineralization can be determined only from direct sampling of bone. The iliac crest is a readily accessible biopsy site and may reflect changes at other clinically relevant sites. A 5 to 8 mm diameter core is obtained transcutaneously under local anesthesia.

In nondecalcified bone sections, osteomalacia is usually characterized by the accumulation of osteoid (unmineralized bone matrix) caused by a defect in the mineralization process. In osteoporosis, the ratio of unmineralized osteoid is normal, but the absolute amount of bone is decreased.

Dynamic tetracycline labeling permits the identification of immature mineral deposits and allows the determination of mineralization rates by autofluorescence. Tetracycline is administered for 3 days, followed by a 14-day interval, and then a second 3-day course of tetracycline is given prior to bone biopsy. The mean distance between the tetracycline labels is divided by the number of days between the two courses of tetracycline to determine the appositional rate. Abnormal patterns of fluorescent label deposition are the hallmark of osteomalacia.

Bone histomorphometry enables the quantitative analysis of undecalcified bone in which the parameters of skeletal remodeling are expressed in terms of volumes, surfaces, and cell numbers. Often, clinical and biochemical studies fail to predict histologic changes. In addition, histologic changes vary regionally and are strongly modulated by local factors including weight-bearing stress (magnitude and direction), blood supply, marrow environment, and type of bone (cortical vs. trabecular).[45]

Bone biopsy is not necessary for most patients with osteoporosis. However, biopsy is an important diagnostic tool in patients (men and women) less than age 50 who have osteopenia; in a patient of any age in whom osteomalacia is suspect; and in patients with chronic renal failure with skeletal symptoms. Because of the inherent problem of regional sample error, bone biopsy should not be used to establish the diagnosis of osteoporosis; rather, it should be used to exclude a diagnosis of osteomalacia or osteitis fibrosa.

OSTEOPENIC DISORDERS

The major osteopenic disorders include osteoporosis, osteomalacia, hyperparathyroidism (osteitis fibrosa), and renal osteodystrophy. Although the last-named entity can present an osteosclerotic picture as well, it will be discussed in this section.

Osteoporosis

Osteoporosis is the most common skeletal disorder in the world and is second only to arthritis as a leading cause of musculoskeletal morbidity in the elderly.[68] It is characterized by a decreased mass per unit volume (density) of normally mineralized bone matrix (osteoid) (Fig. 17–1). The most common type of osteoporosis is due to postmenopausal bone loss (type I), which is the leading cause of fractures in the elderly.[29,120] It is estimated that a third of postmenopausal women will eventually have a major orthopedic problem related to osteoporosis. Age-related (type II) osteoporosis occurs in both men and women and is caused by the slow loss of both trabecular and cortical bone that normally accompanies aging (Table 17–1).

Pathophysiology

Living bone is never completely at rest. Remodeling constantly occurs along lines of stress and is modulated by many systemic and local

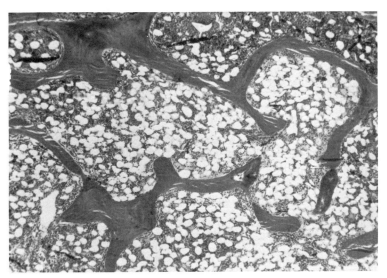

Figure 17–1. Osteoporosis. Histologic section demonstrating decreased bony trabeculae and no osteoid. (Courtesy of Arnold Schwartz, M.D.) (From Borenstein DG, Wiesel SW: Low Back Pain: Medical Diagnosis and Management. Philadelphia, W.B. Saunders, 1989.)

Table 17–1. INVOLUTIONAL OSTEOPOROSIS*

	Postmenopausal (Type I)	Age-Related (Type II)
Epidemiologic Factors		
Age (years)	55–75	>70 (F); >80 (M)
Sex ratio (F/M)	6:1	2:1
Bone Physiology or Metabolism		
Pathogenesis of uncoupling	Increased osteoclast activity; ↑ resorption	Decreased osteoblast activity; ↓ formation
Net bone loss	Mainly trabecular	Cortical and trabecular
Rate of bone loss	Rapid/short duration	Slow/long duration
Bone density	>2 standard deviations below normal	Low normal (adjusted for age and sex)
Clinical Signs		
Fracture sites	Vertebrae (crush), distal forearm, hip (intracapsular)	Vertebrae (multiple wedge), proximal humerus and tibia, hip (extracapsular)
Other signs	Tooth loss	Dorsal kyphosis
Laboratory Values		
Serum Ca^{++}	Normal	Normal
Serum P_i	Normal	Normal
Alkaline phosphatase	Normal (↑ with fracture)	Normal (↑ with fracture)
Urine Ca^{++}	Increased	Normal
PTH function	Decreased	Increased
Renal conversion of 25(OH)-D to 1,25(OH)$_2$-D	Secondary decrease due to ↓ PTH	Primary decrease due to ↓ responsiveness of 1-α-OH$_{ase}$
Gastrointestinal calcium absorption	Decreased	Decreased
Prevention		
High-risk patients	Estrogen or calcitonin supplementation; calcium supplementation; adequate vitamin D; adequate weight-bearing activity; minimization of associated risk factors	Calcium supplementation; adequate vitamin D; adequate weight-bearing activity; minimization of associated risk factors

*From Riggs BL, Melton LJ III: Involutional osteoporosis. N Engl J Med 306:446–450, 1986.

environmental influences. The factors that control bone formation and resorption are not well understood, but under normal circumstances, bone formation is tightly coupled to bone resorption.[112] From birth until the middle of the fourth decade, bone formation slightly exceeds bone resorption and a net accumulation of bone mass occurs until peak bone mass is reached. After that point, the scale tips slightly in favor of bone resorption, and there is a gradual decline in bone mass over time.[118] If the overall rate of bone turnover is slow, this decline is gradual; however, if bone turnover is increased, the loss of bone mass will be more rapid.[47]

Males usually lose between 5 and 8 percent of their bone mass every decade (after age 40), whereas females lose between 10 and 15 percent each decade and even more in the perimenopausal period.[145] In general, males have more bone mass than females, and blacks have more bone mass than whites. Accordingly, the diagnosis of osteoporosis is relative and depends on comparison of an individual to a "normal" population. Some of the more simplistic definitions maintain that osteoporosis is present when BMD is greater than two standard deviations below the mean of a population matched for age, sex, and race.[101]

Using BMD as the sole determinant of osteoporosis is not reliable, as there is a significant overlap between symptomatic and asymptomatic patients. This finding supports the notion that some forms of osteoporosis may involve qualitative rather than simply quantitative defects in bone. The generation of fractures in patients is dependent on other variables such as neurologic dysfunction and the frequency and types of falls for a patient.[74]

The actual cause of osteoporosis in most cases is unknown. Histomorphometric analysis of corticocancellous bone from transiliac biopsies suggests that postmenopausal osteoporosis is a heterogeneous disorder with a spectrum of skeletal kinetics and bone remodeling activity ranging from accelerated to reduced bone turnover. Sometimes excessive osteoclastic activity results in a rapid turnover state. Alternatively, osteoblastic function may be defective.[25] In other cases the rate of turnover may be normal, but a defect in the coupling of formation and resorption may be present. There are hereditary, disuse, nutritional, endocrine, drug-related, and neoplastic causes of osteoporosis (Table 17–2). The person most at risk for osteoporosis is a sedentary, postmenopausal, white or Oriental woman who has a lifelong dietary calcium deficiency. Associated risk factors include small stature, slim body habitus, light-colored hair and freckles, scoliosis, joint hypermobility, cigarette smoking, heavy alcohol intake, early menopause (natural or surgical), and family history.

Clinical Findings

The earliest symptom of osteoporosis may be an episode of acute pain in the middle to low thoracic or high lumbar spine regions while at rest or doing routine daily activities such as standing, bending, or lifting. The episode is often precipitated by activity that under normal circumstances would not be stressful enough to cause a fracture. The onset of

Table 17–2. CAUSES OF OSTEOPOROSIS

Primary	Pharmacologic
Involutional (postmenopausal or senile)	Heparan sulfate
Idiopathic (juvenile)	Anticonvulsants (phenytoin, phenobarbital)
Secondary	Ethanol
Endocrine	Methotrexate
Hypogonadism	Genetic
Adrenocortical hormone excess	Osteogenesis imperfecta
Hyperthyroidism	Homocystinuria
Hyperparathyroidism	Miscellaneous
Diabetes mellitus	Rheumatoid arthritis
Growth hormone deficiency	Chronic liver disease
Nutritional	Chronic renal disease
Calcium deficiency	Immobilization
Phosphate deficiency	Malignancy (multiple myeloma)
Phosphate excess	Metabolic acidosis
Vitamin D deficiency	Cigarette smoking
Protein deficiency	
Vitamin C deficiency	
Intestinal malabsorption	

pain is usually sudden, and most patients can recall the exact moment when it began. They can usually identify the level of originating pain. Spinal movement is severely restricted. Pain is exacerbated with sitting, standing, coughing, sneezing, or straining. Loss of appetite, abdominal distension, and ileus secondary to retroperitoneal hemorrhage may accompany lower thoracic and upper lumbar compression fractures.

Pain is the primary complaint. Generally, there is no neural compression. Spontaneous vertebral compression fractures are stable injuries, although radiculopathies often occur with thoracic or upper lumbar fractures and may cause unilateral or bilateral pain radiating anteriorly along the costal margin of the affected spinal nerve. Spinal cord or cauda equina involvement is even less common and suggests other conditions such as infection or tumor.

During the intervals between compression fractures (often years), most patients are pain-free. However, approximately 30 percent continue to be chronically plagued with dull, aching, postural pain. These compression fractures are in many instances associated with a progressively increasing kyphoscoliosis. As the spinal deformity progresses, there will be a decrease in the patient's height, which can be used to follow the clinical course of the disease.[146]

Extraspinal skeletal manifestations of osteoporosis include fractures caused by minimal trauma. The most common sites of involvement are the proximal femur, distal radius, proximal humerus, and ribs.

Radiographic Findings

Radiographs of the spine provide a traditional method of assessment in osteoporosis or any of the other osteopenic conditions. In general, at least 30 percent of the bone mass must be lost before the change is discernible on plain radiographs.[7] The earliest radiographic evidence of spinal osteopenia is often the resorption of the horizontal trabeculae, which may lead to accentuation of the vertical trabeculae initially, or a hollow-appearing vertebral body in more involved cases. In the most severe cases, the intervertebral disc may appear more dense than the vertebral body, producing a misleading optical illusion.

Before clinically evident vertebral compression fractures occur, the vertebral bodies usually become washed out, and as the subchondral cortical plates weaken, the intervertebral disc space may expand. If the mineral loss is severe, the strength of the vertebral body is decreased and a fracture may occur (Fig. 17–2). Wedging, the reduction in vertical height of the anterior border of a vertebral body, and biconcave compression are the two most common deformities.[14] Symmetric and waferlike collapse of the entire vertebral body is less common with osteoporosis and often suggests metastatic disease, myeloma, lymphoma, or a primary bone tumor. The changes in osteoporotic vertebrae are usually unevenly distributed along the spine.[13] No two affected vertebrae are identical, and roentgenographically normal vertebrae may be found between collapsed levels.

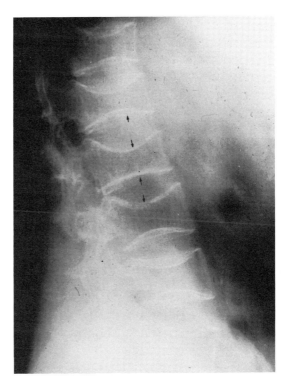

Figure 17-2. Osteoporosis. Radiograph shows generalized loss of bone mineral in multiple vertebral bodies along with thin cortical end plates in a 60-year-old woman with diffuse midline back pain. Disc expansion into vertebral bodies is associated with weakened bone structures (*arrows*). (Courtesy of Anne Brower, M.D.) (From Borenstein DG, Wiesel SW: Low Back Pain: Medical Diagnosis and Management. Philadelphia, W.B. Saunders, 1989.)

Laboratory Findings

There are no specific laboratory findings diagnostic of osteoporosis. In uncomplicated postmenopausal disease, results of routine laboratory tests are normal and do not assess the extent or rate of bone loss or indicate the prognosis. Even in severe postmenopausal disease, serum calcium, inorganic phosphorus, and alkaline phosphatase levels are usually within the normal range, although alkaline phosphatase levels may be elevated for several weeks following a fracture.

Differential Diagnosis

A thorough medical evaluation is desirable before initiating any type of treatment. It is important to rule out other entities that can mimic osteoporosis, including osteomalacia, hyperparathyroidism, hyperthyroidism, primary or metastatic cancer, multiple myeloma, intestinal malabsorption, Cushing's disease, and biliary cirrhosis.[100] Accordingly, a bone biopsy may occasionally be necessary. Osteoporosis should be considered a diagnosis of exclusion.

Treatment

The management of spinal osteoporosis and its complications must address immediate relief of symptoms as well as long-term maintenance of skeletal mass. Spinal compression fractures are painful and can cause significant short-term morbidity. However, they heal quickly, even in severely osteopenic bone. Thus, the initial goals of therapy are to relieve pain, provide comfortable mechanical support for the spine, coordinate a rehabilitation program, and provide encouragement and reassurance to the patient and family.

Bedrest and appropriate analgesics are indicated for several days after an acute spinal compression fracture, until the acute pain begins to subside. A firm mattress prevents spinal flexion, which may aggravate the traumatic kyphosis, and a pillow under the knees will relieve any excessive strain on the lumbar spine. If narcotics are used in the management of acute pain, care must be taken to avoid constipation, urinary retention, and respiratory depression, especially in elderly patients. Occasionally, ileus develops in patients with high lumbar compression fractures, necessitating parenteral fluid therapy for several days.

Once the acute pain begins to subside and the patient can turn in bed comfortably, mobilization should begin. The patient should attempt to sit or stand for periods of no more than 15 minutes several times a day. As more relief is obtained, the patient should increase the frequency and duration of mobilization periods but should continue intermittent bed rest until symptoms disappear.

For severe pain or persistent symptoms following compression fractures in the middle to lower thoracic regions, a rigid thoracolumbar hyperextension orthosis may be used to provide external support. Often rigid braces are not well received and can cause skin problems. In most cases, a custom-fitted elastic corset will give good support to these patients after acute fractures. In severe cases that result in neurologic compromise, surgical intervention may be undertaken to decompress the spinal canal. Between episodes of compression fracture, patients should be encouraged to exercise.[6,79] Walking and swimming are the safest exercises. A cane or walker may be helpful in patients with increased incidence of falls.

Osteoporosis is more effectively prevented than treated. The goals of prevention include (1) achieving as high an initial bone mass as genetically possible by proper nutrition, calcium intake, exercise, and minimization of risk factors prior to skeletal maturity; (2) continuing these beneficial habits through adulthood to help preserve bone mass; and (3) increasing calcium intake with aging and considering the addition of estrogen supplementation at the menopause for those at high risk of developing osteoporosis.

The single most effective measure for prevention of postmenopausal (type I) osteoporosis is estrogen supplementation beginning at the time of the menopause. Estrogen preserves positive calcium balance; however, the mechanism of action of estrogen on bone remains unknown. Only recently have estrogen receptors been found on bone cells, prompting a new search for a direct, rather than indirect, mechanism of action.[38,71,78] The benefits of estrogen therapy are greatest in the perimenopausal period when rates of trabecular bone loss are the highest.

The question of estrogen's effect more than 10 years after menopause remains unanswered. Some work has suggested that estrogen may be beneficial up to age 75.[75]

The increased risk of endometrial cancer with estrogen therapy is about 1 percent per year and can be minimized with the cyclical use of a progestational agent.[39] Estrogen therapy is contraindicated in patients with a strong family history of breast or endometrial cancer or venous thrombosis. Recent work has shown that adequate calcium supplementation may cut the required dose of estrogen in half.[40] The effectiveness of the transdermal estrogen patch is still under investigation.

The hormone calcitonin has been approved by the FDA for use in the treatment (prevention) of postmenopausal osteoporosis. Its major effect is to prevent bone loss by inhibiting bone resorption. Although the medication is expensive and is available only in parenteral forms, calcitonin may provide an alternative for prevention of osteoporosis in the postmenopausal woman in whom estrogen supplementation is contraindicated.

Fluoride was thought to be beneficial in the treatment of established osteoporosis, since it both stabilizes the mineral crystal and stimulates osteoblasts to form new bone matrix. Although newly synthesized bone is radiographically denser, it is not normal. Early research suggested a decreased incidence of vertebral body compression fractures in patients taking sodium fluoride, compared with untreated controls.[54,82,108,121] However, prospective studies have suggested an increased incidence of hip fractures in fluoride-treated patients and no decrease in the rate of spinal fractures.[119] Fluoride therapy without the appropriate intake of calcium and vitamin D, however, can lead to a severe osteomalacic condition. The most frequent complaints in patients taking fluoride include gastrointestinal upset and lower extremity arthralgias.

Adequate lifelong calcium intake may be important in the maintenance of bone integrity.[60] The average postmenopausal woman requires 1500 mg of elemental calcium daily, the equivalent of six glasses of milk. In persons with adequate exposure to sunlight, vitamin D supplements are not necessary. In deficient patients, treatment should not exceed 800 IU daily. It is becoming clear, however, that calcium supplementation alone does not prevent postmenopausal trabecular bone loss and should not be used in place of other therapies.[122]

A recent two-year prospective investigation has shown that intermittent cyclical etidronate therapy significantly increases spinal bone mass and reduces the incidence of new fractures.[151] Etidronate (Didronel) is a bisphosphate that inhibits osteoclast-mediated bone resorption. A daily dose of 400 mg orally (on an empty stomach) is given for 2 weeks (without supplemental calcium) and is followed by 10 weeks of calcium therapy (500 to 1000 mg orally each day); this cycle is then repeated.

Other treatments under investigation include coherence therapy with oral phosphate and calcitonin, diphosphonates, and capacitively coupled electric fields.[19,125]

Osteomalacia

Osteomalacia syndromes are of diverse etiology but are all characterized by a failure of normal mineralization of bone matrix (osteoid). Rickets is characterized by impaired mineralization of cartilage, leading to arrest in the formation of primary spongiosa during endochondral ossification. Rickets, by definition, cannot be present in skeletally mature adults, while osteomalacia can be present at any age once lamellar bone has formed to replace woven bone. The ensuing discussion will focus on osteomalacia and its variants with renal osteodystrophy considered in a separate section.

Pathophysiology

There is a failure of normal mineralization of osteoid in all forms of osteomalacia (Fig. 17–3). Generally, an abnormality in calcium, phosphate, or vitamin D metabolism results in a decreased serum calcium–phosphorus product, which prevents mineralization of newly formed bone matrix.[87] Osteomalacia represents an uncoupling of the pro-

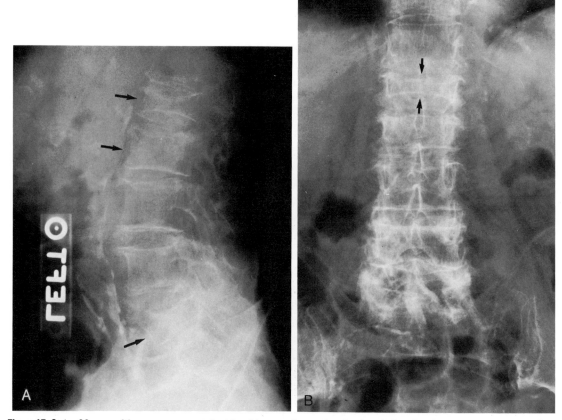

Figure 17–3. An 83-year-old woman presented with a history of acute low back pain localized to the thoracolumbar junction. *A*, Lateral view reveals generalized osteopenia with diminished height of L1, L2, and L5 (*arrows*). *B*, AP view reveals marked loss of height of the L1 vertebral body (*arrows*). (From Borenstein DG, Wiesel SW: Low Back Pain: Medical Diagnosis and Management. Philadelphia, W.B. Saunders, 1989.)

cesses of osteoid synthesis and mineralization. The causes of osteomalacia, although multiple and varied, can be classified into three basic groups: (1) nutritional deficiency, (2) vitamin D–resistant/renal tubular conditions, and (3) renal osteodystrophy (Table 17–3).

The classic and most clearly understood cause of nutritional deficiency osteomalacia is a dietary deficiency of vitamin D, which may be due to lack of precursor intake, inadequate sunlight exposure, or a malabsorption syndrome.[96] In rare cases, the final converting enzyme in the vitamin D pathway may be defective. Regardless, the diminished level of vitamin D results in the decreased synthesis of the active metabolite $1,25(OH)_2$-D with subsequent decreased absorption of calcium from the gastrointestinal tract, and in diminished reabsorption of filtered calcium from the renal tubule. The hypocalcemia may interfere with mineralization of matrix but also results in a mild to moderate secondary hyperparathyroidism, which restores the serum calcium at the expense of further depleting skeletal stores of calcium. The action of parathyroid hormone on the renal tubules causes a marked diuresis and a resultant hypophosphatemia.

In developed communities, genetic or acquired osteomalacic syndromes refractory to therapeutic doses of vitamin D are now more common than those associated with vitamin D deficiencies. A variety of vitamin D–resistant conditions can result from isolated effects on the renal tubules and all cause impaired tubular phosphate reabsorption. The most common condition is familial or X-linked dominant hypophosphatemic vitamin D resistance (type I).[110] Other examples include the Fanconi syndromes, with additional loss of glucose (type II) or of glucose and amino acids (type III), the renal tubular acidosis syndromes, and the hypophosphatemic osteomalacia that can accompany fibrous dysplasia, neurofibromatosis, or other soft-tissue tumors producing putative hypo-

Table 17–3. CAUSES OF OSTEOMALACIA

Nutritional Deficiency
  Vitamin D
  Calcium
  Phosphorus
GI Absorption Defects
  Gastric abnormalities
  Biliary disease
  Enteric absorption defects
Renal Tubular Defects (Vitamin D–Resistant)
  Proximal tubular lesions
  Distal tubular lesions
  Proximal and distal tubular lesions
Renal Osteodystrophy
Osteomalacia Associated with Other
  Conditions
  Fibrous dysplasia
  Neurofibromatosis
  Soft tissue and bone neoplasms (e.g., giant cell
    tumor, nonossifying fibroma)
  Anticonvulsant medication
  Heavy metal ingestion
  Hypophosphatasia

phosphatemic factors.[43] All of these conditions are described as being vitamin D–resistant, and the primary defect is not in the vitamin D pathway but in the body's inability to conserve phosphorus at the kidney. Although serum levels of $1,25(OH)_2$-D are reported as normal in many of these disorders, they are inappropriately low for the level of hypophosphatemia. In these cases, the vitamin D level may reflect decreased renal synthesis of the active metabolite due to feedback inhibition from increased renal phosphorus flux. The calcium-phosphorus product is insufficient for mineralization of newly formed osteoid, and osteomalacia results. In these hypophosphatemic conditions, there is little or no secondary hyperparathyroidism, as the serum calcium is characteristically normal.

In addition to the two major groups of osteomalacia and renal osteodystrophy (discussed later), several less common disorders cause osteomalacia. Hypophosphatasia is a group of disorders resulting from a genetic error in the synthesis of alkaline phosphatase in bone, cartilage, liver, intestinal mucosa, and kidney.[41] In these conditions, the calcium-phosphorus product may actually be high and occasionally manifest life-threatening elevations (infantile form). Owing to the absence of functional bone alkaline phosphatase, inorganic pyrophosphate (a potent inhibitor of mineralization) cannot be degraded, and thus mineralization of osteoid cannot proceed. While infants and children may develop severe changes that mimic rickets, adults may have a milder form that may present like osteomalacia (Fig. 17–4). The ingestion of heavy metals such as cadmium, be-

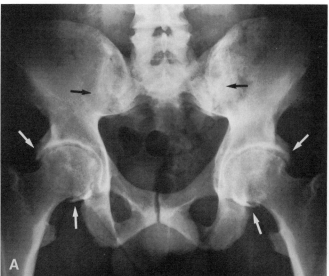
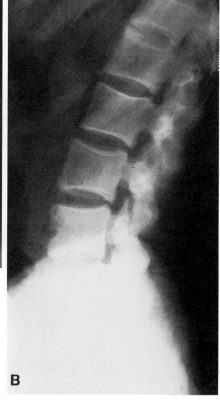

Figure 17–4. Hypophosphatasia. A 37-year-old man presented with marked stiffness of the spine. Laboratory evaluation revealed low serum alkaline phosphatase concentrations. *A*, Pelvic view reveals sclerosis of the sacroiliac joints (*black arrows*) and marked bony overgrowth of both acetabula (*white arrows*). *B*, Lateral view of spine reveals generalized coarsening of vertebral trabeculae. (From Borenstein DG, Wiesel SW: Low Back Pain: Medical Diagnosis and Management. Philadelphia, W.B. Saunders, 1989.)

ryllium, and aluminum can produce an osteomalacic syndrome. Excessive sodium fluoride and diphosphonate ingestion can also cause a similar syndrome. Chronic hyperparathyroidism has also been reported as a rare cause of osteomalacia.[72] Finally, chronic anticonvulsant therapy can decrease serum 25(OH)-D levels and inhibit intestinal calcium absorption enough to result in osteopenia and fractures.[52]

Clinical Findings

The clinical diagnosis of osteomalacia in the adult is considerably more difficult to establish than that of rickets in the child. In the relatively mild forms of the disease, only slowly progressive changes are seen, and the patients may be asymptomatic for years. With more advanced disease, the spinal manifestations of osteomalacia are generalized pain and tenderness beginning in the low back.[43] The patient may also complain of muscular weakness, inability to climb stairs, and poorly localized bone pain with tenderness in the extremities. In some cases, a proximal limb girdle myopathy may result in a waddling gait.

Radiographic Findings

In the spine, the most common radiographic finding is biconcavity of the vertebral bodies, referred to as "codfish vertebrae" (Fig. 17–5).[22] The curves are smooth because the bone is softer than normal, rather than brittle. Vertebrae along the entire spine are usually affected to

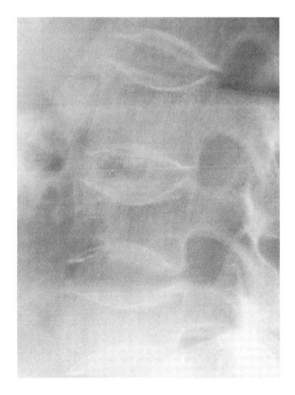

Figure 17–5. Osteomalacia. There is diffuse osteopenia (diminution of bone density) as well as symmetric biconcave deformities at all visible levels. (From Kricun ME: Imaging Modalities in Spinal Disorders. Philadelphia, W.B. Saunders, 1988.)

the same extent. The lumbar vertebrae may show more severe involvement than the thoracic vertebrae, but there is a smooth progression throughout the spine. For the most part, the radiographic appearance is that of osteopenia, indistinguishable from that of hyperparathyroidism or osteoporosis. There may be some subtle loss of end-plate clarity and coarsening of the trabecular pattern not seen in osteoporosis. A slowly progressive kyphosis and shortening of the spine can complicate osteomalacia.[140] Severe spinal deformity may be accompanied by a pigeon chest due to buckling of the sternum. Abrupt changes in height due to vertebral compression fractures do not occur in osteomalacia unless the patient has osteoporosis as well.

The other significant radiographic finding in osteomalacia is pseudofractures. The appearance is that described by Milkman and Looser and consists of a transverse lucency arising spontaneously in a long or flat bone without displacement or callus formation.[99] These defects are often symmetric and painless and do not heal until the underlying metabolic problem is corrected. The transverse radiolucent defects most often occur on the concave side of long bones, the medial aspect of the femoral neck, the ribs, the ischial and pubic rami, and the axillary border of the scapula.

Laboratory Findings

In most patients with osteomalacia, the serum calcium is normal or slightly low, serum inorganic phosphate is diminished, and serum alkaline phosphatase is elevated. The serum calcium is usually not strikingly abnormal because of the secondary hyperparathyroidism that preserves the serum calcium at the expense of bone calcium. Urinary calcium is consistently low (<75 mg/day) in 95 percent of patients with osteomalacia.[103] Renal tubular reabsorption of phosphate (TRP) is also usually diminished.

The only way to definitively diagnose osteomalacia is to perform a bone biopsy.[26] Undecalcified bone obtained at transiliac biopsy reveals both increased thickness in the osteoid seams and increased trabecular bone surface area. Tetracycline labeling will reveal a decrease in the mineral apposition rate and smudging of the label, a diagnostic and pathognomonic feature of osteomalacia. In the nutritional deficiency cases, secondary hyperparathyroidism will result in marrow fibrosis near the bony trabeculae (osteitis fibrosa).

Differential Diagnosis

Osteoporosis and osteomalacia are two commonly confused osteopenic conditions in adults.[102] Osteoporosis involves a decreased density of normally mineralized bone matrix, while osteomalacia may reflect an increased, normal, or decreased mass of insufficiently mineralized bone matrix. While osteoporosis is much more common and occurs mostly in the elderly, osteomalacia may be present at any age.

Osteomalacia is one of many conditions that can present as osteopenia of the spine. All of the osteopenic conditions outlined earlier must be ruled out. Once the diagnosis of osteomalacia is made, the next step is to pinpoint its etiology so that appropriate therapy can be initiated.

Treatment

The management of the various osteomalacic conditions is dependent on the pathophysiology of the underlying disorder. Unlike in osteoporotic fractures, the pseudofractures in osteomalacia will not heal until the primary problem is corrected.

In states of vitamin D deficiency, the treatment is based upon replacement of the lacking vitamin. As long as the hepatic and renal conversions of vitamin D are not impaired, replacement therapy should begin with 400 to 800 IU vitamin D daily, following a loading dose of 50,000 units to replenish body stores. Measurement of the serum 25(OH)-D level is the best single test to assess total body stores of the vitamin.

In the treatment of anticonvulsant osteomalacia,[52] the intermediary hepatic metabolite 25(OH)-D can be used with an initial starting dose of 20/μg orally every other day, followed by carefully titrating therapy to serum levels of 25(OH)-D. Dietary calcium supplementation (500 to 1000 mg/day) is essential. A vitamin D supplement (400 IU/day) should be given to all patients on anticonvulsant therapy.

States of vitamin D resistance are treated primarily with phosphorus therapy (Neutra-phos, 250 mg/day orally in 4 divided doses between meals). However, $1,25(OH)_2$-D must be added to the regimen to help promote absorption of the phosphorus, and to provide direct feedback inhibition to the parathyroid glands, thus preventing secondary hyperparathyroidism. Therapy must be carefully monitored to prevent dangerous hypercalcemia from hypervitaminosis D. Inorganic phosphate and $1,25(OH)_2$-D should be stopped at least 24 hours prior to any surgical intervention for corrective osteotomies and resumed when the patient is ambulatory following surgery. Treatment of vitamin D–resistant states may need to be continued throughout life to prevent symptomatic bone disease.

It is generally not advisable to attempt surgical correction of the spinal deformities in osteomalacia. Mechanical maneuvers consisting of serial traction followed by plaster fixation have been reported in rare cases.[17,110] In general, symptomatic treatment with bracing and pharmacotherapy as outlined above is recommended.

Renal Osteodystrophy

Renal osteodystrophy is a ubiquitous complication of chronic renal failure and is one of the most commonly encountered osteomalacic conditions. Chronic disease of the renal glomerulus results in renal insufficiency, azotemia, and acidosis. These metabolic changes have profound skeletal effects, which may include rickets or osteomalacia, osteitis fibrosa cystica, osteoporosis, osteosclerosis, and metastatic calcification.

Pathophysiology

The pathogenesis of the bone changes in renal osteodystrophy is complex. The two main abnormalities are phosphate retention secondary to uremia and insufficient renal synthesis of $1,25(OH)_2$-D.[27,139] These two abnormalities result in hypocalcemia leading to osteomalacia and subsequently a secondary hyperparathyroidism with bone changes of osteitis fibrosa. In some cases with secondary hyperparathyroidism, the calcium-phosphorus product is exceeded and ectopic calcification may occur in the conjunctivae, blood vessels, periarticular tissues, and skin. As the renal failure progresses and the glomerular filtration rate falls below 20 ml/min, the persistent acidosis further aggravates the negative calcium balance.[30]

Clinical Findings

The skeletal presentation of renal osteodystrophy is similar to that of other forms of rickets/osteomalacia, although more severe.[20] Most of these patients have severe bone pain and pathologic fractures and do not respond to any of the metabolites of vitamin D. In addition, the over-zealous use of aluminum hydroxide gels to control the hyperphosphatemia can aggravate the osteomalacia by deposition of aluminum in bone or can lead to encephalopathy from deposition in the brain.[105]

Radiographic Findings

Long and flat bones show diffuse osteopenia with coarsening of trabeculae and radiolucent cortical defects.[35,51] "Salt and pepper" skull (referring to the speckled appearance of the cranium) is commonly seen, along with erosion of the distal tip of the clavicle. The subperiosteal resorption of the phalanges and distal tuft erosions typical of hyperparathyroidism may also be seen. Osteosclerosis is present in 20 percent of patients (Fig. 17–6) and may be eccentrically located in the long bones or seen as dense and lucent bands in the spine—the "rugger jersey" spine (see Fig. 17–7). Osteosclerosis may not be a true increase in bone deposition, but rather a hypertrabeculation.

Laboratory Findings

Laboratory findings include elevated BUN and creatinine, normal or low serum calcium, and a serum inorganic phosphate usually

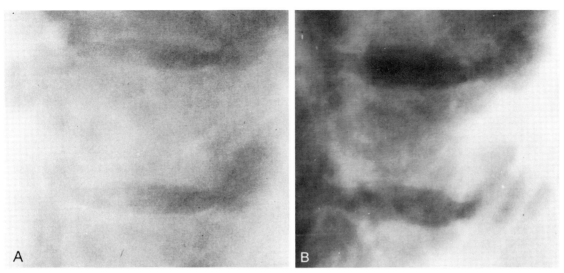

Figure 17-6. Patient with chronic renal failure. *A*, Predialysis. There is mild osteosclerosis. The vertebral margins, although not as well defined as normal, are still sharply but thinly outlined. *B*, Three years after renal dialysis was initiated. There is a central depression deformity ("H" vertebra). The margins of the floor of the central depression are poorly defined. Diffuse osteosclerosis is evident. (From Kricun ME: Imaging Modalities in Spinal Disorders. Philadelphia, W.B. Saunders, 1988.)

over 5.5 mg%. The alkaline phosphatase and PTH levels are almost invariably elevated. For unknown reasons, 20 percent of patients with renal osteodystrophy have relatively normal calcium and phosphorus levels and only slightly increased PTH levels, and yet suffer from profound osteomalacia. In some patients, this may be related to extremely high levels of aluminum deposits in the bone from phosphate binders.

Differential Diagnosis

The diagnosis of renal osteodystrophy is usually straightforward. However, once the condition becomes symptomatic, the individual components of the bone disease must be evaluated with a tetracycline-labeled bone biopsy to guide treatment of the most severe components (i.e., osteomalacia, hyperparathyroidism, and aluminum deposition).[135]

Treatment

The goals of treatment of abnormal mineral metabolism in patients with chronic renal failure include (1) adjustment of the serum calcium and phosphorus levels to normal, (2) suppression of secondary hyperparathyroidism, (3) prevention of extraskeletal deposits of calcium and phosphorus by normalization of the calcium-phosphorus product, and (4) chelating bone aluminum in patients with aluminum-associated osteomalacia.[86] Presently, the only reliable determination of bone aluminum deposition is by analysis of a bone biopsy specimen. Management usually involves chronic dialysis or renal transplantation. Additional measures include calcium acetate to diminish hyperphosphatemia,[129] administration of $1,25(OH)_2$-D to increase calcium absorption and to decrease PTH secretion, and parathyroidectomy to control the sometimes autonomous hyperparathyroidism. Parathyroidectomy in the presence of bone aluminum deposition may actually worsen the bone disease by decreasing bone remodeling rates. Therefore, a bone biopsy is suggested in patients with renal osteodystrophy prior to consideration of parathyroidectomy.

Hyperparathyroidism

Hyperparathyroidism is caused by an increase in the production of parathyroid hormone (PTH). In primary hyperparathyroidism, the excessive production is due to a single enlarged parathyroid gland (adenoma) in 80 percent of the cases, to enlargement of all four glands (hyperplasia) in 20 percent of the cases, and only rarely to cancer.[67,114] In secondary hyperparathyroidism, the stimulation for increased PTH production comes from a state of low serum calcium. In rare instances, hyperparathyroidism can result from ectopic secretion of PTH-like substances from malignant tumors.

Pathophysiology

Pathologic manifestations of hyperparathyroidism result from either a high PTH level or a high serum calcium level. In bone, PTH activates osteoclastic resorption of bone, which can lead to significant bone loss. Although there is a coupled increase in osteoblastic bone formation, resorption exceeds formation. Osteoblasts release alkaline phosphatase, and serum levels are usually elevated in patients with skeletal involvement. In severe cases, large cystic areas in bone are replaced with vascular fibrous tissue interspersed with hemosiderin-laden macrophages and giant cells. The fibrous lesions are referred to as osteitis fibrosa cystica, or Brown tumors.

In the kidney, PTH increases calcium reabsorption in the renal tubule, but this does not compensate for the increased renal filtration due to elevated serum calcium levels; the result is hypercalciuria. Nephrolithiasis occurs in approximately 10 percent of patients, and nephrocalcinosis is extremely rare. Hypercalcemia also decreases the capacity to concentrate urine, which often results in polyuria.

Clinical Findings

Primary hyperparathyroidism is most common in women over age 50, and asymptomatic hypercalcemia is often the presenting scenario.[81] The onset is generally insidious with lethargy, loss of appetite, nausea, vomiting, and polydipsia as the main complaints. Pancreatitis and peptic ulcers may also be seen. Today, most patients with primary hyperparathyroidism never develop osteitis fibrosa cystica because the disease is usually diagnosed early in its course. The skeletal manifestations of secondary hyperparathyroid bone disease are now more commonly seen in patients with chronic renal failure due to the inability to cure the underlying disease process.

The spine is variably affected in hyperparathyroidism. The general disease may be quite severe with only mild spine involvement, or the spine may be the patient's most symptomatic area. However, most patients with clinically significant osteitis fibrosa will have some degree of spinal involvement.[3] The chief complaint is pain with a developing kyphosis. Loss of vertebral height is usually continuous over time and distributed evenly throughout the spine, as in osteomalacia. The loss in height is more rapid than with osteomalacia and may involve the cervical and thoracic spine in addition to the lumbar spine.[2] Although the kyphosis and shortening may be progressive, significant pain is not always an accompanying factor, and neurologic impairment is extremely rare.[134]

Radiographic Findings

Long and flat bones show diffuse osteopenia with coarsening of trabeculae and radiolucent defects. Classic features include subperiosteal resorption of bone in the middle phalanges of the hand, distal digital tufts, and resorption at the margins of some joints (sternoclavicular, acromioclavicular, and sacroiliac). Trabecular resorption in medullary bone results in "salt and pepper" skull.

Changes in the spine may be similar to those seen in renal osteodystrophy. There may be varying combinations of osteitis fibrosa and osteosclerosis. In severe spinal osteitis fibrosa, the vertebrae have coarsened trabeculae and moderate end-plate sclerosis, and are all compressed with mild wedging.[111] As spinal involvement progresses, the picture of "rugger jersey" spine with end-plate sclerosis will emerge (Fig. 17–7).

Laboratory Findings

The most consistent laboratory abnormality in hyperparathyroidism is the elevation of serum alkaline phosphatase. Calcium is usually elevated above 11.5 mg percent but may rarely be normal. Serum phosphate is almost always decreased, and the tubular reabsorption of phosphate (TRP) is usually less than 85 percent. PTH will be elevated in both primary and secondary hyperparathyroidism.

Differential Diagnosis

The differential diagnosis in a patient with a spinal lesion and hypercalcemia (hypercalciuria) must include primary hyperparathyroidism, multiple myeloma, lymphoma, sarcoidosis, humoral hypercal-

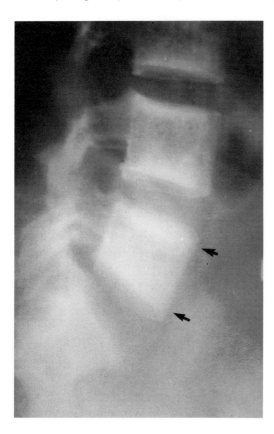

Figure 17–7. Hyperparathyroidism. "Rugger jersey" spine with sclerosis at the superior and inferior margins of the vertebral bodies. This appearance may also be seen with renal osteodystrophy and osteopetrosis. (From Borenstein DG, Wiesel SW: Low Back Pain: Medical Diagnosis and Management. Philadelphia, W.B. Saunders, 1989.)

cemia of malignancy, immobilized Paget's disease, and vitamin D intoxication. The "rugger jersey" spine may be seen in primary hyperparathyroidism, renal osteodystrophy, and osteopetrosis. Each of these entities must be considered and ruled out in an organized evaluation.

Treatment

Surgical intervention is the principal treatment of primary hyperparathyroidism. Once the source of increased PTH is removed, the skeletal lesions will usually heal. Secondary hyperparathyroidism is best managed by treatment of the underlying cause. Specifically for the spine, external support and analgesics should be used as necessary to reduce symptoms.

OSTEOSCLEROTIC DISORDERS

Most metabolic bone disease results in osteopenia of the spine. Less frequently, however, increased radiodensity is seen. This is referred to as hyperostosis when primarily cortical bone is involved and as osteosclerosis if predominantly trabecular bone is affected. Bone of increased density is not always mechanically stronger, since the increase is often due to accumulation of abnormally organized bone.

Osteopetrosis

First described by Albers-Schoenberg, osteopetrosis is a group of closely related disorders characterized by defective osteoclastic resorption of bone. There is a congenital malignant form that usually results in infant or early childhood death as well as a benign, or adult, form. The latter is characterized by an autosomal dominant inheritance, little disability, and normal life expectancy.[66]

The hallmark of congenital osteopetrosis is the complete failure of normal osteoclast activity, which results in a variety of hematologic, neurologic, radiographic, histologic, and metabolic abnormalities.[46] There is a lack of resorption of calcified cartilage and primary bone spongiosa, which results in a decreased marrow space. Despite increased density, the bones are brittle due to a predominance of calcified cartilage.

In the adult form of osteopetrosis, fewer than half the cases are symptomatic. There may be an increased susceptibility to fractures.[57] The radiographic changes are similar to those in the congenital form but are generally less severe.[62] In the spine, there is increased bone density with end-plate widening producing horizontal banding. In the pelvis, long bones, and sometimes the vertebrae, there may be a double cortical outline producing a bone within a bone appearance. The radiographic abnormalities are usually symmetric. Calcium, phosphorus, and alkaline phosphatase are normal; acid phosphatase may be elevated.[66]

The adult form of osteopetrosis rarely requires special management. The congenital form has recently been successfully treated with bone marrow transplantation, resulting in a normalization of the radiographic abnormalities.[69]

Osteofluorosis

This disease results solely from excessive fluoride ingestion. It is seen in areas of the world where the water fluoride content is high (>4 ppm) or with consumption of foods grown in high-fluoride soil.[95,138] Fluorosis is rare now, except in those with extremely high water intake due to diabetes insipidus or those on fluoride therapy for osteoporosis.

Clinical symptoms include back and neck stiffness. Kyphosis and flexion contractures of the hips and knees may also be seen. Rarely, the osteophytes, exostosis, and calcified ligaments may result in neurologic compromise.[138] Radiographs reveal generalized osteosclerosis, especially in the spine. Although the bone is not histologically normal, there is no significant predisposition to fracture.[12,37]

Other Causes of Osteosclerosis

As mentioned earlier, osteosclerosis can occur in Paget's disease, primary hyperparathyroidism, and renal osteodystrophy. Other disorders that should be included in the differential diagnosis are multiple myeloma, metastatic malignancy, lymphoma, heavy metal intoxication, mastocytosis, and myelosclerosis.[58,85]

PAGET'S DISEASE

Paget's disease of bone, or osteitis deformans, was first described by Sir James Paget in 1877, 20 years before X-rays were used in clinical medicine.[107] The disorder is seen in 3 to 6 percent of middle-aged patients, and its incidence increases to 10 percent by the ninth decade.[72,109] It may be monostotic or polyostotic, is frequently asymmetric, and is usually asymptomatic.[110] There is a striking geographic distribution of the disease with the greatest prevalence in England, Western Europe, and Australia.

Pathophysiology

Paget's disease is an idiopathic focal disorder of skeletal remodeling. The primary abnormality appears to be an increase in osteoclastic resorption, with a compensatory increase in coupled bone formation.[4,65] The abnormally remodeled bone consists of a mosaic pattern of lamellar bone with giant multinucleated osteoclasts. It is associated with extensive focal vascularity and increased fibrous tissue in the adjacent marrow.[11]

The pathologic process of Paget's disease can be divided into active and inactive phases. Early in the active phase, intense osteoclastic bone resorption is the predominant activity (lytic phase). Later, compensatory bone formation occurs (mixed phase), and very late in the active phase, bone formation predominates (sclerotic phase). In the inactive or "burnt-out" phase, the cellular activity of osteoblasts and osteoclasts returns to normal; however, the structural bone deformities remain. Although these phases are described in sequence, they may occur simultaneously in different bones.[32]

The etiology of Paget's disease is unknown, but because of its focal nature, it is by strict definition not a metabolic disease. Studies have established the presence of intranuclear inclusions in pagetic osteoclasts that resemble virus particles, suggesting that a virus infection may play an important etiologic role.[137] Pagetic bone cross-reacts antigenically with serum from patients with previous measles infections; however, virus particles have not been isolated from pagetic bone. Repetitive minor trauma in the extremities may also be a causative factor.[141]

Clinical Findings

Since Paget's disease is usually asymptomatic, it is most often detected as an incidental finding on radiographs taken for other purposes. However, when symptoms do occur, the most common complaint is deep aching bone pain.[107] Any bone can be affected by Paget's disease; the most common sites are the spine, pelvis, skull, femur, and tibia. The classic appearance of severe Paget's disease includes dorsal kyphosis, enlarged skull, and bowing of the femur and tibia.[61] In addition to bony deformity, increased skin temperature in affected areas, pseudofractures, and high-output congestive heart failure (with extensive disease) may be seen.

Most patients have some degree of spine involvement. In addition to kyphosis and compression fractures, which usually heal without difficulty, enlarged bones may result in vertebral canal impingement. Cranial neuropathies, spinal radiculopathies, spinal cord compression, and cauda equina syndrome are seen in Paget's disease, but such neurologic problems are rare.[64,76,130] The clinical presentation depends on the level of the disease. Usually weakness and numbness develop gradually in both legs without a definite sensory level, since compression is generally spread out over several vertebrae.[5] Infrequently, when cord compression occurs suddenly from collapse of a single vertebral body, surgical intervention may be required. Finally, sarcomatous degeneration is extremely rare, but should be considered when there is a sudden increase in pain from a quiescent area of involvement.[56,137]

It must be emphasized that even when Paget's disease is diagnosed, low back pain and sciatica are probably due to other causes.

Radiographic Findings

The radiographic appearance in Paget's disease varies with the stage of the disease. In the very early stages, although a bone scan is positive, plain radiographs may show only a slight coarsening of the trabecular pattern. There is often a flame-shaped or blade-of-grass–shaped advancing osteolytic front in the diaphysis of long bones or in the skull (osteogenesis circumscripta). With subsequent compensatory osteoblastic bone formation, the bones become grossly enlarged, with irregular, thickened cortices and coarsened trabeculae. Bowing, incomplete pseudofractures, and complete pathologic fractures are common.[98]

In the spine, the vertebral body is usually expanded, with thickened superior and inferior cortices (Fig. 17–8). The vertebrae may take on a "picture-frame" appearance with irregular and coarse vertical markings.[131] Depending on the balance of resorption and formation, varying

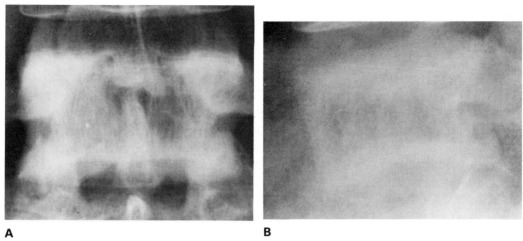

A   B

Figure 17–8. Paget's disease. *A,* Vertebral bodies demonstrate thickened cortices, thickened trabeculae, and widening. *B,* The lateral projection demonstrates the "picture frame" appearance. (From Kricun ME: Imaging Modalities in Spinal Disorders. Philadelphia, W.B. Saunders, 1988.)

degrees of sclerosis may be seen. The most prominent type of sclerosis is referred to as an ivory vertebra.

Laboratory Findings

The most consistent laboratory abnormality is an elevated serum alkaline phosphatase level, which is a reflection of osteoblastic activity. The urinary hydroxyproline level is also elevated, and correlates with collagen breakdown from bone resorption. Both of these parameters correlate fairly well with the activity of the disease, and either can be used to monitor treatment.[150] Occasionally, the acid phosphatase level is also raised, but not to the same extent as in metastatic prostate cancer. The serum calcium and phosphorus are usually normal unless there is coexistent immobilization or hyperparathyroidism.

Differential Diagnosis

The diagnosis of Paget's disease is generally confirmed by plain radiographs. The skull changes may be similar to those in hyperparathyroidism, and the necessary blood test should be done to distinguish the two entities. The spinal changes may resemble those of osteosclerotic metastases from breast or prostate carcinoma. Single or multiple sclerotic vertebrae may also be seen with several of the osteosclerotic disorders discussed earlier.

Treatment

The two major therapeutic agents are diphosphonates and calcitonin. The hormone calcitonin directly blocks bone resorption by inhibiting osteoclastic activity. The hormone is given daily (50 to 100 IU) by subcutaneous injection. Flushing and nausea are common but tolerable side effects. However, resistance to calcitonin may develop in a large proportion of patients. Human-derived calcitonin is less likely to generate antibodies than salmon-derived. Approximately 70 percent of patients have a favorable response to calcitonin therapy within 6 months.

Diphosphonates are pyrophosphate analogues that interfere with bone mineralization and inhibit osteoclast activity. The current recommended dose of ethane hydroxy-diphosphonate (EHDP) does not lead to a significant mineralization defect; however, higher doses or therapy for longer than 6 to 12 months may result in osteomalacia. Pain relief may continue for months after cessation of the treatment.

Although these two medications can be used interchangeably, calcitonin is preferred in patients who are immobilized, have an impending fracture, or have a neurologic deficit. Because diphosphonates may impair mineralization, they should not be used in patients with an impending fracture in a weight-bearing bone.

The medical management of Paget's disease is still evolving. Until recently, suppression of disease activity and symptomatic relief were possible, without improvement in the bone structure. A newer diphosphonate, aminohydroxypropylidene bisphosphonate (APD), does not inhibit mineralization, is more potent, and may be more suitable for long-term administration.[33,55,109,143,148] This parenteral agent has been used extensively in Europe and Australia and is reported to reverse or halt the radiographic osteolytic phase in pagetic bones.[90]

The use of the antibiotic mithramycin, which is cytotoxic to osteoclasts and other marrow cells, should be reserved for severe refractory cases. This drug must be administered intravenously and usually requires hospital supervision.

Bone pain of the spine is best treated initially with controlled physical activity and anti-inflammatory medications. If the discomfort is not relieved, treatment with one of the previously mentioned agents should be initiated. Fractures and kyphosis are best treated symptomatically with rest and support. Neurologic compromise, especially when acute, should be treated with a trial of calcitonin. Surgical decompression may lead to spinal instability and further neurologic compromise.

OCHRONOSIS

Ochronosis is a rare metabolic disorder associated with the deposition of homogentisic acid in connective tissue throughout the body. It is an autosomal recessive disorder with a prevalence of approximately one in ten million.[133,142] The accumulation of homogentisic acid results in darkened pigmentation and progressive degeneration of connective tissue.

Pathophysiology

The cause of this illness is the congenital absence of the enzyme homogentisic acid oxidase, which results in accumulation of homogentisic acid.[80] Alkaptonuria is the disease associated with the excretion of homogentisic acid in the urine. Ochronosis, which is caused by the same enzyme deficiency, is the discoloration of connective tissue from the deposition of a black pigment that is thought to be a polymer of homogentisic acid.[97] The pigment affects the integrity of cartilage matrix and chondrocytes, and results in cartilage damage and degeneration.[132] Pathologic changes in the axial skeleton first occur in the lumbar spine. Pigment is deposited in the nucleus pulposus and in the annulus of the discs, which become secondarily calcified and brittle.

Clinical Findings

Symptoms of ochronosis first appear in the fourth decade of life. Low back pain and stiffness are frequently the initial symptoms of the illness. Herniation of an intervertebral disc, particularly in men, can be the initial symptom in some patients.[94] This disorder may also be seen in association with calcium pyrophosphate dihydrate deposition disease (CPPD).[127]

Physical examination demonstrates limited motion of the lumbar spine and localized tenderness with percussion. Muscle spasm is usually not present. With advanced disease, there is rigidity of the axial skeleton, and chest wall expansion may be limited. Kyphosis may be prominent and is associated with a loss in height. Dark pigmentation may be seen in the nose, ears, sclerae, and fingernails.

Radiographic Findings

Radiographic examination of the lumbar spine in ochronosis demonstrates marked disc space narrowing, osteophyte formation, and disc calcification at multiple levels (Fig. 17–9). Vacuum disc phenomena may be seen and are suggestive of ochronosis when they occur at multiple levels. Disease of long duration may be associated with total obliteration of disc spaces and bony fusion, and may be confused with the axial skeletal changes of ankylosing spondylitis.[136]

Laboratory Findings

The characteristic laboratory finding is the presence of homogentisic acid in the urine. Alkalinization of a urine specimen will cause darkening, indicative of the presence of homogentisic acid. Synovial fluid

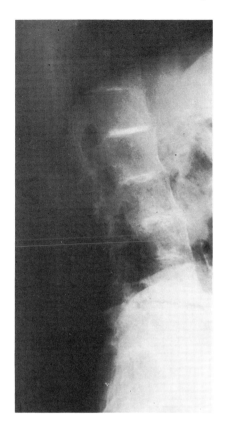

Figure 17-9. Ochronosis of the spine marked by calcification and narrowing of numerous discs. (From Rothman RH, Simeone FA: The Spine, 2nd ed. Philadelphia, W.B. Saunders, 1982.)

analysis may demonstrate a "ground pepper" appearance of the fluid or pyrophosphate crystals.[63]

Differential Diagnosis

A diagnosis of ochronosis is based on the characteristic clinical symptoms and radiographic findings, along with the presence of homogentisic acid in the urine. Other disorders such as CPPD, hemochromatosis, hyperparathyroidism, and acromegaly may involve intervertebral disc calcification and must be considered.[152] Patients with ankylosing spondylitis may have symptoms and signs similar to those of patients with ochronosis but will not have the skin pigmentation or disc calcification.

Treatment

There is no cure for this disease. Symptomatic management includes rest, exercise, analgesics, and anti-inflammatory drugs. Dietary restriction of tyrosine and phenylalanine lowers homogentisic acid levels but has not been shown to produce any significant change in the course of the illness.[132] Ochronosis is generally progressive and variably disabling.[132]

MICROCRYSTALLINE DEPOSITION DISEASE

Microcrystalline disease, gout, and calcium pyrophosphate dihydrate deposition disease (CPPD) are commonly associated with peripheral joint abnormalities. Occasionally, patients with gouty axial skeletal disease may develop episodes of acute low back pain secondary to spinal or sacroiliac joint involvement. The actual prevalence of gout and CPPD is not known. Approximately 5 percent of a large adult population had hyperuricemia, while 6 percent of an elderly population had CPPD in a joint.[53,93]

Pathophysiology

Men develop gout during the fourth or fifth decade, and women after menopause. The etiology is related to the inability of the body to eliminate uric acid due to overproduction or underexcretion through the kidney. The presence of crystals in joints or soft tissues may initiate the inflammatory response that results in acute symptoms. Uric acid can accumulate into large collections, or tophi, that may be located in superficial structures or in deep areas around the joints of the spine.

CPPD causes symptomatic disease half as often as gout.[104] As in gout, men are more commonly affected then women. The disease becomes symptomatic between the sixth and seventh decades. Factors that facilitate the deposition of crystals in cartilage and surrounding articular structures are poorly understood. CPPD may also be associated with a number of metabolic conditions including diabetes mellitus, hyperparathyroidism, hemochromatosis, hypothyroidism, Wilson's disease, and ochronosis.

Clinical Findings

Patients who present with back pain secondary to gout have a long history of peripheral gouty arthritis and are usually over 50 years of age.[53] Most patients have nonradiating low back pain due to chronic gouty arthritis. Occasionally, they may have a sudden onset of low back pain associated with an acute gouty attack in the sacroiliac joints. Tophaceous deposits can affect the spine and neural elements enough to cause radicular symptoms, even in the absence of extraspinal tophi.[147] Physical findings include spinal stiffness, loss of motion, and muscle spasm. Examination of extensor surfaces (triceps and Achilles tendons) may reveal tophaceous deposits.

Patients with CPPD of the spine may also have symptoms of low back pain associated with straightening and stiffening of the spine.[115] They rarely have neurologic symptoms.[36]

Radiographic Findings

Radiographic abnormalities in the sacroiliac joint and axial skeleton are unusual in gout, but there may be joint margin sclerosis with cystic erosions in the ileum and sacrum.[1] Gout may also cause erosions of vertebral end plates, disc space narrowing, and vertebral subluxation (Figs. 17–10 and 17–11). Pathologic fractures in the posterior spinal elements may be seen in patients with extensive gouty involvement.[21] Radiographic manifestations of CPPD in the spine include calcification of the annulus fibrosus, disc space narrowing with osteophytes, and rarely, degenerative spondylolisthesis (Fig. 17–12).[117]

Laboratory Findings and Differential Diagnosis

While laboratory evidence of elevated uric acid may be suggestive of gout, there are no blood studies useful for CPPD. Neither entity can be definitively diagnosed without synovial fluid aspirations for crystals or a clear response to empiric therapy. Crystals from CPPD will reveal positive birefringence under a polarizing microscope, while monosodium urate crystals from gout will demonstrate negative birefringence.

Treatment

Therapy for gout requires immediate control of inflammation during the acute attack and the chronic control of hyperuricemia to prevent further deposits. An acute gouty attack can be controlled with colchi-

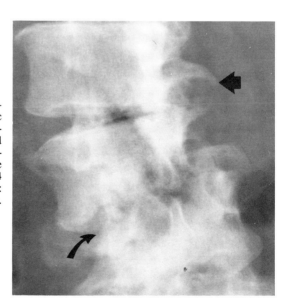

Figure 17–10. Gout. There is marked destruction of the L4-5 intervertebral disc (*curved arrow*) with subluxation of L4 laterally to the right. Large bizarre-shaped bony protrusions (*straight arrow*) resembling overhanging edges seen with gout are present. Degenerative changes at the L3-4 disc are also noted. (From Kricun ME: Imaging Modalities in Spinal Disorders. Philadelphia, W.B. Saunders, 1988.)

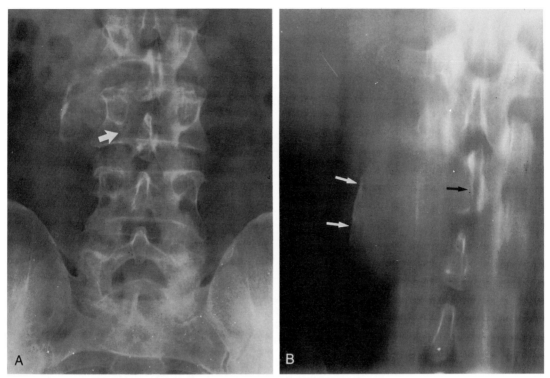

Figure 17–11. A, Huge tophus of gout eroding the lamina (*arrow*) of L2. B, Tomogram shows erosion of the posterior spinous process (*black arrow*). There is a rim of expanding cortex present (*white arrows*). (Courtesy of Anne Brower, M.D.) (From Borenstein DG, Wiesel SW: Low Back Pain: Medical Diagnosis and Management. Philadelphia, W.B. Saunders, 1989.)

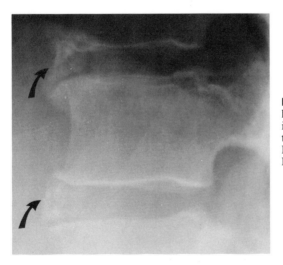

Figure 17–12. Calcium pyrophosphate dihydrate crystal deposition disease. There is calcification of the anterior portion of the annulus (*arrows*). (From Kricun ME: Imaging Modalities in Spinal Disorders. Philadelphia, W.B. Saunders, 1988.)

cine or nonsteroidal anti-inflammatory drugs for 7 to 10 days or until the attack subsides. Once acute inflammation is alleviated, uric acid concentrations can be controlled by increasing uric acid excretion with probenecid or sulfinpyrazone, along with colchicine for prophylaxis. Alternatively, when the patient has renal insufficiency or stones, inhibition of uric acid production with the xanthine oxidase inhibitor allopurinol is the treatment of choice.[77,153]

Therapy for CPPD is primarily directed toward control of inflammation with nonsteroidal anti-inflammatory drugs. Oral colchicine is not very effective at preventing attacks. Controlling the underlying disease associated with the CPPD may help arrest progression, but old deposits are not resorbed.[92]

Summary

In addition to the spine's structural role, it is called upon, with the remainder of the skeleton, to serve as a mineral reservoir for the body's metabolic demands. Therefore, an understanding of the pathophysiology of metabolic bone disease is important when considering problems in the spine. In this chapter, we have focused on only several of the most common principles and disorders of skeletal homeostasis, especially as they relate to the spine.

The metabolic demands of the body's skeletal resources take precedence over anatomic and structural requirements. When all of the physiologic mechanisms regulating normal mineral homeostasis are functioning properly, it is easy to think that the skeleton, including the spine, plays primarily a structural role. Often it is not until the complex regulating system breaks down or is affected by disease that one fully appreciates that the structural integrity of the skeleton rests on a well-balanced physiologic foundation. Accordingly, the majority of treatments for metabolic bone disease of the spine involve symptomatic management coupled with diagnosis and treatment of the underlying systemic physiologic abnormalities.

References

1. Alarcon-Segovia D, Cetina JA, Diza-Jouanen: Sacroiliac joints in primary gout. Clinical and roentgenographic study of 143 patients. Am J Roentgenol 118:438–443, 1973.
2. Albright F: A page out of the history of hyperparathyroidism. J Clin Endocrinol 8:637–657, 1948.
3. Albright F, Aub JC, Bauer W: Hyperparathyroidism: A common and polymorphic condition as illustrated by 17 proved cases from one clinic. JAMA 102:1276–1287, 1934.
4. Albright F, Reifenstein EC: The Parathyroid Glands and Metabolic Bone Disease. Selected Studies. Baltimore, Williams & Wilkins, 1948.
5. Aldren-Turner JW: The spinal complications of Paget's disease. Brain 63:321–349, 1940.
6. Aloia JF, Cohn SH, Ostuni JA, et al: Prevention of involutional bone loss by exercise. Ann Intern Med 89:356–358, 1978.
7. Andran GM: Bone loss not demonstrable by radiography. Br J Radiol 4:107–109, 1951.
8. Austin LA, Heath H: Calcitonin: Physiology and pathophysiology. N Engl J Med 304:269–278, 1981.

9. Avioli L, Haddad JG: Vitamin D: Current concepts. Metabolism 22:507–531, 1973.

10. Azar HA, Wucho CK, Bayyuk SI, et al: Skeletal sclerosis due to chronic fluoride intoxication. Cases from an endemic area of fluorosis in the region of the Persian Gulf. Ann Intern Med 55:193–200, 1964.

11. Barry HC: Paget's Disease of Bone. London, Livingstone, 1969.

12. Baud CA, Lagier R, Boivin G, et al: Value of the bone biopsy in the diagnosis of industrial fluorosis. Virchows Arch 380A:283–297, 1978.

13. Bernett E, Nordin BEC: The radiologic diagnosis of osteoporosis. A new approach. Clin Radiol 11:166–174, 1962.

14. Bick EM, Copel JW: Fracture of vertebrae in the aged. Geriatrics 5:74–81, 1950.

15. Boden SD, Goodenough DJ, Stockham CD, et al: Precise measurement of vertebral bone density using computed tomography without the use of an external reference phantom. J Dig Imag 2:31–38, 1989.

16. Borders J, Kerr E, Sartoris DJ, et al: Quantitative dual-energy radiographic absorptiometry of the lumbar spine: In vivo comparison with dual-photon absorptiometry. Radiology 170:129–131, 1989.

17. Bostrom H, Edgren B, Nilsonne U, et al: Metabolic and orthopedic treatment of a case of adult nonfamilial hypophosphatemia with severe osteomalacia. Acta Orthop Scand 39:238–260, 1968.

18. Breatnach E, Robinson PJ: Repositioning errors in measurement of vertebral attenuation values by computed tomography. Br J Radiol 56:299–305, 1983.

19. Brighton CT, Luessenhop CP, Pollack SR, et al: Treatment of castration-induced osteoporosis by a capacitively coupled electrical signal in rat vertebrae. J Bone Joint Surg 71A:228–236, 1989.

20. Brown DJ, Dawborn JK, Thomas DP, et al: Assessment of osteodystrophy in patients with chronic renal failure. Aust NZ J Med 12:250–254, 1982.

21. Burnham J, Fraker J, Steinbach H: Pathologic fracture in an unusual case of gout. Am J Roentgenol 129:1116–1119, 1977.

22. Caldwell RA: Observation in the incidence, etiology, and pathology of senile osteoporosis. J Clin Pathol 15:421–431, 1962.

23. Cann CE: Low-dose CT scanning for quantitative spinal mineral analysis. Radiology 140:813–815, 1981.

24. Cann CE, Genant HK, Boyd DP, et al: Quantitative computed tomography for prediction of vertebral fracture risk. Bone 6:1–7, 1985.

25. Carasco MG, de Vernejoul MC, Sterkers Y, et al: Decreased bone formation in osteoporotic patients compared with age-matched controls. Calcif Tissue Int 44:173–175, 1989.

26. Chalmers J, Conacher VDH, Gardner DL, et al: Osteomalacia: A common disease in elderly women. J Bone Joint Surg 49B:403–423, 1967.

27. Coburn J, Kanis J, Popovtzer M, et al: Pathophysiology and treatment of uremic bone disease. Calcif Tissue Int 35:712–714, 1983.

28. Collins DH: Paget's disease of bone. Incidence and subclinical forms. Lancet 2:51, 1956.

29. Cummings SR, Black D: Should perimenopausal women be screened for osteoporosis? Ann Intern Med 104:817–823, 1986.

30. Cunningham J, Fraher LJ, Clemens TL, et al: Chronic acidosis with metabolic bone disease. Effect of alkali on bone morphology and vitamin D metabolism. Am J Med 73:199–204, 1982.

31. Dent CE, Hodson CH: Radiological changes associated with certain metabolic bone diseases. Symposium. Generalized softening of bone due to metabolic causes. Brit J Radiol 27:605–617, 1954.

32. Dickson DD, Camp JD, Ghormley RK: Osteitis deformans: Paget's disease of the bone. Radiology 44:449–470, 1945.

33. Dodd GW, Ibbertson HK, Fraser TR, et al: Radiological assessment of Paget's disease of bone after treatment with the bisphosphonates EHDP and APD. Br J Radiol 60:849–860, 1987.

34. Dunn WL, Wahner HW, Riggs BL: Measurement of bone mineral content in human vertebrae and hip by dual photon absorptiometry. Radiology 136:485–487, 1980.

35. Eastwood, JB: Renal osteodystrophy—a radiological review. CRC Crit Rev Diagn Imaging 9:77–104, 1977.

36. Ellman MH, Vazquez T, Ferguson L, et al: Calcium pyrophosphate deposition in ligamentum flavum. Arthritis Rheum 21:611–613, 1978.

37. Epker BN: A quantitative microscopic study of bone remodeling and balance in a human with skeletal fluorosis. Clin Orthop 55:87–95, 1967.

38. Erikson EF, Colvard DS, Berg NJ, et al: Evidence of estrogen receptors in normal human osteoblast-like cells. Science 241:84–86, 1988.

39. Ettinger B: Prevention of osteoporosis: Treatment of estradiol deficiency. Obstet Gynecol 72(Suppl):12S–17S, 1988.

40. Ettinger B, Genant HK, Cann CE: Postmenopausal bone loss is prevented by treatment with low-dosage estrogen with calcium. Ann Intern Med 106:40–45, 1987.

41. Evans GA, Artulanantham D, Gag J: Primary hypophosphatemic rickets. Effect of oral phosphate and vitamin D on growth and surgical treatment. J Bone Joint Surg 62:1130–1138, 1980.

42. Frame B: Metabolic bone disease as a cause of neck ache and back ache. Proceedings of Conference in Neckache and Backache in Association with Neurologic Surgery. Springfield, IL, Charles C Thomas, 1970.

43. Frame B, Parfitt AM: Osteomalacia: Current concepts (a review). Ann Intern Med 89:966–982, 1978.

44. Fraser DR: Regulation of the metabolism of vitamin D. Phys Rev 60:551–604, 1980.

45. Frisch B, Eventov I: Hematopoiesis in osteoporosis: Preliminary report comparing biopsies of the femoral neck and iliac crest. Israeli J Med Sci 22:380–384, 1986.

46. Frost HM, Villanueva AR, Teth J, et al: Tetracycline-based analysis of bone remodeling in osteopetrosis. Clin Orthop 65:203–217, 1969.

47. Garn SM: The course of bone gain and the phases of bone loss. Orthop Clin 3:503–520, 1972.

48. Genant HK, Block JE, Steiger P, et al: Appropriate use of bone densitometry. Radiology 170:817–822, 1989.

49. Genant HK, Steiger P, Block JE, et al: Quantitative computed tomography: Update 1987. Calcif Tissue Int 41:179–186, 1987.

50. Goodsitt MM, Rosenthal DI: Quantitative computed tomography scanning for measurement of bone and bone marrow fat content: A comparison of single- and dual-energy techniques using a sold synthetic phantom. Invest Radiol 22:799–810, 1987.

51. Greenfield GB: Roentgen appearance of bone and soft-tissue changes in chronic renal disease. Am J Roentgenol 116:749–757, 1972.

52. Hahn TJ: Drug-induced disorders of vitamin D and mineral metabolism. Clin Endocrinol Metab 9:107–127, 1980.

53. Hall AP, Barry PE, Dawber TR, et al: Epidemiology of gout and hyperuricemia: A long-term population study. Am J Med 42:27–37, 1967.

54. Hansson T, Roos HT: The effect of fluoride and calcium on spinal osteoporosis: A controlled, prospective (three years) study. Calcif Tissue Int 40:315–317, 1987.

55. Harinck HI, Papapoulos SE, Blanksma HJ, et al: Paget's disease of bone: Early and late responses to three different modes of treatment with aminohydroxypropylidene bisphosphonate (APD). Br Med J 295:1301–1305, 1987.

56. Hartman JT, John DF: Paget's disease of the spine with cord and nerve root compression. J Bone Joint Surg 48A:1079–1084, 1966.

57. Hasenhuttl K: Osteopetrosis. J Bone Joint Surg 44A:359–370, 1962.

58. Havard CW, Scott RB: Urticaria pigmentosa with visceral and skeletal lesions. Quart J Med 28:459–472, 1959.

59. Health and Public Policy Committee, American College of Physicians: Bone mineral densitometry. Ann Intern Med 107:932–936, 1987.

60. Heaney RP: Management of osteoporosis: Nutritional considerations. Clin Invest Med 5:185–187, 1982.

61. Herwitz SH: Osteitis deformans, Paget's disease. Bull Johns Hopkins Hosp 24:263–274, 1913.

62. Hinkle CL, Beiler DD: Osteopetrosis in adults. Am J Roentgenol 74:46–64, 1955.

63. Hunter T, Gordon DA, Ogryzlo MA: The ground pepper sign of synovial fluid. A new diagnostic feature of ochronosis. J Rheumatol 1:45–53, 1974.

64. Jardon OM, Burney DW, Fink RL: Hypophosphatasia in an adult. J Bone Joint Surg 52A:1477–1484, 1970.

65. Johnson LC: Morphologic analysis in pathology: The kinetics of disease and general biology of bone. In Frost HM (ed): Bone Biodynamics. Boston, Little, Brown, 1964, pp. 543–654.

66. Johnston CC, Lavy N, Lord T, et al: Osteopetrosis. A clinical, genetic, metabolic, and morphologic study of the dominantly inherited benign form. Medicine 47:149–167, 1968.

67. Juler GL, Kutas A, Skowsky WR: Primary hyperparathyroidism: A pleomorphic disease. Arch Surg 118:483–487, 1983.

68. Kaplan FS: Osteoporosis. Clin Symp 39:1–32, 1987.

69. Kaplan FS, August CS, Fallon MD, et al: Successful treatment of infantile malignant osteopetrosis by bone-marrow transplantation. A case report. J Bone Joint Surg 70A:617–623, 1988.

70. Kaplan FS, Dalinka M, Karp JS, et al: Quantitative computed tomography reflects vertebral fracture morbidity in osteopenic patients. Orthopedics 12:949–955, 1989.

71. Kaplan FS, Fallon MD, Boden SD, et al: Estrogen receptors in bone in a patient with polyostotic fibrous dysplasia (McCune-Albright syndrome). N Engl J Med 319:421–425, 1988.

72. Kaplan FS, Soffer SR, Fallon MD, et al: Osteomalacia as a very late manifestation of primary hyperparathyroidism. Clin Orthop 228:26–32, 1988.

73. Kelly TL, Slovik SM, Schoenfeld DA, et al: Quantitative digital radiography versus dual photon absorptiometry of the lumbar spine. J Clin Endocrinol Metab 67:839–844, 1988.

74. Kelsey JI, Hoffman S: Risk factors for hip fracture. N Engl J Med 316:404–406, 1987.

75. Kiel DP, Felson DT, Anderson JJ, et al: Hip fracture and the use of estrogen in postmenopausal women. The Framingham study. N Engl J Med 317:1169–1174, 1987.

76. Klenerman L: Cauda equina and spinal cord compression in Paget's disease. J Bone Joint Surg 48B:365–370, 1966.

77. Klinenberg JR, Goldfinger S, Seegmiller JE: The effectiveness of the xanthine oxidase inhibitor allopurinol in the treatment of gout. Ann Intern Med 62:639–647, 1965.

78. Komm BS, Terperning CM, Benz DJ, et al: Estrogen binding, receptor mRNA, and biologic response in osteoblast-like osteosarcoma cells. Science 241:81–84, 1988.
79. Krolner B, Toft B, Nielsen PS, et al: Physical exercise as prophylaxis against involutional vertebral bone loss: A controlled trial. Clin Sci 64:541–546, 1983.
80. LaDu BN, Zannoni VG, Laster L, et al: The nature of the defect in tyrosine metabolism in alkaptonuria. J Biol Chem 230:251–260, 1958.
81. Lafferty FW: Primary hyperparathyroidism: Changing clinical spectrum, prevalence of hypertension, and discriminant analysis of laboratory tests. Arch Intern Med 141:1761–1766, 1980.
82. Lane JM, Healey JH, Schwartz E, et al: Treatment of osteoporosis with sodium fluoride and calcium: Effects on vertebral fracture incidence and bone histomorphometry. Orthop Clin North Am 15:729–745, 1984.
83. Lange SM, Moyle DD, Berg CEW, et al: Correlation of mechanical properties of vertebral trabecular bone with equivalent mineral density as measured by computed tomography. J Bone Joint Surg 70A:1531–1538, 1988.
84. Laval-Jeantet AM, Roger B, Bouysse S, et al: Influence of vertebral fat content on quantitative CT density. Radiology 159:463–466, 1986.
85. Leonard BJ, Israels MC, Wilinson JF: Myelosclerosis: A clinicopathologic study. Q J Med 26:131–148, 1957.
86. Malluche HH, Smith AJ, Abreo H, et al: The use of desferoxamine in the management of aluminum accumulation in bone in patients with renal failure. N Engl J Med 311:140–144, 1984.
87. Mankin HJ: Review article: Rickets, osteomalacia, and renal osteodystrophy. J Bone Joint Surg 56A:101–128, 1974.
88. Mazess RB: Errors in measuring trabecular bone by computed tomography due to marrow and bone composition. Calcif Tissue Int 35:148–152, 1983.
89. Mazess RB: Bone density in diagnosis of osteoporosis: Thresholds and breakpoints. Calcif Tissue Int 41:117–118, 1987.
90. Mautalen CA, Gonzalez D, Ghiringhelli G: Efficacy of the bisphosphonate APD in the control of Paget's bone disease. Bone 6:429–432, 1985.
91. McBroom RJ, Hayes WC, Edwards WT, et al: Prediction of vertebral body compressive fracture using quantitative computed tomography. J Bone Joint Surg 67A:1206–1214, 1985.
92. McCarty DJ: Calcium pyrophosphate dihydrate crystal deposition disease (pseudogout syndrome)—clinical aspects. Clin Rheum Dis 3:61–89, 1977.
93. McCarty DJ, Hogan JM, Gatter RA, et al: Studies on pathological calcifications in human cartilage. Part I. Prevalence and types of crystal deposits in the menisci of 215 cadavers. J Bone Joint Surg 48A:309–325, 1966.
94. McCollum DE, Odom GL: Alkaptonuria, ochronosis, and low back pain: A case report. J Bone Joint Surg 47A:1389–1392, 1965.
95. McGeown MG: Severe hyperparathyroid bone disease without apparent involvement of the kidneys. Lancet 2:199–202, 1962.
96. Meredith SC, Rosenberg IH: Gastrointestinal-hepatic disorders and osteomalacia. Clin Endocrinol Metab 9:177–205, 1980.
97. Milch RA: Biochemical studies on the pathogenesis of collagen tissue changes in alkaptonuria. Clin Orthop 24:213–229, 1962.
98. Milgram JW: Orthopedic management of Paget's disease of bone. Clin Orthop 127:63–69, 1977.
99. Milkman LA: Pseudofractures (hunger osteopathy, late rickets, osteomalacia). Am J Roentgenol 24:29–37, 1930.
100. Morgan DB: Osteomalacia, Renal Osteodystrophy, and Osteoporosis. Springfield, IL, Charles C Thomas, 1973.
101. Nordin BEC: The definition and diagnosis of osteoporosis. Calcif Tissue Int 40:57–58, 1987.
102. Nordin BEC, Heyburn PJ, Peacock M, et al: Osteoporosis and osteomalacia. Clin Endocrinol Metab 9:177–205, 1980.
103. Nordin BEC, Hodgkinson A, Peacock M: The measurement and the meaning of urinary calcium. Clin Orthop 52:293–322, 1967.
104. O'Duffy JD: Clinical studies of acute pseudogout attacks: Comments on prevalence, predispositions and treatment. Arthritis Rheum 19:349–352, 1976.
105. Ott SM, Maloney NA, Coburn JW, et al: Prevalence of bone aluminum deposition in renal osteodystrophy and its relation to the response to calcitriol therapy. N Engl J Med 307:709–713, 1982.
106. Pacifici R, Rupich R, Vered I, et al: Dual energy radiography (DER): A preliminary comparative study. Calcif Tissue Int 43:189–191, 1988.
107. Paget J: On a form of chronic inflammation of bone (osteitis deformans). Clin Orthop 49:3–16, 1966.
108. Pak CYC, Sakhaee K, Zerwekh JE, et al: Safe and effective treatment of osteoporosis with intermittent slow release sodium fluoride: Augmentation of vertebral bone mass and inhibition of fractures. J Clin Endocrinol Metab 68:150–159, 1989.
109. Papapoulos SE, Harinck HI, Bijvoet OL, et al: Effects of decreasing serum calcium on circulating parathyroid hormone and vitamin D metabolites in normocalcaemic and hypercalcaemic patients treated with APD. Bone Min 1:69–78, 1986.

110. Parfitt AM: Hypophosphatemic vitamin D refractory rickets and osteomalacia. Orthop Clin North Am 3:653–680, 1972.

111. Parfitt AM: The clinical and radiographic manifestations of renal osteodystrophy. In David DJ (ed): Perspectives in Hypertension and Nephrology. Calcium Metabolism in Renal Failure and Nephrolithiasis. New York, John Wiley & Sons, 1977.

112. Parfitt AM: The coupling of bone formation to bone resorption: A critical analysis of the concept and of its relevance to the pathogenesis of osteoporosis. Metab Bone Dis Rel Res 4:1–6, 1982.

113. Potts JT, Kronenberg HM, Habener JR, et al: Biosynthesis of parathyroid hormone. Ann NY Acad Sci 343:38–55, 1980.

114. Pyrah LN, Hodgkinson A, Anderson CK: Primary hyperparathyroidism. Br J Surg 53:245–316, 1966.

115. Reginato A, Valenzuela F, Martinez V, et al: Polyarticular and familial chondrocalcinosis. Arthritis Rheum 13:197–213, 1970.

116. Reichel H, Koeffler HP, Norman AW: The role of the vitamin D endocrine system in health and disease. N Engl J Med 320:980–991, 1989.

117. Resnick D, Niwayama G, Goergen TG, et al: Clinical, radiographic, and pathologic abnormalities in calcium pyrophosphate dihydrate deposition disease (CPPD): Pseudogout. Radiology 122:1–15, 1977.

118. Richelson LS, Wahner HW, Melton LJ III, et al: Relative contribution of aging and estrogen deficiency to postmenopausal bone loss. N Engl J Med 311:1273–1275, 1984.

119. Riggs BL, Hodgson SF, Wahner HW, et al: Effect of long-term fluoride therapy in bone metabolism, bone density, and fracture rate in type I (postmenopausal) osteoporosis: Final results of prospective, controlled, double-blind clinical trial. J Bone Min Res 4(Suppl 1):S418, 1989.

120. Riggs BL, Melton LJ III: Involutional osteoporosis. N Engl J Med 306:446–450, 1986.

121. Riggs BL, Seeman E, Hodgson SF, et al: Effect of fluoride/calcium regimen on vertebral fracture occurrence in postmenopausal osteoporosis: Comparison with conventional therapy. N Engl J Med 306:446–450, 1982.

122. Riis B, Thomsen K, Christiansen C: Does calcium supplementation prevent postmenopausal bone loss? N Engl J Med 316:173–177, 1987.

123. Root AW, Harrison HE: Recent advances in calcium metabolism. I. Mechanisms of calcium homeostasis. J Pediatr 88:177–199, 1976.

124. Rosenthal DI, Ganott MA, Wyshak G, et al: Quantitative computed tomography for spinal density measurement: Factors affecting precision. Invest Radiol 20:306–310, 1985.

125. Rubin CT, McLeod KJ, Lanyon LE: Prevention of osteoporosis by pulsed electromagnetic fields. J Bone Joint Surg 71A:411–417, 1989.

126. Ruegsegger P, Anliker M, Dambacher M: Quantification of trabecular bone with low dose computed tomography. J Comput Assist Tomogr 5:384–390, 1981.

127. Rynes RI, Sosman JL, Holdsworth DE: Pseudogout in ochronosis. Report of a case. Arthritis Rheum 18:21–26, 1975.

128. Sartoris DJ, Andre M, Resnick C, et al: Trabecular bone density in the proximal femur: Quantitative CT assessment. Radiology 160:707–712, 1986.

129. Schiller LR, Santa Ana CA, Sheikh MS, et al: Effect of the time of administration of calcium acetate on phosphorus binding. N Engl J Med 320:1110–1113, 1989.

130. Schmidek HH: Neurologic and neurosurgical sequelae of Paget's disease of bone. Clin Orthop 127:70–77, 1977.

131. Schreiber MH, Richardson LA: Paget's disease confined to one lumbar vertebra. Am J Roentgenol 90:1271–1276, 1963.

132. Schumacher HR, Holdsworth DE: Ochronotic arthropathy. I. Clinicopathologic studies. Semin Arthritis Rheum 6:207–246, 1977.

133. Seradge H, Anderson MG: Alkaptonuria and ochronosis: Historic review and update. Orthop Rev 7:41–46, 1978.

134. Shaw MT, Davies M: Primary hyperparathyroidism presenting as spinal cord compression. Br Med J 4:230–231, 1968.

135. Sherrard DJ, Baylink DJ, Wergedal JE, et al: Quantitative histological studies on the pathogenesis of uremic bone disease. J Clin Endocrinol 39:119–135, 1974.

136. Simon G, Zorab PA: The radiological changes in alkaptonuric arthritis: A report of 3 cases (one an Egyptian mummy). Br J Radiol 34:384–386, 1961.

137. Singer FR, Schiller AL, Pyle EB, et al: Paget's disease of bone. In Avioli LV, Krane SM (eds): Metabolic Bone Disease, Vol II. New York, Academic Press, 1978.

138. Singh A, Jolly SS: Endemic fluorosis with particular reference to fluorotic radiculomyelopathy. Quart J Med 30:357–372, 1961.

139. Slatopolsky E, Rutherford WE, Hruska K, et al: How important is phosphate in the pathogenesis of renal osteodystrophy? Arch Intern Med 138:848–852, 1978.

140. Smith R: Biochemical Disorders of the Skeleton. London, Butterworth, 1979.

141. Solomon LR, McKusick V, Rebel A, et al: Billiard-player's fingers: An unusual case of Paget's disease of bone. Br Med J 2:931, 1979.

142. Srsen S: Alkaptonuria. Johns Hopkins Med J 145:217–226, 1979.

143. Theibaud D, Jaeger P, Burckhardt P: Paget's disease of bone treated in five days with AHPrBP (APD) per os. J Bone Min Res 2:45–52, 1987.
144. Tinetti ME, Speechley M: Prevention of falls among the elderly. N Engl J Med 320:1055–1059, 1989.
145. Trotter M, Broman GE, Peterson RR: Densities of bone of white and negro skeletons. J Bone Joint Surg 42A:50–58, 1960.
146. Urist MR, Gurvey MS, Fareet DO: Long-term observations on aged women with pathologic osteoporosis. In Barzel US (ed): Osteoporosis. New York, Grune & Stratton, 1970, pp. 3–37.
147. Varga J, Giamphole C, Goldenberg DL: Tophaceous gout of the spine in a patient with no peripheral tophi: case report and review of the literature. Arthritis Rheum 28:1312, 1985.
148. Vellenga CJ, Mulder JD, Bijvoet OL: Radiological demonstration of healing in Paget's disease of bone treated with APD. Br J Radiol 58:831–837, 1985.
149. Wahner HW, Dunn WL, Mazess RB, et al: Dual-photon Gd-153 absorptiometry of bone. Radiology 156:203–206, 1985.
150. Walton RJ, Preston CJ, Bartlett M, et al: Biochemical measurements in Paget's disease of bone. J Clin Invest 7:37–39, 1977.
151. Watts NB, Harris ST, Genant HK, et al.: Intermittent cyclical etidronate treatment of postmenopausal osteoporosis. N Engl J Med 323:73–79, 1990.
152. Weinberger A, Myers AR: Intervertebral disc calcification in adults. A review. Semin Arthritis Rheum 8:69–75, 1978.
153. Yu TF, Gutman AB: Principles of current management of primary gout. Am J Med Sci 254:893–907, 1967.

CHAPTER 18

Arthritis and the Aging Spine

Rheumatologic disorders of the spine are common causes of back pain. These diseases affect the bones, joints, ligaments, tendons, and muscles of the spine. While mechanical problems such as muscle strain, degenerative disc disease, spinal stenosis, and osteoarthritis are frequent causes of pain, there are a number of other inflammatory and noninflammatory disorders that can cause symptoms in the aging spine.

The most important rheumatic disorders that cause inflammation in the joints of the axial skeleton are the seronegative spondyloarthropathies. This group of diseases is characterized by sacroiliac joint involvement, peripheral large joint disease, and the absence of serum rheumatoid factor. The seronegative spondyloarthropathies include ankylosing spondylitis, Reiter's syndrome, psoriatic arthritis, enteropathic arthritis, familial Mediterranean fever, Behçet's syndrome, Whipple's disease, and arthritis associated with hidradenitis suppurativa. While most of the disorders are diagnosed before the fifth decade of life, the sequelae are present as the patients continue to age and are frequently coexistent with mechanical problems of a degenerative etiology.

ANKYLOSING SPONDYLITIS

Ankylosing spondylitis is a chronic inflammatory disease characterized by a variable symptomatic course and progressive involvement

of the sacroiliac and axial skeletal joints. It is the prototype of the seronegative spondyloarthropathies. The disease complex is characterized by
axial skeletal arthritis, absence of rheumatoid factor in the serum, lack of
rheumatoid nodules, and presence of HLA-B27—a histocompatibility
marker on host cells. Ankylosing spondylitis affects about 1 percent of the
white population, a prevalence equal to that of rheumatoid arthritis. The
male to female ratio is thought to be about 3:1.[17]

Pathophysiology

The etiology of ankylosing spondylitis is unknown. Previous
theories of bacterial or traumatic origin have not been substantiated.[24,25]
In the patients predisposed to this disease, significant tissue injury may
result in an inflammatory process that promotes tissue calcification and
joint ankylosis.[62]

There is a genetic predisposition to ankylosing spondylitis and
to the seronegative spondyloarthropathies in general. HLA-B27 is present
in over 90 percent of white patients with ankylosing spondylitis, compared to a frequency of 8 percent in a normal population.[67] HLA-B27 is
present in 50 percent of blacks with ankylosing spondylitis with a prevalence of 4 percent in the normal population.[31] Blacks in Africa do not have
the HLA-B27 antigen and rarely develop ankylosing spondylitis. It is clear
that environmental factors must also play a role in the development of the
disease.[36]

Ankylosing spondylitis is a disease of the synovial and cartilaginous joints of the axial skeleton. The large appendicular joints may also be
affected in 30 percent of patients. The inflammatory process is characterized by chondritis or osteitis at the junction of cartilage and bone in the
spine. Inflammatory granulation tissue forms and erodes the vertebral
body margins. Ankylosing spondylitic inflammation results in ankylosis
of joints and ossification of ligaments surrounding the vertebrae (syndesmophytes), in contrast to rheumatoid arthritis, in which osteopenia is an
early manifestation.

Clinical Findings

The typical patient is a man, aged 15 to 40 years, with intermittent low back pain and stiffness that has progressed slowly over several
months.[55] Back pain occurs in 95 percent of patients and is worst in the
morning and after periods of inactivity. The back pain usually abates with
exercise. In some cases, the pain may be severe, with radiation into the
legs, simulating a lumbar disc herniation. The usual patient has a moderate degree of intermittent aching pain in the lumbosacral area with loss of
the normal lumbar lordosis. With progression of the disease, pain develops in the cervical spine and costovertebral joints and may affect chest excursion and pulmonary function. Peripheral joint arthritis and extra-

articular abnormalities (iritis, cardiac defects, constitutional symptoms) may also be present.[32]

Over time, ankylosing spondylitis results in two significant changes in the spine: osteopenia due to decreased spinal motion and loss of flexibility due to ankylosis of the spine. The ankylosed spine is brittle and fractures may occur, but they should exhibit normal healing potential.[37] In some older patients with the disease, cauda equina compression syndrome may develop.

Radiographic Findings

The typical radiographic features include symmetric involvement of the sacroiliac joints with a loss of subchondral bone, joint widening, reactive sclerosis, and eventual ankylosis (Fig. 18–1). In the spine, radiographic abnormalities include squaring of the vertebral bodies, symmetric marginal syndesmophyte formation, and apophyseal joint fusion, which proceeds from the sacrum to the neck (Figs. 18–2 and 18–3). These characteristic changes may be difficult to visualize in the early stages of the disease.[51] It is also important to realize that the inflammatory sacroilitis does not always result in ankylosis.[48]

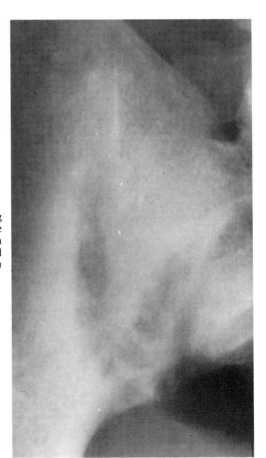

Figure 18–1. Ankylosing spondylitis. Widening of the sacroiliac joint is caused by erosions. The margins of the joint are poorly defined. (From Kricun ME: Imaging Modalities in Spinal Disorders. Philadelphia, W.B. Saunders, 1988.)

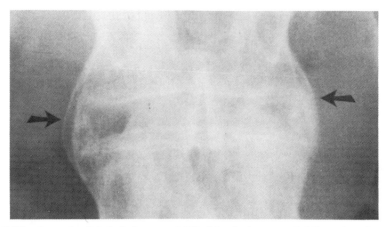

Figure 18–2. "Bamboo spine." Ankylosing spondylitis. Marginal symmetric bilateral syndesmophytes bridge the lateral vertebral margins (*arrows*). (From Kricun ME: Imaging Modalities in Spinal Disorders. Philadelphia, W.B. Saunders, 1988.)

Laboratory Findings

Laboratory results are nonspecific and add little to the diagnosis of ankylosing spondylitis. Erythrocyte sedimentation rate is elevated in 80 percent of patients with active disease.[43] The rheumatoid factor and antinuclear antibody are characteristically absent. A minority of patients will have a mild anemia. Histocompatibility antigen HLA-B27 is present in 90 percent of the patients with ankylosing spondylitis, but it is not diagnostic.

Differential Diagnosis

The differential diagnosis of low back pain with sacroiliac changes, and lumbar spine stiffness that improves with activity, recurrent radicular pain that alternates from side to side, or a history of iritis, must include the other spondyloarthropathies. Also to be considered are herniated disc, diffuse idiopathic skeletal hyperostosis, osteitis condensans ilii,

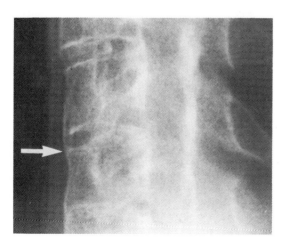

Figure 18–3. Ankylosing spondylitis. Cervical spine. There is fusion of all apophyseal joints. In addition, thin calcification of the anterior longitudinal ligament is noted (*arrow*). (From Kricun ME: Imaging Modalities in Spinal Disorders. Philadelphia, W.B. Saunders, 1988.)

osteoarthritis, rheumatoid arthritis, fibrositis, and malignancy (Table 18–1).

Osteitis condensans ilii results in a triangular area of sclerosis on the iliac side of the sacroiliac joint and does not cause joint erosions or sacral involvement. It is important to distinguish this disorder from ankylosing spondylitis since it is benign and is nonprogressive.

Treatment

The goals of therapy are to control pain and stiffness, reduce inflammation, maintain function, and prevent deformity. Patients should be educated about the disease and encouraged to continue with as normal a lifestyle as possible. Aspirin or other nonsteroidal anti-inflammatory drugs may be quite effective in mild or moderate disease. Systemic corticosteroids are rarely needed and are of limited benefit. A spinal brace to prevent forward flexion in the back or neck may be useful in appropriate patients. Surgical procedures on the spine, such as a lumbar osteotomy, are limited to patients who have such severe kyphosis that they cannot see where they are walking or have decreased pulmonary function.[68] These procedures have multiple potential complications and are viewed as a last resort.[12]

REITER'S SYNDROME

Reiter's syndrome is associated with the triad of urethritis, arthritis, and conjunctivitis.[6] It is the most common cause of arthritis in young men and primarily affects the joints of the lower extremity and spine. The course of the illness, while usually benign, may be chronic and remitting, resulting in significant long-term disability.

Reiter's syndrome occurs throughout the world, and there is no associated racial or ethnic predilection. Approximately 1 percent of patients with nongonococcal urethritis will develop the syndrome. It may also be seen in up to 3 percent of patients with enteric infections secondary to *Shigella, Salmonella, Campylobacter,* and *Yersinia.* The venereal infection occurs predominantly in males (10:1), while the outbreaks secondary to enteric infection or unknown causes affect males and females with equal frequency.[56]

Pathophysiology

The etiology of Reiter's syndrome is unknown. The disease results from the interaction of an environmental factor, usually venereal or enteric infection, and a genetically predisposed host. Between 60 and 80 percent of the patients are positive for HLA-B27 or a related HLA-B antigen.[2] Whether urethritis is an initiating event or a manifestation of the

Table 18–1. DIFFERENTIAL DIAGNOSIS OF ANKYLOSING SPONDYLITIS*

	Ankylosing Spondylitis	Reiter's Syndrome	Psoriatic Arthritis	Enteropathic Arthritis	Reactive Arthropathy	Herniated Nucleus Pulposus	Osteitis Condensans Ilii	Osteoarthritis of the Spine	Rheumatoid Arthritis	Fibrositis	Infection	Tumors
Sex	Male	Male	=	=	=	=	Female	=	Female	Female	=	=
Age at onset (years)	15–40	20–30	30–40	15–45	Any age	20–40	30–40	40–50	20–60	30–50	Any age	Young—benign Older—malignant
Presentation	Back pain	Arthritis Urethritis Conjunctivitis	Extremity arthritis Psoriasis Back pain	Abdominal pain	GI, GU infection	Radicular pain	Back pain	Back pain	Peripheral arthritis	Generalized fatigue Sleeplessness Tender points	Acute, severe unilateral back pain	Slowly progressive, insidious pain
Sacroiliitis	Symmetric	Asymmetric	Asymmetric	Symmetric	Symmetric	–	Asymmetric	–	Symmetric	–	Asymmetric	Asymmetric
Axial skeleton	+	+/–	+/–	+	+/–	–	–	+	(Cervical spine)	–	–	–
Peripheral joints	Lower	Lower	Upper	Lower	Lower	–	–	Lower	Upper and lower	–	–	–
Enthesopathy	+	+	+	–	+/–	–	–	–	–	–	–	–
Erythrocyte sedimentation rate	Elevated	Elevated	Elevated	Elevated	Elevated	Normal	Normal	Normal	Elevated	Normal	Elevated	Elevated (malignant)
Rheumatoid factor	–	–	–	–	–	–	–	–	80%	–	–	–
HLA-B27	90%	80%	60% (spondylitis)	50% (spondylitis)	90%	8%	8%	8%	8%	8%	8%	8%
Course	Continuous	Relapsing	Continuous	Continuous	Self-limited or continuous	Episodic	Self-limited	Relapsing	Continuous	Continuous	Episodic	Continuous
Therapy	Nonsteroidals Exercise	Nonsteroidals Gold Methotrexate	Nonsteroidals Gold Methotrexate	Nonsteroidals Corticosteroids Antibiotics	Nonsteroidals Antibiotics	Nonsteroidals Muscle relaxants Surgery	Bed rest Bracing Nonsteroidals	Nonsteroidals	Nonsteroidals Gold Methotrexate	Tricylic antidepressants Nonsteroidals	Antibiotics Bracing	En bloc excision Chemotherapy Radiotherapy
Disability	Hip	Lower extremity	Lower extremity	Hip		Neurologic dysfunction	Neurologic dysfunction	Neurologic dysfunction	Generalized joint deformities (sacroiliitis late in disease)	Muscle pain	Neurologic dysfunction	Local invasion— benign Metastases— malignant

*From Borenstein DB, Wiesel SW: Low Back Pain: Medical Diagnosis and Comprehensive Management. Philadelphia, W.B. Saunders, 1989.

syndrome is unclear.[59] The syndrome can develop in patients who deny enteric or venereal infection and may be related to joint trauma.[1,17,18]

Clinical Findings

The typical patient in North America is a young man who develops urethritis and a mild conjunctivitis, followed by the onset of a predominantly lower extremity oligoarthritis.[28] The weight-bearing joints (knees, ankles, and feet) are most commonly affected in an asymmetric pattern. Back pain is a frequent symptom, occurring in 30 to 90 percent of the patients. [28,57,61] The pain is of an aching quality and is improved with activity. The pain may radiate into the posterior thigh, often unilaterally, corresponding to the asymmetric involvement of the sacroiliac joints. This pattern is in contrast to the symmetric involvement seen with ankylosing spondylitis.[66] Involvement of the lumbar, thoracic, and cervical portions of the spine occurs less commonly than sacroiliitis.[30]

Radiographic Findings

Radiographic changes may be helpful in confirming the diagnosis in patients who do not manifest the complete triad of Reiter's syndrome.[50] Joint destruction is most severe in the feet, with sparing of the hips and shoulders. The enthesopathy of Reiter's syndrome results in periosteal new bone formation at the attachments of the plantar fascia and Achilles tendon into the calcaneus. Sacroiliac involvement is asymmetric early in the disease but may later become bilateral, as in ankylosing spondylitis (Fig. 18–4).[57] Spondylitic involvement of the axial skeleton is dis-

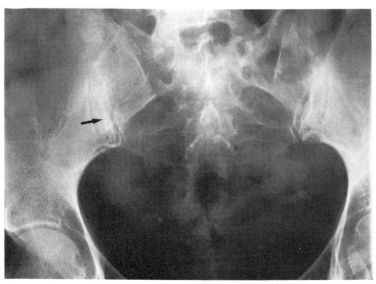

Figure 18–4. Reiter's syndrome. Spot view of the pelvis reveals greater involvement of the right sacroiliac joint characterized by joint sclerosis (*arrow*) predominantly on the ilium. (From Borenstein DG, Wiesel SW: Low Back Pain: Medical Diagnosis and Management. Philadelphia, W.B. Saunders, 1989.)

continuous with skip areas and is characterized by nonmarginal bony bridging of vertebral bodies (Fig. 18–5). These vertical hyperostoses are markedly thickened compared to the syndesmophytes of ankylosing spondylitis.

Laboratory Findings

Laboratory studies are nonspecific and not helpful in making the diagnosis. A mild anemia of chronic disease, leukocytosis, and thrombocytosis can be seen in one third of patients.[1] The erythrocyte sedimentation rate is frequently elevated, but it does not follow the clinical course of the disease. Synovial fluid analysis demonstrates a nonspecific inflammatory fluid. *Chlamydia* can sometimes be cultured from the synovial fluid, urethra, and conjunctiva.

Differential Diagnosis

Patients with Reiter's syndrome are distinguished from patients with other spondyloarthropathies and gonococcal arthritis by an episode

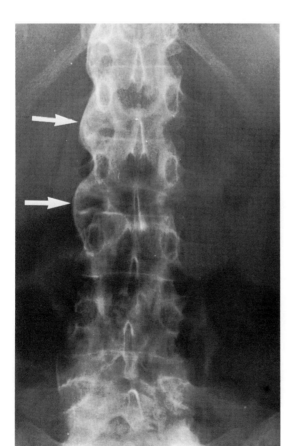

Figure 18–5. Reiter's syndrome. A 35-year-old man with midline back pain has asymmetric nonmarginal syndesmophytes on the right side (more common on the nonaortic side) of the lumbar spine (*arrows*). A similar pattern may be seen with psoriatic spondylitis. (Courtesy of Anne Brower, M.D.) (From Borenstein DG, Wiesel SW: Low Back Pain: Medical Diagnosis and Management. Philadelphia, W.B. Saunders, 1989.)

of peripheral arthritis of more than 1 month's duration occurring in association with urethritis and/or cervicitis.[76] The differential diagnosis of the patient who presents with low back pain and no other manifestations of Reiter's syndrome is the same as that presented earlier for ankylosing spondylitis.

Treatment

The therapeutic regimen includes patient education, medications, and physical therapy. The association of this syndrome with venereal disease must be explained. Acute joint symptoms are treated with nonsteroidal anti-inflammatory drugs and physical therapy modalities. The role of antibiotic therapy in the acute phase of Reiter's syndrome remains controversial.[41] Gold salt therapy may be helpful in patients with progressive, destructive peripheral joint disease. Methotrexate is reserved for patients with uncontrolled progression of disease.[26]

There is no cure for Reiter's syndrome. The illness is self-limited in 30 to 40 percent of patients; and another 30 to 50 percent develop a pattern of relapsing illness with periods of complete remission. The remaining 10 to 25 percent have chronic, unremitting disease associated with significant disability.[28,29] Patients who are HLA-B27–positive have more frequent back pain, longer duration of disease, and more frequent chronic low back symptoms and sacroiliitis.[47]

PSORIATIC ARTHRITIS

Patients with psoriasis who develop a characteristic pattern of joint disease have psoriatic arthritis. The typical patterns include asymptomatic oligoarthritis, symmetric polyarthritis, and spondylitis. The arthritis is slowly progressive but is rarely associated with significant disability. Psoriatic arthritis occurs in 5 to 7 percent of individuals with psoriasis and in 0.1 percent of the general population.[35]

Pathophysiology

The basic abnormality, which results in the increased metabolic activity of the skin, is unknown, and there is no agreement as to whether the problem lies in the peridermal or dermal layers of the skin. A genetic predisposition for psoriasis and psoriatic arthritis exists, with one third of patients reporting a positive family history.[54] Patients with psoriatic arthritis have an increased frequency of HLA-BW38, HLA-DR4, and HLA-DR7 antigens.[25] As with ankylosing spondylitis and Reiter's syndrome, environmental factors such as trauma and bacterial infection have been thought to play a role in the development of psoriatic arthritis.[15,45,49,75]

Clinical Findings

The clinical forms of psoriatic arthritis can be divided into three patterns: asymmetric oligoarthritis (54%); symmetric arthritis (25%); and spondyloarthritis (21%).[39] Distal interphalangeal joint involvement occurs most commonly in asymmetric oligoarthritis. Symmetric polyarthritis, which affects the small joints of the hands and feet, resembles rheumatoid arthritis.

The typical patients who develop axial skeletal disease, sacroiliitis, or spondylitis are men who have onset of psoriasis later in life.[44] Low back pain, which is indistinguishable from the pain associated with other spondyloarthropathies, is present in the vast majority of patients with axial skeletal disease. Between 10 and 20 percent of patients will have arthritis prior to the appearance of psoriatic skin changes.

Radiographic Findings

While the radiologic features of psoriatic and rheumatoid arthritis may be somewhat similar, certain deformities of the interphalangeal joints in psoriatic arthritis are distinctive.[3,77] The involvement is oligoarticular with erosive changes in the distal interphalangeal joint and distal phalanx. The "pencil-in-cup" deformity (osteolysis of the proximal phalanx and widening of the distal phalanx) is characteristic.

Axial skeletal involvement is manifested by sacroiliitis, which can be unilateral or bilateral.[51] Spondylitis is characterized by asymmetric involvement of the vertebral bodies and nonmarginal syndesmophytes (Fig. 18–6). Some patients have been described as having axial skeletal in-

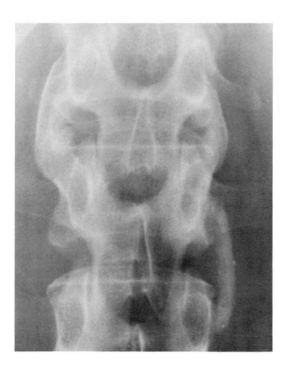

Figure 18–6. Psoriatic spondylitis. Large asymmetric paravertebral ossifications (syndesmophytes) are noted. (From Kricun ME: Imaging Modalities in Spinal Disorders. Philadelphia, W.B. Saunders, 1988.)

volvement quite similar to that of ankylosing spondylitis. Paravertebral ossification not in contact with the vertebral body may occur in the thoracolumbar region.[16] The cervical spine may also be affected in psoriatic spondylitis with joint space sclerosis and narrowing as well as calcification of the anterior longitudinal ligament (Fig. 18–7).[40]

Laboratory Findings

The findings of anemia, mild leukocytosis, and elevated erythrocyte sedimentation rate occur in a minority of patients.[5] Hyperuricemia due to increased metabolic activity of the skin can be detected in 20 percent of patients. HLA-B27 is found in 35 to 60 percent of patients with axial skeleton disease.[13] Synovial fluid is nondiagnostic.

Differential Diagnosis

The diagnosis of psoriatic arthritis is easily made when the patient already has skin lesions. In patients in whom arthritis precedes cutaneous involvement, the differential diagnosis should include Reiter's syndrome, gout, erosive osteoarthritis, and rheumatoid arthritis. Psoriatic arthritis can be distinguished from these other entities by the absence of urethritis, monosodium urate crystals, osteophytes/sclerosis/cysts in the interphalangeal joints, or serum rheumatoid factor.

Treatment

Treatment of the cutaneous and peripheral joint symptoms is similar to that for Reiter's syndrome. In addition to nonsteroidal anti-inflammatory drugs, gold salts may be useful.[22,39] In patients with extensive disease, immunosuppressive therapy with methotrexate, 6-mercaptopurine, or azothiaprine is indicated.[7,8,23] The course of

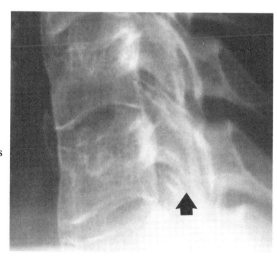

Figure 18–7. Psoriatic spondylitis. Cervical spine. There are thin calcification of the anterior longitudinal ligament and very mild indistinctness of apophyseal joints (*arrow*) caused by the inflammatory process. (From Kricun ME: Imaging Modalities in Spinal Disorders. Philadelphia, W.B. Saunders, 1988.)

psoriatic arthritis is unpredictable.[65] Patients who develop spondylitis acquire varying degrees of restriction of spinal motion. There is poor correlation between the severity of axial and peripheral disease. As in ankylosing spondylitis, fusion of the axial skeleton makes it more vulnerable to fracture from minimal trauma.

RHEUMATOID ARTHRITIS

Rheumatoid arthritis is a chronic systemic inflammatory disease that results in varying degrees of pain, heat, swelling, and destruction in synovial joints. The joints characteristically affected include the small joints of the hands and feet as well as the wrists, elbows, hips, knees, ankles, and cervical spine. The prevalence of rheumatoid arthritis is 1 to 3 percent of the United States population.[58]

Pathophysiology

The etiology of rheumatoid arthritis is probably multifocal, including genetic and environmental factors. Histologic patterns in affected synovium and the clinical course suggest that immunologic factors play an important role in its pathogenesis.[72] An unknown antigen localized to the synovial surface is theorized to initiate formation of antibodies directed against it. The subsequent formation of antigen-antibody complexes binds complement and attracts polymorphonuclear leukocytes into the joint space. The accumulation of leukocytes results in the release of lysosomal enzymes that are responsible for some of the inflammatory changes. Periarticular erosions result in ligamentous instability and joint subluxation.

Clinical Findings

Radiographic studies of the cervical spine in rheumatoid patients have demonstrated atlantoaxial subluxations in 25 percent.[19,53] Subluxation may be anterior, posterior, or vertical (settling of the skull in relation to the atlas). Horizontal anterior subluxations are the most common, the vertical type is less common, and the horizontal posterior variety is very rare. Pain localized to the upper neck or radiating to the occiput, forehead, or eye is the most frequent symptom of atlantoaxial subluxation. Generally, pain will increase with neck motion, particularly rotation. Involvement of the spinal cord or medulla may be associated with complaints of weakness, paresthesias, vertigo, and dysuria. Signs of upper motor neuron involvement, such as weakness, spasticity, and hyperreflexia, are the most frequently encountered neurologic findings in rheumatoid patients with atlantoaxial instability.

The clinical manifestations of rheumatoid arthritis in the subaxial (below C1-2 level) cervical spine reflect inflammation of synovial tissue and ligaments, destruction of the zygoapophyseal joints, and secondary involvement of nerve roots and the spinal cord. The root/cord symptoms may result from compression of neural elements from synovial pannus or vertebral subluxation with subsequent impingement. Vascular ischemia of the anterior spinal cord may also play a role when myelopathy is present. Pain is generally localized to the neck but may radiate to the intrascapular area, shoulder, arm, or chest. Neck motion is likely to be limited and painful. The most common neurologic findings with subaxial rheumatoid spondylitis are weakness, spasticity, hyper-reflexia, Babinski signs, and a hemisensory deficit for pain.

The lumbar spine is rarely involved in the rheumatoid process. The clinical manifestations of rheumatoid spondylitis in the lumbar spine include local and referred pain (to the thighs), which is accentuated by motion, pain on forced motion of the spine, and spinous process tenderness.[70] Neurologic examination is generally normal. Patients with rheumatoid arthritis of the lumbar spine usually have a history of extensive involvement of long duration. The sacroiliac joints are usually asymptomatic.

Radiographic Findings

Radiographs of the cervical spine will delineate atlantoaxial subluxation if optimal views are obtained in flexion and extension. Normally, there is less than 3 to 4 mm of space between the dens and the anterior ring of the axis on a lateral radiograph (Fig. 18–8).[11] Detection of vertical subluxation may require tomograms or a CT scan. Erosions in C1-2 will also be visualized and may contribute to instability (Fig. 18–9).

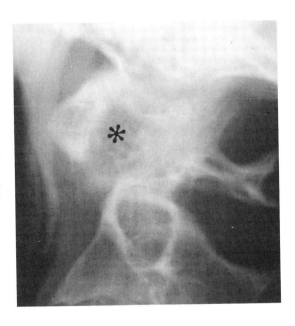

Figure 18–8. Rheumatoid arthritis. Atlantoaxial subluxation. There is widening of the space between the odontoid process and the anterior arch of the atlas (*asterisk*). (From Kricun ME: Imaging Modalities in Spinal Disorders. Philadelphia, W.B. Saunders, 1988.)

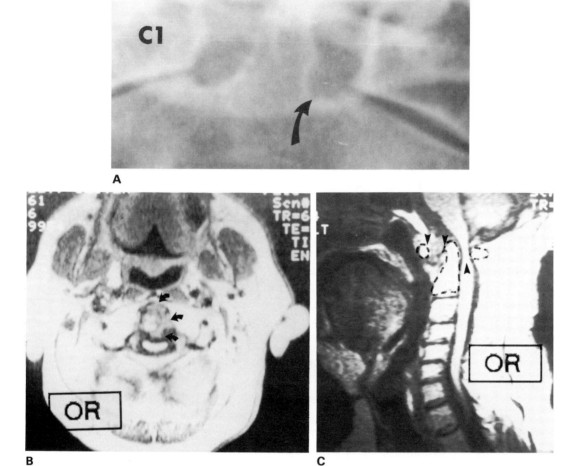

Figure 18-9. *A,* Rheumatoid arthritis. There are erosions about the odontoid process (*arrow*). (From Kricun ME: Imaging Modalities in Spinal Disorders. Philadelphia, W.B. Saunders, 1988.) *B* and *C,* This 62-year-old male has rheumatoid arthritis, pannus erosion of the dens, atlantoaxial instability, and compressive myelopathy. *B,* Axial MRI shows mass effect and cord compression from pannus (*arrows*). *C,* Sagittal MRI shows 17-mm atlantoaxial interval with occipital flexion and cord compression (*arrows*).

Radiographic evidence of rheumatoid spondylitis in the subaxial portion of the cervical spine is marked by dislocations, subluxations, disc narrowing, osteopenia, and erosions (Fig. 18–10). Multiple subluxations, and particularly subluxations at C2-3, are suggestive of rheumatoid disease.[53] Multiple level involvement with disc narrowing in the absence of osteophytes is also common.[19]

Radiographic signs of rheumatoid spondylitis in the lumbar spine are difficult to visualize. Involvement of the apophyseal or costovertebral joints is marked by osteopenia, erosions, and joint space narrowing.[21,46,70] Subluxations, osteopenia, and disc space narrowing without hypertrophic osteophytes may signify rheumatoid involvement of the intervertebral joints. These findings, however, may be superimposed upon or complicated by degenerative disc disease. Sacroiliac joint changes include asymmetric involvement with mild narrowing without any erosions, sclerosis, or fusion.[4]

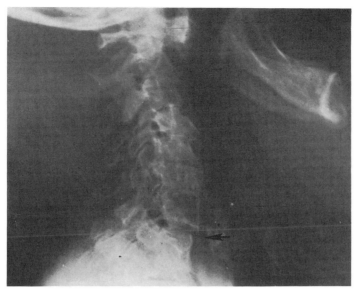

Figure 18–10. Advanced rheumatoid spondylitis with marked narrowing of multiple discs and subluxation of C7 on T1. (From Rothman RH, Simeone FA: The Spine, 2nd ed. Philadelphia, W.B. Saunders, 1982.)

Laboratory Findings

Abnormal laboratory findings include anemia, increased erythrocyte sedimentation rate, and increased serum globulins. Rheumatoid factors are present in 80 percent and antinuclear antibodies are present in 30 percent of rheumatoid arthritis patients.[72] Histologic analysis of affected synovium demonstrates an inflammatory, hyperplastic tissue, characterized by mononuclear cell infiltration, synovial cell proliferation, fibrin deposition, and necrosis.[40]

Differential Diagnosis

Rheumatoid arthritis is a clinical diagnosis and may be confirmed by the classic radiographic findings in the peripheral joints or cervical spine. In the patient who develops back pain in the setting of long-standing rheumatoid disease, the diagnosis of rheumatoid spondylitis is possible. However, since involvement of the lumbar spine is rare, other possibilities such as herniated disc, local infection, and the seronegative spondyloarthropathies should be considered.

Treatment

Therapy for rheumatoid arthritis affecting the spine is similar to that for generalized disease. Patient education, physical therapy, nonsteroidal anti-inflammatory drugs, remittive agents (gold, penicillamine), corticosteroids, and immunosuppressive agents may be indicated.[38]

Rheumatoid patients should also have systemic rest as a general supportive measure and joint rest.

Rheumatoid spondylitis requires special attention. The treatment of atlantoaxial horizontal subluxations must be individualized based on the patient's age, general health, and severity of symptoms. Cervical collars can help temporarily but may not change the long-term progression of deformity. If there is rapid deterioration in neurologic function or progressive deformity, surgical stabilization should be considered. Vertical subluxation is a more serious problem and warrants more active consideration of surgery.

In the remainder of the cervical spine, rheumatoid spondylitis may be superimposed upon degenerative disc disease in older patients. Again, nonoperative symptomatic management is preferred unless a neurologic deficit develops. In some cases, the cervical spine will ankylose and stabilize itself.

Rheumatoid spondylitis affecting the lumbar spine can in most cases be managed with the general rheumatoid therapeutic schema outlined above.

DIFFUSE IDIOPATHIC SKELETAL HYPEROSTOSIS (DISH)

Diffuse idiopathic skeletal hyperostosis (DISH), originally described by Forestier,[27] is a disease characterized clinically by spinal stiffness and pain and radiographically by exuberant calcification of spinal and extraspinal structures. The disorder is common and is found in 6 to 28 percent of autopsy populations.[9,64,74] The typical patient is a male between the ages of 50 and 85 years.[73]

Pathophysiology

The etiology of DISH is unknown. Occupational stress, spinal trauma, acromegaly, hypoparathyroidism, and diabetes mellitus have all been suggested as associated factors, but hard evidence is lacking.[63,73] A specific genetic predisposition has not been identified. HLA-B27 positivity was found in about a third of one DISH study population and found to have no association in another investigation.[69,71]

Clinical Findings

The most common musculoskeletal symptom, spinal stiffness, occurs in 80 percent of DISH patients.[73] The duration of back symptoms may be 10 to 20 years. Typically, morning stiffness resolves within an hour and recurs in the late evening.[27] Back pain in the thoracolumbar spine is the initial complaint in 57 percent of patients.[63] Occasionally, patients may have cervical spine pain as their initial complaint, and dysphagia occurs in 17 to 28 percent due to constriction of the esophagus by anterior spinal osteophytes.[73] Physical examination reveals little more than minimally limited spinal motion unless there is also extraspinal ossification.

Radiographic Findings

Radiographic findings include flowing calcification along the anterior aspect of at least four contiguous vertebral bodies, preservation of intervertebral disc height, and absence of apophyseal joint ankylosis (Fig. 18–11).[63,64] The posterior spinal elements are not affected and, as in ankylosing spondylitis, the vertebral foramina are uninvolved. Although it is rare to have pain syndromes as a result of this disease, dysphagia due to the osteophytes posterior to the esophagus may occur (Figs. 18–12 and 18–13).

Although quite common in Japan, ossification of the posterior longitudinal ligament (OPLL) of the cervical spine occurs rarely in this country but may be associated with DISH.[10] In contrast to DISH, OPLL can produce encroachment in the cervical spinal canal and can result in neural compression. The radiographic appearance of OPLL is diagnostic and consists of a linear band of ossified tissue along the posterior margin of some or all of the vertebral bodies in the cervical spine (Fig. 18–14).

Laboratory Findings

Laboratory findings are entirely normal in patients with DISH.[33] Occasionally, a mild elevation in erythrocyte sedimentation rate may be seen.

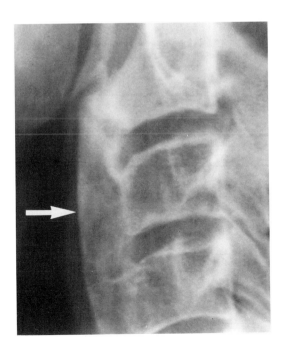

Figure 18–11. Diffuse idiopathic skeletal hyperostosis (DISH). Cervical spine. Thick bony mass that appears fused with the vertebral bodies and is characteristic of more advanced DISH (*arrow*). (From Kricun ME: Imaging Modalities in Spinal Disorders. Philadelphia, W.B. Saunders, 1988.)

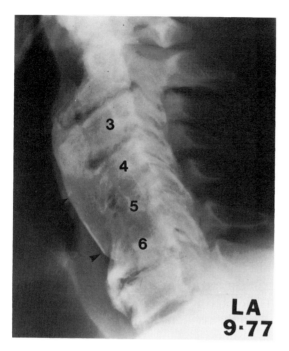

Figure 18–12. Lateral roentgenogram of a patient with long-standing osteoarthritis of the cervical spine and DISH. Note the flowing ossification along the anterior borders of the third through sixth vertebral bodies (*arrows*). (From Bohlman HH: Osteoarthritis of the cervical spine. In Moskowitz RW, Howell DS, Goldberg VM, Mankin HJ, eds: Osteoarthritis, Diagnosis and Management. Philadelphia, W.B. Saunders, 1984.)

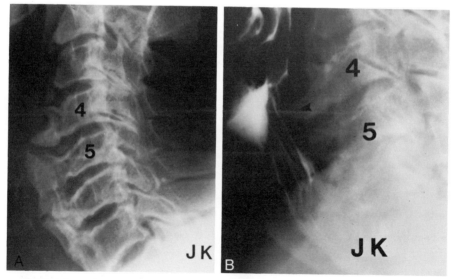

Figure 18–13. *A*, Lateral roentgenogram of the cervical spine in a patient with DISH and large anterior osteophytes at the C4 and C5 levels. The patient complained of severe dysphagia. *B*, Lateral roentgenogram demonstrating the barium swallow and marked esophageal impingement by the anterior fourth cervical osteophyte (*arrow*). This was removed successfully with relief of dysphagia. (From Bohlman HH: Osteoarthritis of the cervical spine. In Moskowitz RW, Howell DS, Goldberg VM, Mankin HJ, eds: Osteoarthritis, Diagnosis and Management. Philadelphia, W.B. Saunders, 1984.)

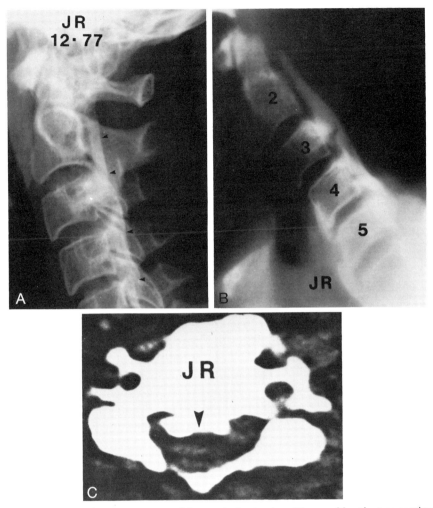

Figure 18–14. *A*, Lateral roentgenogram of the cervical spine in a 55-year-old patient presenting with cervical myeloradiculopathy. Note the thickened ossified posterior longitudinal ligament (OPLL) extending from the second through the sixth cervical vertebrae, severely compromising the diameter of the cervical spinal canal (*arrows*). *B*, Lateral tomograms of the cervical spine further define the ossified posterior longitudinal ligament and additional osteoarthritis of the atlantoaxial complex. *C*, Computed axial tomogram demonstrating severe compromise of the cervical spinal canal by the ossified posterior ligament, anterior to the spinal cord (*arrow*). (From Bohlman HH: Osteoarthritis of the cervical spine. In Moskowitz RW, Howell DS, Goldberg VM, Mankin HJ, eds: Osteoarthritis, Diagnosis and Management. Philadelphia, W.B. Saunders, 1984.)

Differential Diagnosis

The diagnosis of DISH is based upon the presence of characteristic radiographic changes as previously described. Other diseases that can result in bony outgrowths of the spine include the spondyloarthropathies, acromegaly, hypoparathyroidism, fluorosis, ochronosis, neuropathic arthropathy, and trauma.

Treatment

Treatment is directed at relieving pain and maximizing function. In patients with back pain and stiffness, nonsteroidal anti-inflammatory drugs may be helpful. Exercise programs are prescribed to encourage maximum range of motion throughout the axial skeleton. Local steroid/lidocaine injections may be helpful in extraspinal, peripheral areas of bone overgrowth.

Patients with significant dysphagia may require removal of the offending hyperostosis.[52] Exostoses can recur after surgical removal. In patients with associated OPLL and neural compression, surgical intervention is necessary to decompress the spinal cord.

OTHER SPONDYLOARTHROPATHIES

Several other disorders are associated with a seronegative spondyloarthropathy. Ulcerative colitis and Crohn's disease are inflammatory bowel disorders that are associated with extraintestinal manifestations including arthritis. Axial skeletal disease is similar to ankylosing spondylitis and follows a course independent of bowel symptoms.[20]

Familial Mediterranean fever is a hereditary disorder seen in individuals of Middle Eastern descent that is characterized by recurrent brief episodes of fever, peritonitis/pleuritis, and arthritis. Sacroiliitis, frequently asymptomatic, has been described in patients with familial Mediterranean fever, with between 10 and 17 percent of patients having either unilateral or bilateral disease.[14,34] Lumbar spine changes occur less commonly.

Behçet's syndrome is a chronic relapsing systemic disease characterized by the triad of oral and genital ulcers and iritis. Peripheral arthritis is common and is asymmetric, recurrent, and nondeforming. Axial skeletal disease, back pain, and sacroiliitis have been reported in about 10 percent of patients.[60,78]

Whipple's disease, or intestinal lipodystrophy, is a rare disorder characterized by granulomatous inflammation and subsequent multiorgan system dysfunction. In addition to peripheral joint arthritis, back pain due to axial skeleton involvement, spondylitis, or sacroiliitis may be seen in up to 19 percent of patients.[42]

Summary

All patients with persistent neck or back complaints that are unexplained by mechanical disorders in the spine should undergo a rheumatologic evaluation. In managing patients with spinal complaints, the physician must remember to inquire about and examine other joints that may be symptomatic. This step will often lead to discovery of an underlying etiology of back or neck pain that might otherwise have been missed. The inflammatory spondyloarthropathies are not an uncommon cause of spinal complaints and frequently respond to systemic treatment.

References

1. Arnett FC: Reiter's syndrome. Johns Hopkins Med J 150:39–44, 1982.
2. Arnett FC, Hochberg MD, Bias WB: Cross-reactive HLA antigens in B27-negative Reiter's syndrome and sacroiliitis. Johns Hopkins Med J 141:193–197, 1977
3. Avila R, Pugh DG, Slocumb CH, et al: Psoriatic arthritis: a roentgenologic study. Radiology 75:691–701, 1960.
4. Baggenstoss AH, Bickel WH, Ward LE: Rheumatoid granulomatous nodules as destructive lesions of vertebrae. J Bone Joint Surg 34A:601–609, 1952.
5. Baker H, Golding DH, Thompson M: Psoriasis and arthritis. Ann Intern Med 58: 909–925, 1963.
6. Bauer W, Engleman EP: A syndrome of unknown etiology characterized by urethritis, conjunctivitis, and arthritis (so-called Reiter's disease). Trans Assoc Am Phys 57:307–313, 1942.
7. Baum J, Hurd E, Lewis D, et al: Treatment of psoriatic arthritis with 6-mercaptopurine. Arthritis Rheum 16:139–147, 1973.
8. Black RL, O'Brien WM, Van Scott EJ, et al: Methotrexate therapy in psoriatic arthritis: double-blind study in 21 patients. JAMA 189:743–747, 1964.
9. Boachie-Adjii O, Bullough PG: Incidence of ankylosing hyperostosis of spine (Forestier's disease) at autopsy. Spine 12:739–743, 1987.
10. Bohlman HH: Osteoarthritis of the cervical spine. In Moskowitz RW, Howell DS, Goldberg VM, Mankin HJ, eds: Osteoarthritis, Diagnosis and Management. Philadelphia, W.B. Saunders, 1984, pp. 443–459.
11. Boyle AC: The rheumatoid neck. Proc Royal Soc Med 64:1161–1165, 1971.
12. Bradford PS, Schumacher WL, Lonstein JE, et al: Ankylosing spondylitis: experience in surgical management of 21 patients. Spine 12:238–243, 1987.
13. Brewerton DA, Coffrey M, Nicholls A, et al: HLA-B27 and arthropathies associated with ulcerative colitis and psoriasis. Lancet 1:956–958, 1974.
14. Brodey PA, Wolff SM: Radiographic changes in the sacroiliac joints in familial Mediterranean fever. Radiology 114:331–333, 1975.
15. Buckley WR, Raleigh RL: Psoriasis with acaro-osteolysis. N Engl J Med 261:539–541, 1959.
16. Bywaters EGL, Dixon ASJ: Paravertebral ossification in psoriatic arthritis. Ann Rheum Dis 24:313–331, 1965.
17. Calin A, Fries JF: Striking prevalence of ankylosing spondylitis in "healthy" W27 positive males and females: a controlled study. N Engl J Med 293:835–839, 1975.
18. Cohen LM, Mittal KK, Schmid FR, et al: Increased risk for spondylitis stigma in apparently healthy HLA-W27 men. Ann Intern Med 84:1–7, 1976.
19. Conlon PW, Isdale IC, Rose BS: Rheumatoid arthritis of the cervical spine. Ann Rheum Dis 25:120–126, 1966.
20. Dekher-Saeys BJ, Meuwissen SG, van der Berg-Loonen EM, et al: Prevalence of peripheral arthritis, sacroiliitis and ankylosing spondylitis in patients suffering from inflammatory bowel disease. Ann Rheum Dis 37:33–35, 1978.
21. Dixon ASJ, Lience E: Sacroiliac joint in adult rheumatoid arthritis and psoriatic arthropathy. Ann Rheum Dis 20:247–257, 1961.
22. Dorwart BB, Gall EP, Schumacher HR, et al: Chrysotherapy in psoriatic arthritis: efficacy and toxicity compared to rheumatoid arthritis. Arthritis Rheum 21:513–515, 1978.
23. DuVivier A, Munro DD, Verboy J: Treatment of psoriasis with azathioprine. Br Med J 1:49–51, 1974.
24. Edmonds J, Macauley D, Tyndall A, et al: Lymphocytotoxicity of anti-Klebsiella antisera in ankylosing spondylitis and related arthropathies: patient and family studies. Arthritis Rheum 24:1–7, 1981.
25. Espinoza LR, Vasey FB, Oh JH, et al: Association between HLA-BW38 and peripheral psoriatic arthritis. Arthritis Rheum 21: 72–75, 1978.
26. Farber GA, Forshner JG, O'Quinn SE: Reiter's syndrome: treatment with methotrexate. JAMA 200:171–173, 1967.
27. Forestier J, Lagier R: Ankylosing hyperostosis of the spine. Clin Orthop 74:65–83, 1971.
28. Fox R, Calin A, Gerber RC, Gibson D: The chronicity of symptoms and disability in Reiter's syndrome: an analysis of 131 consecutive patients. Ann Intern Med 91:190–193, 1979.
29. Good AE: Involvement of the back in Reiter's syndrome: follow-up study of thirty-four cases. Ann Intern Med 57:44–59, 1962.
30. Good AE: Reiter's syndrome: Long-term follow-up in relation to development of ankylosing spondylitis. Ann Rheum Dis 38:39–45, 1979.
31. Good AE, Kawaniski H, Schultz JS: HLA-B27 in blacks with ankylosing spondylitis or Reiter's disease. N Engl J Med 294:166–167, 1976.

32. Graham DC, Smythe HA: The carditis and aortitis of ankylosing spondylitis. Bull Rheum Dis 9:171–174, 1958.
33. Harris J, Carter AR, Glick EN, et al: Ankylosing hyperostosis: I. Clinical and radiological features. Ann Rheum Dis 33:210–215, 1974.
34. Heller H, Gafni J, Michaeli D, et al: The arthritis of familial Mediterranean fever. Arthritis Rheum 9:1–17, 1966.
35. Hellgren L: Association between rheumatoid arthritis and psoriasis in total populations. Acta Rheum Scand 15:316–326, 1969.
36. Hochberg MC, Bias WB, Arnett FC: Family studies in HLA-B27 associated arthritis. Medicine 57:463–475, 1978.
37. Hunter T, Dubo H: Spinal fractures complicating ankylosing spondylitis. Ann Intern Med 88:546–549, 1978.
38. Jacobs RP: Update on the treatment of rheumatoid arthritis. Primary Care 6:483–503, 1979.
39. Kammer GM, Soter WA, Gibson DJ, et al: Psoriatic arthritis: a clinical, immunologic and HLA study of 100 patients. Semin Arthritis Rheum 9:75–97, 1979.
40. Kaplan D, Plotz CM, Nathanson L, et al: Cervical spine in psoriasis and in psoriatic arthritis. Ann Rheum Dis 23:50–55, 1964.
41. Keat AC, Maini RN, Nkwazi GC, et al: Role of Chlamydia trachomatis and HLA-B27 in sexually acquired reactive arthritis. Br Med J 1:605–607, 1978.
42. Kelley JJ, Weisiger BB: The arthritis of Whipple's disease. Arthritis Rheum 6:615–632, 1963.
43. Kendal MJ, Lawrence DS, Shuttleworth GR, et al: Hematology and biochemistry of ankylosing spondylitis. Br Med J 2:235–237, 1973.
44. Lambert JR, Wright V: Psoriatic spondylitis: a clinical radiological description of the spine in psoriatic arthritis. Q J Med 46:411–425, 1977.
45. Landau JW, Gross BG, Newcomer VD, et al: Immunologic response of patients with psoriasis. Arch Dermatol 91:607–610, 1965.
46. Lawrence JS, Sharp J, Ball J, et al: Rheumatoid arthritis of the lumbar spine. Ann Rheum Dis 23:205–217, 1964.
47. Leirisalo M, Skylv G, Kousa M, et al: Follow-up study on patients with Reiter's disease and reactive arthritis, with special reference to HLA-B27. Arthritis Rheum 25:249–259, 1982.
48. Lindvall W: Early x-ray diagnosis of sacroiliitis. Scand J Rheumatol 32:(Suppl):98–102, 1979.
49. Mansson I, Olhagen B: Intestinal Clostridium perfringens in rheumatoid arthritis and other connective tissue disorders: Studies of fecal flora, serum antitoxin levels, and skin hypersensitivity. Acta Rheum Scand 12:167–174, 1966.
50. Martel W, Braunstein EM, Borlaza G, et al: Radiologic features of Reiter's disease. Radiology 132:1–10, 1979.
51. McEwen C, DiTata D, Ling GC, et al: Ankylosing spondylitis and spondylitis accompanying ulcerative colitis, regional enteritis, psoriasis, and Reiter's disease: A comparative study. Arthritis Rheum 14:291–318, 1971.
52. Meeks LW, Renshaw TS: Vertebral osteophytosis and dysphagia. J Bone Joint Surg 55A:197–201, 1973.
53. Meikle JAK, Wilkenson M: Rheumatoid involvement of the cervical spine. Ann Rheum Dis 30:154–161, 1971.
54. Moll JMH, Wright V: Familial occurrence of psoriatic arthritis. Ann Rheum Dis 32:181–199, 1973.
55. Neustadt DH: Ankylosing spondylitis. Postgrad Med 61:124–135, 1977.
56. Neuwelt CM, Borenstein DG, Jacobs RP: Reiter's syndrome: A male and female disease. J Rheumatol 9:268–272, 1982.
57. Oates JK, Young AC: Sacroiliitis in Reiter's disease. Br Med J 1:1013–1015, 1959.
58. O'Sullivan JB, Cathcart ES: The prevalence of rheumatoid arthritis: Follow-up evaluation of the effect of criteria on rates in Sudbury, Massachusetts. Ann Intern Med 76:573–577, 1972.
59. Paronen I: Reiter's disease: A study of 344 cases observed in Finland. Acta Med Scand 212(Suppl): 1–112, 1948.
60. Perkins ES: Behçet's disease. Ophthalmological aspects. Proc Royal Soc Med 54:106–107, 1961.
61. Popert AJ, Gill AJ, Laird SM: A prospective study of Reiter's syndrome: An interim report on the first 82 cases. Br J Vener Dis 40:160–165, 1964.
62. Resnick D, Dwosh IL, Goergen TG, et al: Clinical and radiographic "reankylosis" following hip surgery in ankylosing spondylitis. Am J Roentgenol 126:1181–1188, 1976.
63. Resnick D, Niwayama G: Radiographic and pathologic features of spinal involvement in diffuse idiopathic skeletal hyperostosis (DISH). Radiology 119:559–568, 1976.
64. Resnick D, Shaul SR, Robins JM: Diffuse idiopathic skeletal hyperostosis (DISH): Forestier's disease with extraspinal manifestations. Radiology 115:513–524, 1975.
65. Roberts MET, Wright V, Hill AGS, et al: Psoriatic arthritis: follow-up study. Ann Rheum Dis 35:206–212, 1976.
66. Russel A, Davis P, Percy JS, et al: The sacroiliitis of acute Reiter's syndrome. J Rheumatol 4:293–296, 1977.
67. Schlosstein L, Terasaki PI, Bluestone R, et al: High association of an HL antigen, W27, with ankylosing spondylitis. N Engl J Med 288:704–706, 1973.

68. Scudese VA, Calabro JJ: Vertebral wedge osteotomy: Correction of rheumatoid (ankylosing) spondylitis. JAMA 186:627–631, 1963.
69. Shapiro RF, Utsinger PD, Wiesner KB, et al: The association of HLA-B27 with Forestier's disease (vertebral ankylosing hyperostosis). J Rheumatol 3:4–8, 1976.
70. Sims-Williams H, Jayson MIV, Baddeley H: Rheumatoid involvement of the lumbar spine. Ann Rheum Dis 36:524–531, 1977.
71. Spagnola AM, Bennett PH, Terasaki PI: Vertebral ankylosing hyperostosis (Forestier's disease) and HLA antigens in Pima Indians. Arthritis Rheum 21:467–472, 1978.
72. Stastny P: Immunogenetic factors in rheumatoid arthritis. Clin Rheum Dis 3:315–332, 1977.
73. Utsinger PD, Resnick D, Shapiro R: Diffuse skeletal abnormalities in Forestier's disease. Arch Intern Med 136:763–768, 1976.
74. Vernon-Roberts B, Pirie CJ, Trenwith V: Pathology of the dorsal spine in ankylosing hyperostosis. Ann Rheum Dis 33:281–288, 1974.
75. Williams KA, Scott JT: Influence of trauma on the development of chronic inflammatory polyarthritis. Ann Rheum Dis 26:532–537, 1967.
76. Willkens RF, Arnett FC, Bitter T, et al: Reiter's syndrome: Evaluation of preliminary criteria for definite disease. Bull Rheum Dis 32:31–34, 1982.
77. Wright V: Psoriatic arthritis: A comparative study of rheumatoid arthritis and arthritis associated with psoriasis. Ann Rheum Dis 20:123–131, 1961.
78. Wright VA, Chamberlin MA, O'Duffy JD: Behçet's syndrome. Bull Rheum Dis 29:972–979, 1979.

Compensation-Related Spinal Disorders

CHAPTER 19

Workers' Compensation and Its Effects on Treatment of the Aging Spine

Low back pain has challenged health care systems dating back to at least the ancient Egyptians 5000 years ago.[81] Today, low back pain is one of the most common medical conditions in the Western world, afflicting up to 85 percent of all persons at some time during their lives.[71] As an increasing number of people remain actively employed into their seventh, eighth, and ninth decades, back and neck problems in the workplace will become even more common. Although neck injuries do occur in industry, the majority are due to motor vehicle accidents. As a result, many neck injuries have both a compensation and a litigation component.[37,47]

Low back pain, and especially neck pain, are illnesses of all people, not just workers. However, these problems pose special challenges in the industrial setting, and back pain has become the most common disabling musculoskeletal symptom in the Western work force. Despite the magnitude of the problem, surprisingly little has been done to provide an organized approach to the management of low back or neck pain in industry. As a result, the potential for misuse and abuse of the workers' compensation system persists.[33]

In this chapter, the epidemiology and impact of compensation-related spinal disorders are outlined to establish a basis for the setting in which control strategies must function. Preventive efforts as well as standardized evaluation and treatment programs are discussed that may help to reduce the impact of this ubiquitous problem.

COMPENSATION LOW BACK PAIN

Prevalence and Impact

The exact incidence and prevalence of low back pain in industry are unknown; however, it has been estimated that annually, 2 percent of the United States' work force incurs industrially related back injuries.[46] Several population studies in Sweden have demonstrated a prevalence of 60 to 80 percent.[38] Rowe reviewed data from a large group of employees just before their retirement at the Eastman Kodak Company and found that at some time during their career 56 percent had severe enough low back pain to require medical care.[64]

The impact of low back pain in the workplace is formidable. Kelsey and associates reported that back symptoms were the most common chronic condition resulting in decreased work capacity and reduced leisure time activities for people below the age of 45 years.[43] Over a 10-year period in Sweden (1960–1971), back pain was responsible for 12.5 percent of all sickness absence days; of all available workdays, 1 percent were lost each year because of back complaints (an average of 2.5 days for each working person yearly).[35] In Great Britain, Benn and Wood found that between 1969 and 1970, of all workdays 3.6 percent were lost due to low back pain.[7] In 1974, they reported that 1011 days per 1000 working persons were lost each year for the same reason.[80]

In the United States, based on estimates derived from the Bureau of Labor Statistics' Annual Survey of Injuries and Illnesses, about 1,000,000 workers suffered back injuries in 1980. Back injuries accounted for almost one out of every five injuries and illnesses in the workplace, although the frequency is variable depending on the industry.[14] This ratio is similar to that reported in Great Britain and Canada.[3] Data from the National Health Survey indicate that in 1983 back impairment and intervertebral disc disorders were reported as chronic conditions by 8,000,000 currently employed persons.[17] Only heart conditions and hypertension had a higher prevalence.

The most recent data from the Department of Labor Injury and Illness Survey demonstrate that back injuries comprised 23 percent of all cases in 1983 involving disability in the 18 states surveyed.[19] The majority of these disability cases (87%) were sprains or strains, with 4 percent dislocations and 2 percent bruises and contusions. Although lumbosacral sprain is the most common diagnosis rendered in the compensation setting, herniated intervertebral discs, spinal stenosis, and spondylolisthesis are also seen. In addition, Rowe reported that inflammatory arthritis may be responsible for up to 20 percent of "nonspecific" low back pain.[63]

The financial impact of compensation for low back pain is estimated to surpass 30 billion dollars in annual expenditures by the year 2000.[69] One study of a large industrial manufacturer found that claims related to back injuries constituted 19 percent of all workers' compensation claims, but were responsible for 41 percent of the total injury costs.[71] Furthermore, it has been shown that the small percentage of claimants who receive permanent total or partial disability payments are responsible for a disproportionate amount of the total costs associated with back pain or injury. It is estimated that less than 10 percent of back pain cases account for nearly 75 percent of lost days, medical costs, and indemnity payments.[1] Careful evaluation of these cases will likely provide the greatest conservation of resources and increase in productivity.

Risk Factors

It would be ideal if risk factors could be used to identify persons at high risk for low back pain or at risk for prolonged symptoms once injury occurs. Unfortunately, the complex epidemiology of this problem makes early identification and screening somewhat difficult. Although as many as 65 percent of low back pain patients are unaware of any specific causative factor, several risk factors have been identified.[25,63]

Low back pain typically begins in young adulthood, affecting the most productive years of life in an industrial worker. There is a rising prevalence with age until the fourth and fifth decades, after which there is a leveling off or decrease in prevalence.[63] Attacks of low back pain seem to be more common among those who have had back pain before. Buckle found that among 68 patients, over 70 percent reported at least one prior episode.[12] Rowe similarly noted that 85 percent of low back pain patients had a history of intermittent episodes.[63]

Several studies have examined sex differences in the risk of low back injury.[4,31] Women represent about 40 percent of the working population but develop only 20 percent of the industrial low back problems. This may be because women are typically employed in less physically demanding jobs. In a review of 31,000 manufacturing employees, Bigos and colleagues found that women had statistically fewer injuries than men but were more likely to become high-cost injury claimants.[10] In occupations demanding strenuous physical efforts, Magora reported that women had a higher incidence of low back pain than men.[48] Other investigators report equal prevalences of back pain in men and women.[8] After age 60, however, the incidence of low back pain in women increases due to osteoporosis and vertebral crush fractures.

Many investigators have examined the association between various radiographic abnormalities and the occurrence of back pain, usually concluding that no association exists.[29] Rowe reported that the prevalence of leg length differences, increased lumbosacral angle, spondylolisthesis, transitional lumbosacral vertebrae, and spina bifida occulta among low back pain patients was not significantly different from that among a control group.[63] In a cohort study of 321 men, Frymoyer and co-workers found no correlation between back pain and transitional vertebrae, Schmorl's nodes, or the vacuum disc sign.[25] However, when there were traction spurs or disc space narrowing between the fourth and fifth lumbar vertebrae, an increased incidence of severe low back pain was evident.

At least two studies have found low back pain to be more prevalent in cigarette smokers than in nonsmokers.[26,68] It is not clear whether this association is a result of increased intradiscal pressure from chronic coughing and straining or if nicotine itself has a direct biochemical role in the pathophysiology of back injury.

Poor physical fitness may be a predisposing factor for back pain. In a prospective study of firefighters, Cody and colleagues found that the least fit group of employees was ten times more susceptible to developing back pain than the most fit group.[13]

One of the more well-studied risk factors for industrial low back pain is job type; however, the data are inconsistent. The Bureau of Labor Statistics has identified construction and mining as the industries with the highest incidence of back injuries, followed closely by the trucking industry and the nursing profession.[44] Workers in government and finance were least likely to be affected. Accordingly, it has been hypothesized that the worker in heavy industry is most susceptible to a back injury. Sairanen and associates, however, found no significant difference between lumberjacks and controls doing light work with regard to low back pain occurrence.[66] Nachemson has also maintained that there is not a higher incidence among heavy laborers.[56] In a retrospective study of 2000 workers, Rowe found that 35 percent of sedentary workers and 45 percent of heavy handlers had made visits to physicians for low back pain within a 10-year period.[63] Eastrand reported a survey of Swedish workers that suggested that the number of years spent doing heavy labor had a cumulative effect on predisposition to low back problems.[21]

Despite contradictory data, it does seem likely that certain tasks in the workplace are important in the development of low back pain. Snook found that handling tasks were responsible for 70 percent of low back injuries, and Klein later reported similar findings.[44,70] The weight of the object lifted has been implicated in lifting injuries. In a recent study, more than half the injured workers had lifted objects weighing at least 60 pounds.[18] The risk for low back pain is thought to be increased by prolonged sitting and exposure to vibration.[42] Less physically stressful but boring and repetitive jobs (assembly-line work) have also been linked to increased incidence of back pain.[9]

Magora reported that workers who were dissatisfied with their present occupation, place of employment, or social situation had a high incidence of low back pain.[49] This was also true of workers who felt that a high degree of responsibility and concentration was required of them. A correlation between back injuries and poor employee appraisal ratings by the supervisor has been demonstrated by Bigos.[10] Frymoyer has shown an association of diminished spinal motion with specific abnormalities on formal psychological testing in back pain patients.[27] It is difficult, however, to determine whether any unusual psychological characteristics in the low back patient are primary problems or secondary to medical illness. Certainly, it is clear that many job and workplace factors other than mechanical loading of the spine play a role in development of industrial low back pain.

Prevention

In view of the elusive etiology of industrial low back pain, it is not surprising that attempts at prevention in industry have not met with great success. Previous efforts have focused on careful selection of workers, training in proper lifting techniques, and designing the job to fit the worker.

The goal of careful worker selection is to screen job applicants with the hope of identifying and bypassing those at increased risk for developing low back pain. The most commonly used screening tool is the pre-employment history and physical examination. Rowe, reviewing injuries at Kodak, found that only 10 percent of workers who would subsequently develop low back problems could be identified from a pre-employment medical history and examination.[64] He found the best predictor was a history of back problems, but often potential employees will not volunteer such information.

Pre-employment lumbar spine radiography has been advocated in the past,[52] but most recent investigations have shown little value to this procedure.[54,65] The American Occupational Medical Association has recommended that the lumbar spine roentgenographic examination should not be used as a routine screening procedure for back problems but should be reserved as a diagnostic tool when there are appropriate clinical indications. Techniques such as biplanar radiography and dynamic measurements on flexion-extension radiographs may prove to be more sensitive indicators of early spine dysfunction.[11,62] Further investigation with these methods will determine their role in prediction of low back disorders.

Pre-employment strength testing is based on the premise that careful matching of the worker's strength to the requirements of the job will help prevent low back injuries. The only strength testing method proved to be effective in industry is isometric simulation of the job, as advocated by Chaffin and co-workers.[15] In a series of studies, they found that a worker's likelihood of sustaining a back injury or musculoskeletal illness increased when job lifting requirements approached or exceeded the strength capacity demonstrated on an isometric simulation of the job.

Education and training in lifting methods have been allocated much time, effort, and expense, but despite endorsement from the National Safety Council, there is little evidence that such programs can reduce the incidence of low back problems.[81] Snook found that back injuries were as common among workers who had participated in such an instructional program as among those who had not received training.[70]

Finally, it may be possible to alter the workplace and the job to better fit the abilities of the worker. Matching the job to the worker, rather than the reverse, can be accomplished by defining work loads rather than selection of workers. Ergonomic redesign of the job, such as reducing the size of loads to allow them to be lifted between the legs or modifying the working methods involved, has been considered the most promising method for the prevention of low back injuries.[81]

Factors Affecting the Duration of Work Loss

Once a low back pain episode has occurred, efforts must be concentrated on returning the employee to work as soon as possible and identifying patients who will require a permanent adjustment of their work duties. While 90 percent of patients will return to work within 6 weeks of onset of the back pain, the importance of early return to employment cannot be overemphasized. Longer delays in return are clearly associated with a decreased likelihood of ever returning to the work force. McGill reported that workers with back complaints who are absent from work for more than 6 months have only a 50 percent possibility of ever returning to productive employment.[52] If they are off work more than 1 year this possibility drops to 25 percent, and after 2 years it is almost zero. Accordingly, Frymoyer and Cats-Baril have hypothesized that intensive rehabilitation early in the course of a low back disabling episode can prevent long-term disability and is cost effective.[24]

Although a multivariate model to predict disability from low back pain has not yet been developed, several factors have been shown to affect the duration of work absenteeism. First is the severity and type of injury. This may be difficult to evaluate because the history provided by the patient may be consciously or unconsciously biased. Patients who have a potential for compensation will typically identify the onset of a problem as acute rather than chronic. Most injuries, however, produce few objective physical findings.

Because objective findings are usually absent, other factors must be considered. Gallagher and associates concluded that psychological rather than physical factors predict return to work among patients with low back pain.[28] Waddell and co-workers estimated that objective physical impairment accounts for only one half the total disability, suggesting that psychological reactions such as emotional distress play a large role.[75] Similar conclusions were reached by Deyo and Tsio-Wu, who found that low educational level and low income were strongly correlated with work absenteeism.[20]

The role that the secondary gain of compensation plays in the length of disability is an issue that remains unresolved. Sander found that patients injured on duty had a statistically significantly longer period of disability than those injured off duty.[67] Evaluation of the compensation patient may be complicated by malingering or by conscious exaggeration and creation of symptoms with subconscious amplification of the injury and symptoms. Conscious manipulators often arrive at the physician's office with extensive documentation and with above-average command of the medical jargon pertinent to their injury. These patients are often persistently defensive and hostile and may selectively withhold vital information. In contrast, documentation is less important to the subconscious exaggerator, whose defensive attitude is more transient, who rarely and only briefly expresses anger, and who does not knowingly withhold useful information.

Another factor affecting time off from work in industrial low back pain is financial compensation. The Federal government and the individual states have developed their own regulations, and compensation payments can amount to as much as 100 percent of the worker's wage. Increased settlements for compensation claims and increases in the dollar value of compensation are closely associated with a subsequent increase in the number of claims made for alleged injury. Several investigations have concluded that a higher level of benefits prolonged the duration of back-related work loss.[76] The presence of compensation claims is also associated with a reduced rate of successful rehabilitation, as well as less successful surgical results.[24]

Workers' compensation laws influence diagnostic evaluation, treatment, and recovery from injury.[76] Beals suggested that paradoxically, financial compensation may discourage return to work; the appeal process may increase disability; an open claim may inhibit return to work; and recovering patients may be unable to return to work.[6] Although one study has concluded that personal injury litigants do not describe their pain as more severe than nonlitigants,[53] other studies have shown that if a lawyer becomes involved in the claim process there is a greater probability of chronic pain and disability.[24,32]

Health care providers also share responsibility for delaying return to work and escalating costs. Some physicians are less comfortable treating back pain and continue to see the injured worker at unnecessarily frequent intervals. Others take advantage of the third-party fee-for-service payment system by liberally utilizing their own radiographic and physical therapy facilities with questionable medical benefit to the patient. The result is a highly variable quality of health care and unnecessary financial expenditures, both of which have served as the impetus for development of standardized approaches to the diagnosis and treatment of industrial low back pain.

Standardized Approach to Diagnosis and Treatment of Industrial Low Back Pain

The vast majority of low back injuries are not serious, and most employees can return to work in a short time. However, employees return to work sooner and incur lower medical and compensation costs if an organized approach to evaluation, diagnosis, and treatment is used.[58,77] Unfortunately, there are few standardized diagnostic or treatment protocols available in industry.

The authors recently evaluated the effect of such an organized approach in two industries. The study was prompted by a 1980 review of employee work loss at a public utility company that revealed that 45 percent of all lost time was due to back injuries.[5] In addition, the number of back operations performed on these employees was much higher than in a noncompensation setting.

Under a newly developed program, the clinical approach to every patient was standardized by using an algorithm for low back pain diagnosis and treatment similar to the one presented in Chapter 11. The algorithm was derived from information on previous patients in whom treatment was successful as well as on those who failed to respond to treatment. This protocol enabled the treating physician to make decisions based on well-delineated rules rather than on intuition or emotion. The monitoring physicians were unbiased because they were not allowed to become involved in the patient's ongoing care. The algorithm has been modified to incorporate new data and technology since it was originally published.[77] We regard the use of a systematic and standardized approach as being the critical element, even as we expect the pathways of the algorithm to evolve.

Two employee populations were studied with monitoring programs of differing intensity. "Passive" surveillance was used to follow back pain patients from the U.S. Postal Service, which employs 14,000 people in the Washington, D.C., area. These patients were evaluated by one of the investigators (all orthopedic surgeons) after the initial episode of back pain. Computer forms were completed and, based on diagnostic data and impressions, a prediction was made regarding when the patient could return to work. This estimate was based in part on previous averages for specific diagnostic entities. The patient was seen again only if return to work was not achieved within 5 days of the predicted date or if surgical intervention was subsequently proposed by the treating physician. The study was conducted for 1 year (1982–1983) and resulted in a 41 percent decrease in the number of low back pain patients, a 60 percent decrease in days lost from work, and a 55 percent decrease in compensation costs.

A second group of patients was "actively" followed. The Potomac Electric Power Company (PEPCO) employs 5380 employees, 75 percent of whom are blue collar workers. Under the "active" monitoring program, PEPCO patients with back pain were seen weekly or biweekly by one of the investigators until their return to work. If there was any disagreement between the monitoring orthopedic surgeon and the treating physician regarding management according to the algorithm, the latter was contacted for discussion. If an acceptable agreement could not be reached, a third physician was consulted for an independent medical opinion.

PEPCO patients have been followed in this "active" fashion for 5 years (1981–1986). Using the standardized approach, there was an average decrease of 56 percent in the number of low back cases (from 98 per year prior to the study to 42 per year in the last study year). There was also a 54 percent average decrease in days lost (from 3640 per year prior to the study to 2118 per year in the last year). The cost savings were dramatic; nearly $2,000,000 was saved over the 5-year study (costs based on time lost from work—direct medical cost savings not included). The number of surgical procedures decreased from nine in the year before the study to only nine over the next 4 years. Perhaps more significant is that the surgical procedures performed under the algorithm criteria had a much higher rate of success in terms of patient return to work.[79]

Both the passive and active surveillance systems produced important savings and reductions in work disability. Although many of the reductions were greater in the active system, such a program is more expensive to employ. A cost-effectiveness study is needed to resolve this issue.

The etiology of these large reductions seen with the standardized approach remains speculative. Workers may have realized that they were being closely observed by low back experts and that they would not receive time off work without legitimate problems. Light duty was made available to recovering patients, and although records prior to the study years were unavailable concerning light duty availability, this alternative may have contributed to the savings. Finally, the acceptance of the fact that surgical procedures would never return workers to very heavy duty and recognition that surgical indications were limited helped decrease the number of surgical procedures.

The employee response to this program has been enthusiastic. This standardized approach to the diagnosis and treatment of low back pain has certainly accomplished the goals required of any health care system in industry: (1) early return to normal activity, (2) avoidance of unnecessary surgery, (3) efficient and precise use of diagnostic studies, and (4) a treatment format with affordable costs to society.

COMPENSATION NECK PAIN

Incidence of Neck Injuries

Various types of trauma can result in neck pain; however, the most common etiology is a hyperextension injury. The precise number of neck injuries is difficult to determine, but it is estimated that over one half million cases of hyperextension occur each year.[61] These patients represent 2.8 percent of all occupants in police-reported automobile accidents. It is estimated that 85 percent of all neck injuries result from motor vehicle accidents, and the majority involve rear-end collisions.[39,40,72]

Litigation in Acute Neck Injuries

The effect of litigation in acute neck injury has been the subject of several investigations. In the typical accident leading to a hyperextension injury, the striking vehicle is held at fault. In addition, the injured person rarely has an objective abnormality and appears as a blameless victim incapacitated by subjective symptoms that are difficult to prove or disprove. In this setting, it is not surprising that more than half of the accident victims receive some type of settlement.[60]

Several studies have investigated the relationship between litigation and ultimate relief of symptoms. Gotten studied 100 patients whose whiplash injuries prompted them to sue; 88 percent were asymptomatic after settlement.[30] Approximately 80 percent of the patients satisfied with their settlement had no further symptoms, while only 25 percent of those who were dissatisfied experienced complete relief. MacNab reported that 45 percent of his study population (mostly hyperextension injuries) had persistent symptoms, even after settlement.[47] Although most reports maintain that litigation is a major negative influence on recovery from neck injuries, some studies have found no relationship between the presence or settlement of litigation and the ultimate relief of symptoms.[37,59]

Standardized Approach to Diagnosis and Treatment of Neck Pain in Industry

Despite the prevalence of neck pain, industry has no standardized diagnostic and treatment protocols. Although most episodes of neck pain are self limited, it has been shown that employees receive better care and return to work sooner if an organized approach to evaluation and treatment of their neck problems is used.

A cervical spine algorithm has been developed and implemented in the same public utility company (PEPCO) in which the low back pain protocol described earlier was used.[78] Each injured employee was seen within 1 week of injury, and recovery was monitored using the algorithm. If a patient's clinical progress differed from that predicted by the algorithm, an independent medical examination was obtained.

The initial analysis indicated that 8 percent of all time lost from work was caused by neck injuries. Results with the cervical spine algorithm were encouraging after the first year. Days lost from work and light-duty days due to neck injuries were reduced by 65 percent, and there were 50 percent fewer acute neck accidents than during the previous (baseline) year. The number and type of automobile accidents reported were unchanged.

The benefits of the standardized approach were similar to those for the low back pain algorithm. In comparing the two populations, neck cases were only 20 percent as frequent as low back cases, but the amount of lost time and light-duty time per case was substantially higher for the neck patients.

Impairment Determination

Despite success in the diagnosis and management of low back and neck problems with these standardized approaches, some patients are unable to return to their preinjury level of function. Any physical injury that occurs in the work-related setting must be quantitated, especially if the patients are unable to return to their previous level of employment. For example, a laborer who undergoes back or neck surgery should not be expected to return to a position requiring heavy lifting. Such workers must be given a permanent partial impairment rating, a task for which there are few satisfactory or accepted guidelines.

It is imperative to understand the distinction between physical impairment and physical disability. Physical impairment is an objective anatomic or pathologic dysfunction leading to loss of normal body ability.[74] Permanent impairment is an objective assessment of functional abnormality or loss after the acute injury phase and after maximum medical rehabilitation. Physical disability is a measure of reduced capacity to engage in gainful everyday activity as a result of some impairment.

Assessment of physical impairment is solely a medical responsibility.[73] However, the assignment of the more subjective disability rating should be made by someone independent of the treating physician. Disability rating is best calculated by administrative, vocational, or legal specialists from impairment ratings generated by the physician.[55]

A major problem for the orthopedic surgeon is the paucity of useful guidelines for determining physical impairment ratings for the spine. One source is the American Medical Association's *Guides to the Evaluation of Permanent Impairment.*[22] The AMA *Guides* uses the concept of the "whole man," with each part of the body representing a part of the whole, based on functional use. In this system the (lumbar) spine contributes a maximum of 90 percent of the whole man. The AMA *Guides* originally used loss of motion as the sole criterion for impairment and considered pain only when it could be substantiated by clinical findings. Measurement of spinal motion, however, has a poor correlation with physical impairment, owing to large variations in normals as well as poorly reproducible measurement techniques.[16,73] The recent third edition of the *Guides* has replaced goniometer measurements with inclinometer readings, which may prove to be more reliable.[22,41,51]

The other commonly cited source is the *Manual for Orthopaedic Surgeons in Evaluating Permanent Physical Impairment,* published by the American Academy of Orthopaedic Surgeons (AAOS).[3] The AAOS *Manual* gives suggested impairment ratings for several diagnostic entities but relies extremely heavily on subjective symptoms. Because patients with low back or neck pain frequently have few or no objective clinical findings, many physicians take into consideration age, degree of pain, motivation, intelligence, education, and social factors, and are thereby actually rating disability rather than impairment.[31,50]

The current smorgasbord of impairment guidelines and the vast spectrum of interpretations generate tremendous variation in ratings.[82] Clark and colleagues have recently developed a new impairment schedule based on a comprehensive literature review and the collected opinions of a large number of back specialists.[16] Their goal was to develop a system that would give more consistent results by incorporating more objective and fewer subjective data. Preliminary results with a small number of cases have been favorable, and more extensive data are awaited.

Perhaps one of the most workable guidelines available for evaluating the low back was described by Feffer.[23] This scheme uses a consensus of diagnosis-related impairment ratings compiled from a survey of members of the International Society for Study of the Lumbar Spine (ISSLS). The ISSLS ratings for a standardized set of diagnostic situations were then matched to the physical exertion requirements developed by the Social Security Administration. The result is a logical and integrated system of diagnosis-related low back evaluation guidelines (Table 19–1). A survey of members of the Cervical Spine Research Society has facilitated compilation of a similar data base for neck injuries.

In general, the physician should treat the back pain patient conservatively and wait up to 6 weeks for a response. The worker with an acute back strain should be able to return to work within 2 weeks; a heavy laborer may require 3 to 4 weeks of treatment. At the time of initial return to work, there should be some activity restrictions such as the elimination of repeated bending, stooping, and twisting. Three weeks after return, these restrictions can be dropped and most patients will have complete recovery.

Treatment of the patient with an acute neck sprain, defined as a soft tissue injury of an otherwise normal neck, should permit return to normal activities within 2 to 3 weeks. The recovery period for hyperextension injuries from vehicular accidents depends on the severity of symptoms and the type of work to which the patient must return. Often, busy professional patients return to work after 1 week, nonmanual laborers can usually return in 2 weeks, and patients employed in positions involving heavy manual labor may require 3 to 4 weeks of treatment. Generally, most patients are able to return to work by 6 weeks after injury and should be encouraged to do so, even if mild symptoms persist.

The majority of the small group of patients who remain symptomatic will have continuing complaints without objective findings. In this

Table 19–1. WORK RESTRICTION CLASSIFICATION OF COMPENSABLE LOW BACK AND NECK INJURIES*

Work Category	Work Restriction	PPPI†	Relevant Low Back Diagnosis	Relevant Neck Diagnosis
Very Heavy	Occasional lifting in excess of 100 pounds	0%	Recovered acute back strain	Neck strain with complete recovery
	Frequent lifting of 50 pounds or more		Herniated nucleus pulposus treated conservatively with complete recovery	Hyperextension injury with complete recovery
Heavy	Occasional lifting of 100 pounds	0%	Healed acute traumatic spondylolisthesis	Herniated nucleus pulposus treated conservatively, with complete recovery
	Frequent lifting of up to 50 pounds		Healed transverse process fracture	Pre-existing degenerative disease or cervical canal stenosis with secondary neck strain, with complete recovery

Table 19–1. WORK RESTRICTION CLASSIFICATION OF
COMPENSABLE LOW BACK AND NECK INJURIES* *Continued*

Work Category	Work Restriction	PPPI†	Relevant Low Back Diagnosis	Relevant Neck Diagnosis
Medium	Occasional lifting of 50 pounds	<5%	Chronic back strain Degenerative lumbar intervertebral disc disease under reasonable control	Chronic back strain Degenerative cervical disc disease under reasonable control
	Frequent lifting of 25 pounds		Herniated nucleus pulposus treated by surgical discectomy and completely recovered Spondylolysis/spondylolisthesis under reasonable control Healed compression fracture with 10% residual loss of vertebral height	Herniated nucleus pulposus treated by surgical discectomy with complete recovery Hyperextension injury with residual pain Healed odontoid/hangman's fracture treated nonoperatively Pre-existing radiologically evident degenerative disease with secondary hyperextension injury, with moderate pain and restriction
Light	Occasional lifting of no more than 20 pounds	10% to 15%	Degenerative lumbar intervertebral disc disease with chronic pain and restriction Herniated nucleus pulposus treated conservatively or operatively, but left with some discomfort, restriction, and neurologic deficit	Degenerative cervical disc disease with chronic pain and restriction Herniated nucleus pulposus treated conservatively or operatively, with residual discomfort, restriction, and neurologic deficit
	Frequent lifting of up to 10 pounds		Acute traumatic spondylolysis/spondylolisthesis, treated conservatively or operatively, but with residual discomfort and restriction Lumbar canal stenosis Moderately severe osteoarthritis accompanied by instability Healed compression fracture with 25% to 50% residual loss of vertebral height	Hyperextension injury with chronic pain and restriction Cervical canal stenosis Moderately severe osteoarthritis accompanied by instability
	No overhead work			Hangman's fracture treated with fusion Odontoid fracture treated with fusion Burst/compression fracture of lower cervical spine with no neurologic deficit treated with external fixation or fusion
Sedentary	Occasional lifting of 10 pounds Frequent lifting of no more than lightweight articles and dockets	20% to 25%	Multiply operated back (failed back syndrome)	Multiply operated neck (constant pain) Pre-existing cervical stenosis with neck injury treated by surgery, with patient subjectively and objectively worse

*Adapted from Social Security Administration Regulations.
†PPPI = permanent partial physical impairment.

case if the physician believes the patient, a 5 to 10 percent impairment rating is fair; otherwise, no impairment should be assigned. In either case the physician should encourage early, gradual, biomechanically controlled return to activity and work for these patients with no objective findings.[57] Patients with a true radiculopathy should never be expected to return to very heavy work, nor should an operation be expected to qualify them for heavy work. After discectomy, impairment typically ranges from 10 percent with an excellent operative result to 20 percent if the patient has continued symptoms. An employee who is given a permanent partial impairment rating must have a restructuring of work duties based on the new physical exertion restriction.

Summary

Compensation low back and neck pain is a significant health care problem. As our population continues to work longer, degenerative aging of the spine will play a larger role in the compensation setting, and injuries due to "normal" degenerative changes in the spine will need to be distinguished from other spinal disorders. Specific risk factors that have been implicated in spine problems in industry have been discussed. Although many studies on risk factors are contradictory, it is evident that persons who have had back pain before are likely to have it again. It is important to understand how the relationship of pain, impairment, and subsequent disability may be different in compensation patients. Accordingly, specially designed strategies for standardized evaluation and treatment of lumbar and cervical spine pain in the industrial setting have proved to be effective at delivering quality care, decreasing the costs of medical treatment, and minimizing the amount of lost productivity.

References

1. Abenhaim L, Suissa S: Importance and economic burden of occupational back pain: A study of 2,500 cases representative of Quebec. J Occup Med 29(8):670–674, 1987.
2. Akeson WH, Murphy R: Editorial comments: Low back pain. Clin Orthop 129:2–3, 1977.
3. American Academy of Orthopaedic Surgeons: Manual for Orthopaedic Surgeons in Evaluating Permanent Physical Impairment. Chicago, AAOS, 1960, pp. 28–29.
4. Andersson GBJ: Low back pain in industry: Epidemiological aspects. Scand J Rehabil Med 11:163–168, 1979.
5. Bauer W: Scope of industrial low back pain. In Wiesel SW, Feffer H, Rothman R (eds): Industrial Low Back Pain. Charlottesville, VA, The Michie Co., 1985, pp. 1–35.
6. Beals RK: Compensation and recovery from injury. West J Med 140(2):233–237, 1984.
7. Benn R, Wood P: Pain in the back. Rheumatol Rehabil 14:121–128, 1975.
8. Bergenudd H, Nilsson B: Back pain in middle age; occupational workload and psychologic factors: An epidemiologic survey. Spine 13:58–60, 1988.
9. Bigos SJ, Spengler DM, Martin NA, et al: Back injuries in industry: A retrospective study II. Injury factors. Spine 11:246–251, 1986.
10. Bigos SJ, Spengler DM, Martin NA, et al: Back injuries in industry: A retrospective study III. Employee-related factors. Spine 11:252–256, 1986.
11. Boden SD, Wiesel SW: Lumbosacral segmental motion in normal individuals. Spine 15:571–576, 1990.
12. Buckle P, Kember P, Wood AD, et al: Factors influencing occupational back pain in Bedfordshire. Spine 5:254–258, 1980.
13. Cady L, Bischoff D, O'Connell E, et al: Strength and fitness and subsequent back injuries in fire-fighters. J Occup Med 21:269–272, 1979.

14. California, State of: Disabling Work Injuries Under Workers' Compensation Involving Back Strain Per 1,000 Workers, by Industry, California 1979. San Francisco, Department of Industrial Relations, Division of Labor Statistics and Research, 1980.
15. Chaffin D, Herin G, Keyserling W: Pre-employment strength testing: An updated position. J Occup Med 20:403–409, 1978.
16. Clark WL, Haldeman S, Johnson P, et al: Back impairment and disability determination. Another attempt at objective, reliable rating. Spine 13:332–341, 1988.
17. Department of Health and Human Services: Disability Days United States, 1983. Publication No. (PHS) 87-1586. Hyattsville, MD, National Center for Health Statistics, 1986.
18. Department of Labor Bureau of Labor Statistics: Back Injuries Associated with Lifting. Bulletin 2144. August 1982.
19. Department of Labor Bureau of Labor Statistics: Injury and Illness Data Available From 1983 Workers' Compensation Records. Announcement 86-1. March 1986.
20. Deyo RA, Tsio-Wu YJ: Functional disability due to back pain: A population-based study indicating the importance of socioeconomic factors. Arthritis Rheum 30(11):1247–1253, 1987.
21. Eastrand N: Medical, psychological, and social factors associated with back abnormalities and self reported back pain: A cross sectional study of male employees in a Swedish pulp and paper industry. Br J Ind Med 44:327–336, 1987.
22. Engelberg AL: Guides to the Evaluation of Permanent Impairment, 3rd ed. Chicago, American Medical Association, 1988, pp. 71–94.
23. Feffer HL: Evaluation of the low back diagnosis related impairment rating. In Wiesel SW, Feffer HL, Rothman RH (eds): Industrial Low Back Pain. Charlottesville, VA, The Michie Co., 1985, pp. 642–665.
24. Frymoyer JW, Cats-Baril W: Predictors of low back pain disability. Clin Orthop 221:89–98, 1987.
25. Frymoyer JW, Newberg A, Pope MH, et al: Spine radiographs in patients with low-back pain. J Bone Joint Surg 66A:1048–1055, 1984.
26. Frymoyer JW, Pope MH, Clements JH, et al: Risk factors in low-back pain. J Bone Joint Surg 65A:213–218, 1983.
27. Frymoyer JW, Rosen JC, Clements JH, et al: Psychologic factors in low-back-pain disability. Clin Orthop 195:178–184, 1985.
28. Gallagher RM, Rauh V, Langelier R, et al: Psychological, but not physical, factors predict return to work in low back pain. Psychosom Med 48(3/4):296, 1986.
29. Gibson ES: The value of preplacement screening radiography of the low back. In Deyo RA (ed): Occupational Medicine: State of the Art Reviews, Vol. 3, No. 1. Philadelphia, Hanley & Belfus, 1988, pp. 91–107.
30. Gotten N: Survey of one hundred cases of whiplash injury after settlement of litigation. J Am Med Assoc 162:856–857, 1956.
31. Greenwood JG: Low-back impairment-rating practices of orthopaedic surgeons and neurosurgeons in West Virginia. Spine 10:773–776, 1985.
32. Haddad GH: Analysis of 2932 workers' compensation back injury cases: The impact on the cost to the system. Spine 12:765–769, 1987.
33. Hadler NM: Industrial rheumatology: The Australian and New Zealand experience with arm pain and back ache in the workplace. Med J Aust 144:191–195, 1986.
34. Hansson T, Bigos S, Beecher P, Wortley M: The lumbar lordosis in acute and chronic low-back pain. Spine 10:154–155, 1985.
35. Helander E: Back pain and work disability. Social Med T 50:398–404, 1973.
36. Hirsch C: Etiology and pathogenesis of low back pain. Int J Med Sci 2:362–370, 1966.
37. Hohl M: Soft tissue injuries of the neck in automobile accidents: Factors influencing prognosis. J Bone Joint Surg 56A:1675–1682, 1974.
38. Hult L: Cervical, dorsal, and lumbar spine syndromes. Acta Orthop Scand 17(Suppl):1–102, 1954.
39. Jackson R: The positive findings in alleged neck injuries. Am J Orthop 6:178–187, 1964.
40. Jackson R: Crashes cause most neck pain. Am Med News, December 5, 1966.
41. Keeley J, Mayer TG, Cox R, et al: Quantification of lumbar function. V. Reliability of range-of-motion measures in the sagittal plane and an in vivo torso rotation measurement technique. Spine 11:31–35, 1986.
42. Kelsey JL, Godlen AL: Occupational and workplace factors associated with low back pain. In Deyo RA (ed): Occupational Medicine: State of the Art Reviews, Vol. 3, No. 1. Philadelphia, Hanley & Belfus, 1988, pp. 7–16.
43. Kelsey JL, Pastides H, Bisbee G: Musculoskeletal Disorders: Their Frequency of Occurrence and Their Impact on the Population of the United States. New York, Neale Watson Academic Publications, 1978.
44. Klein BP, Jensen RC, Sanderson LM: Assessment of workers' compensation claims for back strains/ sprains. J Occup Med 26:443–448, 1984.
45. Laubach LL: Comparative muscular strength of men and women; a review of the literature. Aviat Space Environ Med 47:534–572, 1976.
46. Leavitt S, Johnston T, Beyer R: The process of recovery: Patterns in industrial back injury. I. Cost and other quantitative measures of effort. Indust Med 40:7–14, 1971.
47. MacNab I: Acceleration injuries of the cervical spine. J Bone Joint Surg 46A:1797–1799, 1964.

48. Magora A: Investigation of the relation between low back pain and occupation. I. Age, sex, community, education and other factors. Indust Med Surg 39:465–471, 1970.
49. Magora A: Investigation of the relation between low back pain and occupation. V. Psychological aspects. Scand J Rehab Med 5:191–196, 1973.
50. Mayer TG: Assessment of lumbar function. Clin Orthop 221:99–109, 1987.
51. Mayer TG, Tencer AF, Kristoferson S, et al: Use of noninvasive techniques for quantification of spinal range-of-motion in normal subjects and chronic low-back dysfunction patients. Spine 9:588–595, 1984.
52. McGill CM: Industrial back problems: A control program. J Occup Med 10:174–178, 1968.
53. Mendelson G: Compensation, pain complaints, and psychological disturbance. Pain 20:169–177, 1984.
54. Montgomery C: Pre-employment back x-ray. J Occup Med 18:495–498, 1976.
55. Mooney V: Impairment, disability, and handicap. Clin Orthop 221:14–25, 1987.
56. Nachemson A: Low back pain: Its etiology and treatment. Clin Med 78:18–24, 1971.
57. Nachemson A: Work for all—for those with low back pain as well. Clin Orthop 179:77–85, 1983.
58. National Safety Council: Accident Facts. Chicago, National Safety Council, 1978, p. 26.
59. Norris SH, Watt I: The prognosis of neck injuries resulting from rear end vehicle collisions. J Bone Joint Surg 65B:608–614, 1983.
60. O'Neill B, Haddon W, Kelley AN, et al: Automobile head restraint—frequency of neck injury claims in relation to the presence of head restraint. Am J Pub Health 62:399–406, 1972.
61. Partyka S: Whiplash and other inertial force neck injuries in traffic accidents. Paper for the Mathematical Analysis Division, National Center for Statistics and Analysis, Washington, D.C., December 1981.
62. Pearcy M, Portek I, Shepherd J: Three-dimensional X-ray analysis of normal movement in the lumbar spine. Spine 9:294–297, 1984.
63. Rowe ML: Low back pain in industry: A position paper. J Occup Med 11:161–169, 1969.
64. Rowe ML: Low back disability in industry: Updated position. J Occup Med 13:476–478, 1971.
65. Rowe ML: Are routine spine films on workers in industry cost or risk benefit effective? J Occup Med 24:41–43, 1982.
66. Sairanen E, Brushaber L, Kaskinen M: Felling work, low back pain, and osteoarthritis. Scand J Work Environ Health 7:18–30, 1981.
67. Sander RA, Meyers JE: The relationship of disability to compensation status in railroad workers. Spine 11:141–143, 1986.
68. Sivensson H, Andersson G: Low back pain in 40 to 47 year old men, work history and environment factors. Spine 8:272–276, 1983.
69. Snook SH: The costs of back pain in industry. In Deyo RA (ed): Occupational Medicine: State of the Art Reviews, Vol. 3, No. 1. Philadelphia, Hanley & Belfus, 1988, pp. 1–5.
70. Snook SH, Campanelli RA, Hart JW: A study of three preventive approaches to low back injury. J Occup Med 20:478–481, 1978.
71. Spengler DM, Bigos SJ, Martin NA, et al: Back injuries in industry: A retrospective study I. Overview and cost analysis. Spine 11:241–245, 1986.
72. States JD, Korn MW, Masengill JB: The enigma of whiplash injuries. NY State J Med 70:2971–2978, 1970.
73. Waddell G: Clinical assessment of lumbar impairment. Clin Orthop 221:110–120, 1987.
74. Waddell G, Main CJ: Assessment of severity of low-back disorders. Spine 9:204–208, 1984.
75. Waddell G, Main CJ, Morris EW, et al: Chronic low-back pain, psychologic distress, and illness behavior. Spine 9:209–213, 1984.
76. Walsh NE, Dumitru D: The influence of compensation on recovery from low back pain. In Deyo RA (ed): Occupational Medicine: State of the Art Reviews, Vol. 3, No. 1. Philadelphia, Hanley & Belfus, 1988, pp. 109–121.
77. Wiesel SW, Feffer HL, Rothman RH: Industrial low-back pain: A prospective evaluation of a standardized diagnostic and treatment protocol. Spine 9:199–203, 1984.
78. Wiesel SW, Feffer HL, Rothman RH: The development of a cervical spine algorithm and its prospective application to industrial patients. J Occup Med 27:272–276, 1985.
79. Wiesel SW, Feffer HL, Rothman RH: Low back pain: Development and five-year prospective application of a computerized quality-based diagnostic and treatment protocol. J Spinal Dis 1:50–58, 1988.
80. Wood P, Badley M: Epidemiology of back pain. In Jeyson M (ed): The Lumbar Spine and Back Pain. London, Pitman, 1980, pp. 29–33.
81. Yu TS, Roht LH, Wise RA, et al: Low-back pain in industry: An old problem revisited. J Occup Med 26:517–524, 1984.
82. Ziporyn T: Disability evaluation—a fledgling science? JAMA 250:873–874, 879–880, 1983.

Index

Note: Page numbers in *italics* refer to illustrations; page numbers followed by t refer to tables.